Naturally Supporting Cancer Treatment

Evidence-based ways to help prevent cancer formation and recurrence, and assist treatment

JENNY GRAVES

Advanced Diploma of Naturopathy

First published in 2021

Published by Kamberry Press, Canberra, 2021

ISBN: 978-0-6452932-0-3

A catalogue record for this book is available from the National Library of Australia

Typesetting and cover design by Working Type

Disclaimer

The information in this book is not intended as medical advice. It has been thoroughly researched but it is limited to being general information which you should only use with professional guidance and in consultation with your treatment team. The author does not claim that this information will help to cure or heal cancer or any associated medical condition. It is essential that you conduct your own research, seek advice from appropriately qualified professionals and make informed choices about what is right for you in your specific circumstances.

If you are a naturopath or health service practitioner, note that that this information is provided as resource material for your information and professional development. You take full responsibility for any advice or treatment you provide to your clients.

Foreword

Meeting Jenny, a fellow Naturopath, was a breath of fresh air in my ongoing education as a Naturopath working in the field of oncology support.

Our profession is one of lifelong learning and in my pursuit to maintain up to the minute knowledge to support my patients from diagnosis through to treatment and long-term prevention, I read a lot!

Yet Jenny's unique position as a Naturopath and cancer survivor has enabled her to provide a very different, one of a kind book. A unique, incredibly powerful and empathetic educational resource. Thus Jenny's book, *Naturally supporting cancer treatment*, is so well placed to support cancer patients and their loved ones through the 'journey' that is cancer.

When Jenny introduced me to her book, she said this was "the kind of book I wanted when I was on my journey". Having had the pleasure of reading through Jenny's book and learning from her journey these words have rung true, Jenny has created this book!

Jenny enables patients and their loved ones to clearly and simply understand the benefits of using natural and complementary medicines through any stage, from prevention to treatment and post cancer. Sharing her story, tips and successful solutions that worked for her, from dietary and lifestyle advice right through to advanced herbal and nutritional support. Jenny provides confident, clear and actionable steps full of evidence-based references.

Whether you are like me and have read extensively on this topic or you are brand new to cancer education and natural medicine, Jenny has you covered with actionable steps and a big dose of inspiration.

Holistic, insightful – a must read! Let Jenny guide you back to wellness.

Thank you, Jenny, for sharing your passion.

Carla Wrenn
BHSc (Naturopathy)
Integrative Naturopathic Practitioner

Supporting oncology patients to prosper before, during and after cancer treatment using evidence based complementary natural medicines, dietary and lifestyle advice.

carlawrenn.com

Dedication

*To the memory of all my friends
who have succumbed to cancer.*

Contents

Testimonials

'I am amazed at the amount of information that the author has gathered and I think that it will help all people who read this book to eat healthier, whether they are sick or not. For this reason, I would recommend this book to all people who are interested in how to recover as easily as possible during and after hospital treatment, but also to those who are interested in how to live healthier in this fast-paced world where the least thought is given to health until you get sick.'—**Stjepan Cobets, poet, author, and Goodreads reviewer**

'I received my electronic copy of this book as my daughter is undergoing chemo for breast cancer and I am living after colon cancer. The information contained is helpful and backed by research, which the author uses extremely well. Cancer seems to touch everyone's world somehow and this is a great reference and resource site for all questions relating to food, chemicals, exercise and guided imagery. I have signed up to get the author's newsletter.'—**Kimberley, Goodreads reviewer**

'It offers support and alternatives, but also hope as much as as (sic) anything else. And I intend to use for myself and my family as a guide to help prevent the disease. I will be referring to it often. A definite must read.'—**Art Isaacs, author and Goodreads reviewer**

' I need this book in paperback now, so that I can earmark pages and return often to all the fabulous lists... because this book isn't a fad... it is a book for life. It is a manual for looking after your body all the time, so don't wait until you may have cancer to read it, take all of the authors advice to heart.'—**T.N. Traynor, author and Goodreads reviewer**

'The author combines her own experience with evidence-based insights, providing guidance on topics like diet, stress reduction, exercise, sleep, and cutting down on household toxins. This book is an invaluable resource for cancer patients and caregivers, offering hope and empowerment through knowledge. It is also a good manual to follow for cancer prevention. The writing style is clear, concise, and easy to understand. It's an uplifting guide that bridges the gap between natural and conventional healing methods and shows how they can work together to improve outcomes.' —**Scott Peters, author and Goodreads reviewer**

'NATURALLY SUPPORTING CANCER TREATMENT is simply excellent. It is a straightforward, well-written, simply written, and extensively researched handbook on ways to prevent, mitigate, and potentially heal cancer (but also, I'd other (sic), other forms of disease brought upon by everyday toxins). She won me over as a credible and compassionate narrator, and I enjoyed learning more about this topic through her findings.' — **Angela Panayotopulos, author and Goodreads reviewer**

'I'd give this book ten stars if the option was available. It was well written – concise, easy to follow and well categorised. It was fantastically researched – informative, includes empirical evidence and references given at the end of each chapter. It was all encompassing – looking at diet, stress, exercise, sleep and other health related subjects. It was written by a qualified naturopath AND cancer survivor. It was, in conclusion, so worth the read.' **—Ellie Hearts Books, Goodreads reviewer**

'A large percentage of the book concerns preventing cancer. It alerts us to cancer-causing substances in our everyday lives, healthier substitutes for those products, and foods and supplements that help prevent cancer or make us more resilient if we do get sick. It is worth reading cover to cover, but is best kept as a reference book as you make changes in your lifestyle. Even if you only follow about 25% of the advice here, you could be making a tremendous difference in your and your family's health.' – **Amani Jesu, author and Goodreads reviewer**

'What I really like is that the writing is concise, easy to understand, and includes documented references if the reader wants to do additional research on their own. I would recommend getting a hard copy of this book over an electronic version because after you've read the book you will want to go back and access specific advice. Also it has a lot of helpful charts that are easier to view on a paper version of the material.' — **S.D., author and Goodreads reviewer**

Preface

It all started on Boxing Day 2008 with a sore throat. I've always used natural medicines to treat myself when I get a cold, so I dosed myself up with echinacea, took some extra Vitamin C and gargled with antiseptic. But the sore throat didn't go away. Over the next few weeks, I had a series of infections: cystitis, a boil (on my bottom!), a spot on my face, a huge mouth ulcer, and all of them took ages to heal. Then I got a really bad earache, so I went to the doctor.

The doctor couldn't find anything wrong but he sent me away with some antibiotics and powerful painkillers. They didn't touch the pain. A few days later I went back. He injected me with penicillin. That didn't help either. So I went back again and got another penicillin shot. Still no joy. So he sent me to an ear, nose and throat specialist who also said he couldn't find anything wrong. After I refused to leave without a diagnosis, he pressed on my tonsil and I almost hit the ceiling with pain. He decided that I had tonsillitis and tried to book me in to have them taken out. There were no signs of tonsillitis, so I politely declined and went back to work.

When I reached the office, I rang my husband in tears. He suggested I try another doctor. So, I made an appointment for later that day. I told her the whole story and her eyes got wider and wider. I said I thought I had something wrong with my immune system. She examined me, and couldn't find anything either, but she gave me a blood test form. I just had time to get to the pathology lab and get the blood taken before it closed.

At 9.30 that night the phone rang. It was the doctor, wanting to know whether I had any preference for a haematologist, as she needed to refer me to a specialist. I said no, but now I was worried. When I asked her what was wrong, she told me that my white blood cell count was very low. I asked what could cause it and she said that it was usually a problem with the bone marrow.

My heart sank as I got off the phone. I had studied biology at high school and I had an inkling that it was leukaemia. I didn't dare tell my husband because I thought he would just think I was being hysterical. But I figured the doctor wouldn't have called me so late at night unless it was something serious.

I went to bed, but tossed and turned for hours, with all sorts of thoughts going around in my head. In my mind, I had my funeral planned and composed a farewell letter to my husband, and I cried my eyes out. It was about 2 am before I finally decided to abandon the worrying until I got a firm diagnosis, and eventually drifted off to sleep.

I went to work later that morning, thinking that if I got a phone call from the haematologist early in the morning then it was definitely leukaemia. I got that call at about 2 minutes past 9. The rest of the day was surreal. Yes, it was leukaemia. The haematologist took me through what was actually happening in my body. She was surprised I wasn't more shocked, until I explained that I'd already worked out what the disease was and had experienced my initial reactions. She asked me whether I would have chemotherapy (chemo) and in response I asked her whether there was an alternative. She gave me the stark answer that some people tried natural therapies but they usually died quite quickly. Apparently my life expectancy without chemo would be about 6 weeks! That was quite a shock! I agreed that I would have the chemo, and after some further tests that afternoon she wheeled me over to the ward which would become my second home for the next 3 months or so.

Your own story is probably just as dramatic. For me, it was as though it was happening to someone else. It just didn't seem real. Looking back, it still feels a bit like that.

I had packed a bag to take into hospital, including my vitamin supplements, glucosamine for my joints and my bioidentical hormone replacement therapy (HRT). A different doctor was going to look after me and when she came to see me she asked what medication I was on. To my surprise, when I showed her my stash, she told me I would have to stop taking it all. I had thought the supplements would be helpful, or at least not harmful, alongside the chemo treatment. I was really upset, as it felt that my attempts to help myself were being taken away. I did understand, though, that she genuinely thought that they might interfere with the effectiveness of the drugs and I agreed to stop taking them.

Things got worse. The food in hospitals is never all that tasty, but because my immune system was so weak I wasn't allowed anything uncooked, apart from a cheese sandwich. Chemo gave me really severe nausea, and even the smell of hot food triggered it. I asked for a cheese sandwich, which I thought I could manage to keep down. It arrived, made with white bread (something I never ate at home) and processed cheese. There was no chutney, salad or sauce with it and the wretched thing just stuck to the roof of my mouth like glue. I didn't try that again. I couldn't keep hot food down, so I ended up eating cereal, milk, toast and jam, jelly and desserts but I realised this really wasn't a healthy diet for me. I can remember dreaming about eating mountains of salad and fresh fruit!

One of my friends in England phoned me in hospital every few days to give moral support. I was complaining to her about my lack of vitamins and the appalling food that I was being given. She was really sympathetic and suggested I should write a book, and that was how the seeds for this book were sown.

It has taken me a few years. I had a bone marrow transplant, which caused some complications to work through, but I came out the other side in remission and have stayed there ever since. I do appreciate the care that I received from the doctors, but as soon as possible I started taking my vitamins and some herbs I'd identified as helpful from my own research. I made a very good recovery but I had pretty bad 'chemo brain'. Oh yes, it is a real thing. Just ask my poor long-suffering husband. My memory was appalling for a year or 2. I went back to work, but kept thinking about the book I should write, the one that I would have liked to read when I was going through treatment.

I wouldn't have very much credibility without some sort of knowledge about how to carry out research, and an understanding of the human body. So I decided to study naturopathy, or natural medicine. It took 4 years to complete those studies, and over this time I learned how the body works, about the chemistry and biochemistry involved in its processes, nutrition, herbal medicine and some of the more common diseases. I also learned how to read scientific papers and how to distinguish which research was good and which wasn't.

Please don't think I'm suggesting you should use only natural therapies. It's true that some people do, and some make a full recovery. But my research shows that natural therapies alone aren't usually as successful as regular medical treatment, and that medical treatment along with carefully chosen natural therapies is more effective still. The ideas in this book can certainly make a difference but personally, I wouldn't stake my life on them alone, and I don't recommend that you do either. Surgery, chemotherapy (chemo) and radiation (also known as cut, poison and burn) are certainly brutal, but, despite what some websites say, they are effective for most people, depending on how far the cancer has progressed and how aggressive it is. With the support of natural therapies, though, the results can be better and the side-effects reduced.

Naturopaths specialise in individualised treatment plans. Obviously, I can't do that here because I don't know your particular problems. My aim is to show you some of the things you can safely use alongside regular medical treatment that will increase your odds of surviving cancer and the research that supports them. If you choose to use any of the ideas here, I strongly recommend that you talk to your oncologist about them first. With the references to the science behind them, presented here, you'll be able to show medical professionals that they are safe and effective add-ons to your regular treatment. Ideally, I'd recommend that you consult a naturopath to get a personalised plan and ask them to liaise directly with your oncologist to ensure that everyone is fully aware of the range of treatments being used.

It would be close to impossible to cover in one book every possible natural therapy that's effective. So I've tried to pick out the ones I believe are most effective based on current research, bearing in mind that research is constantly giving new information. The book will help guide you and your healthcare practitioner on:

- how the natural therapy works
- whether the therapy interacts with any of the best-known medical treatments available
- any medical conditions it shouldn't be used with
- the evidence for its effectiveness.

Much of the advice appears to be preventive, but it's just as important during and after your treatment as before it because it will give your body the chance to heal itself.

Where I've used medical terms, acronyms and abbreviations in bold type, you'll find them in the Glossary on page xxi. Please also refer to the Index on page 329, which provides details of research on different types of cancer.

Glossary, acronyms and abbreviations

Adaptogen	A herb that improves the body's response to stress.
AGE	Advanced glycation end-product.
AICR	American Institute of Cancer Research.
Angiogenesis	The formation of new blood cells by a tumour.
Apoptosis	The programmed death of a cell.
ATP	Adenosine triphosphate, used by the body to produce energy.
B cell	A type of white blood cell that produces antibodies.
BMI	Body mass index, a measure commonly used to determine health based on weight and height.
BPA	Bisphenol A, a hormone disruptor found in plastics.
Cachexia	Loss of weight and muscle mass that often occurs in advanced cancers.
Carcinogen	Something that encourages cancers to form. Carcinogenic is the adjective. Carcinogenesis is the first stage of cancer formation.

Control group	A group used in a research study that does not receive the material being tested.
Cytokine	A chemical messenger released by white blood cells which can cause inflammation.
DHA	Docosahexaenoic acid, a type of omega 3 fatty acid.
DEA	Diethanolamine, a chemical used in personal care products.
DNA	Deoxyribonucleic acid, the structure in our chromosomes that carries our genetic code.
EPA	Environmental Protection Agency.
Epidemiological study	Study that measures disease outcomes in a particular population.
EWG	Environmental Working Group, a non-profit organisation committed to empowering people to live healthier lives.
FDA	Food and Drug Administration in the USA.
g	Gram, a metric unit of weight, 1/1,000th of a kilogram.
GABA	Gamma aminobutyric acid, a neurotransmitter that relaxes the body.
Gene	The unit of DNA that controls a particular characteristic of the body.
Glycolysis	The first step in producing energy in a cell.
HDL cholesterol	High-density lipid cholesterol, commonly known as 'good' cholesterol because it takes cholesterol away from the cells.

IARC	International Agency for Research on Cancer.
In vitro	Research conducted outside a living body, in an artificial environment.
kg	Kilogram, a metric measure of weight.
LDL cholesterol	Low-density lipid cholesterol, commonly known as 'bad' cholesterol because it carries cholesterol out to the cells.
Litre	A metric measure of volume.
Lymph	Fluid that bathes the body's cells and is pumped around the body with movement.
MEA	Monoethanolamine, a chemical used in personal care products.
Meta-analysis	A statistical summary of a group of trials on a particular research question.
Metastasis	The spread of cancer cells to another part of the body.
Microgram	1/1,000,000th of a kilogram, a metric unit of weight.
mg	Milligram, 1/1,000th of a kilogram, a metric unit of weight.
ml	Millilitre, 1/1,000th of a litre, a metric unit of volume.
MTHFR	A gene that regulates the breakdown of folate.
Mucositis	A chemo and radiotherapy side-effect that causes extreme soreness throughout the digestive tract.

Mutation	An error in DNA copying.
NAC	N-acetyl cysteine, an antioxidant nutritional supplement.
Neutrophil	A type of white blood cell important for immunity.
NK cells	Natural killer cells, which target cancer cells and destroy them.
NSAID	Non-steroidal anti-inflammatory drug.
NSLC	Non-small cell lung cancer.
NTP	National Toxicology Program.
p53 gene	This gene manages apoptosis, the process of destroying faulty cells. Mutations of the gene can result in cancer.
PAH	Polycyclic aromatic hydrocarbons, which are chemical pollutants.
PCE	Perchloroethylene, a chemical used in making hydrofluorocarbons and refrigerants. Also known as TCE.
PFC	Perfluorocarbon, a compound containing carbon and fluorine, often referred to as a 'greenhouse gas'.
Prospective cohort study	A study where the subjects are recruited and baseline data is collected at the beginning of the study, then followed up to see whether the outcome of interest has occurred.
RDA	Recommended daily allowance.

ROS	Reactive oxygen species, also known as free radicals, which cause damage to the body. Antioxidants act to mop them up.
Systematic review	A summary of the evidence found for a particular research question.
T cell	A type of white blood cell that secretes chemicals that kill cancer cells directly.
TCE	Trichoroethylene, a chemical used in making hydrofluorocarbons and refrigerants. Also known as PCE.
TEA	Triethanolamine, a chemical used in personal care products.
Topically	Used on the skin, not internally.
VOC	Volatile organic compound, a harmful chemical that easily turns into a gas that can be inhaled.
WCRF	World Cancer Research Fund.
WHO	World Health Organization.

Summary

My general advice to healthcare practitioners and anyone either currently going through treatment or wanting to prevent cancer forming or returning is summarised in the bullet points below. The page number after each point takes you to more information and a description of why it's important. This summary does not include any of the nutritional supplements and herbs, which you'll find in Chapters 7 and 8. They should be looked at on an individual basis depending on the cancer being treated and the individual circumstances. The relevant research for each cancer type is in the Index at the back of the book, and you should consult a natural health practitioner for advice.

Key points are:

- Eat regularly and enjoy food, so that you're relaxed when eating (page 9).
- Where possible, eat organic foods and especially avoid genetically modified (GMO) foods (page 9).
- Eat plenty of fresh vegetables and some fruit every day. Aim to eat at least one green, one yellow, one red, one orange and one purple vegetable or fruit every day (page 13).

- Eat no more than one or 2 meals of red meat per week and avoid processed meat (page 16).
- Avoid cooking meat at high temperatures, such as by barbecuing and frying (page 18).
- Include fermented dairy products in your diet (page 20).
- Avoid full-fat dairy products, such as whole milk, high-fat cheeses and full-fat yoghurt and use low-fat dairy instead, such as cottage cheese and low-fat ricotta and low-fat yoghurt (page 22).
- Avoid dairy milk and cut down on butter (page 23).
- Eat plenty of healthy fats such as avocado, nuts, and fresh (non-rancid) olive and coconut oils (page 23).
- Drink plenty of water, tea (especially green tea) and herbal teas, but avoid carbonated drinks, both sugary and artificially sweetened, and alcohol (page 26).
- Avoid sugary foods, salt or artificial sweeteners (page 30).
- Eat dark chocolate with at least 70% cocoa but avoid milk or white chocolate (page 32).
- Eat fermented foods like yoghurt, sauerkraut, kimchi, kefir and kombucha (page 33).
- Avoid eating or drinking anything that interferes with your sleep, such as caffeine-laden drinks (page 36).
- Avoid using non-stick (Teflon® coated) pans for cooking (page 38).
- Don't store your foods in plastic (page 39).
- Follow an alkalising diet (page 53).

- Find ways to reduce your stress, such as:
  - Meditation (page 71)
  - Yoga (page 74)
  - T'ai chi and Qi Gong (page 77)
  - Hypnosis (page 77)
  - Massage (page 78)
  - Acupuncture (page 79)
  - Pet therapy (page 80)
  - Journaling (page 81)
  - Earthing (page 82)
  - Laughter (page 84)
  - Prayer (page 86)
  - Cognitive behaviour therapy (page 87)
  - Visualisation (page 87).
- Find some sort of exercise that you enjoy doing and move as much as possible (Chapter 4).
- Get plenty of sleep. Tips to improve your sleep include:
  - Train your body clock by going to bed and getting up at the same time each day (page 110).
  - Make your bedroom as comfortable as possible (page 111).
  - Avoid stimulants like caffeine, chocolate, nicotine and alcohol in the evening (page 112).
  - Relax by using meditation and muscle relaxation techniques, avoid worrying at night, and read something soothing at bedtime (page 113).
  - Avoid exercise for 2 hours before sleep (page 114).
  - Avoid blue light by dimming lights in the evening and

  avoiding watching TV, or using your phone, computer or tablet (page 114).
  - Limit daytime naps to 30 minutes (page 115).
  - In the evening, eat small snacks of foods that will help you sleep, such as eggs, fish, small amounts of wholegrain cereals, nuts and seeds, tart cherries and their juice, legumes like chickpeas and lentils, oily fish such as salmon or mackerel, bananas and green leafy vegetables (page 115).
  - Diffuse essential oils into the air in the evening. Lavender, bergamot, sandalwood, frankincense and mandarin all help to promote sleep (page 116).
  - Cognitive behaviour therapy, which is provided by psychologists, can help cancer patients improve their sleep (page 120).
  - You can buy herbal medicines that help with sleep in health food stores. These include valerian, kava, lemon balm and passionflower (page 121).
  - Melatonin is available from your GP in Australia and can be bought over the counter in some other countries (page 128).
- Avoid using toxic products, such as:
  - Personal care products (page 156)
  - House cleaning chemicals (page 166)
  - Pesticides and herbicides (pages 170 and 178).

- Minimise your exposure to:
    - Chemicals in furniture (page 177)
    - Electromagnetic radiation in your environment, as much as possible (page 182).

Within each chapter, items are not necessarily listed in order of importance. You might find some of the ideas here a little too extreme. They all work, but it's up to you whether you choose to use them or not. The more of these strategies you use, the more you can help your body to heal. Remember too that it's what you do the majority of the time that matters. So if you go away on holiday and don't follow the dietary advice for a couple of weeks, for example, don't think you've completely blown it. Just return to healthy eating when you get back.

Research and recommendations are constantly changing. You can keep up to date on the latest research, get useful information, and find links to other helpful sites on my website at:

www.NaturallySupportingCancerTreatment.com.au and my Facebook page at **www.facebook.com/NaturallySupportingCancerTreatment.**

On my website, you can sign up for my newsletter that lets you know about new blog posts too. I encourage you to do that so that you don't miss anything. You can also send me messages through the website and Facebook pages. I am not currently taking clients but I do have access to many experienced naturopaths who can help you if you want individualised help, and I'd be glad to put you in touch with them.

I sincerely hope that the ideas in this book help you back to wellness and keep you healthy so that you can lead a long and happy life.

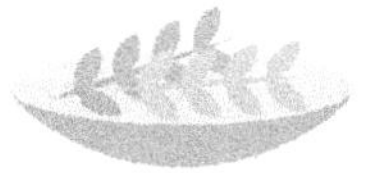

Chapter 1

What is cancer and how does it start?

It's important for you to have an idea of how cancer starts and progresses so that you can understand how the things I'm suggesting might help you. Please don't skip this.

Cancer isn't like an infection, where a microbe has invaded the body. It doesn't start outside the body. It happens when one of our own cells has a glitch. The cells in our bodies aren't immortal. Our **DNA** governs when they're supposed to self-destruct, a process called **apoptosis**. When cells divide, the strands of **DNA** are copied and sometimes a 'typo' happens, known as a **mutation**. The strands of **DNA** contain our **genes**, and each **gene** controls a particular characteristic. If a **mutation** is on a **gene** that manages **apoptosis**, then the cell can become immortal, as it does not self-destruct. Instead, it replicates itself and creates more immortal cells, producing a tumour.

The most common **gene** managing **apoptosis** is called **p53** and **mutations** of it are involved in about half of all cancers. As an example, you might have come across the BRCA1 and BRCA2 **genes**. BRCA stands for BReast CAncer and these **genes** manage

apoptosis in breast and ovarian tissue. If **p53** mutates, sometimes it doesn't suppress tumours any more, which raises the risk of developing breast and ovarian cancers. This **mutation** can be inherited from either of your parents. If you have the **mutation**, your risk of breast cancer by the age of 70 rises from about 7% to about 50%, and your risk of ovarian cancer by the age of 70 rises from about 1% to about 30%.[1]

Genetic changes aren't reversible, but epigenetics is a relatively new science that shows that our behaviour, like diet and exercise, can change how our **genes** work.[2]

The body has several processes to prevent **mutation**s from creating a problem. Firstly, **DNA** has a proof-reader that usually picks up any typos and causes the defective cell to self-destruct. If it manages to get past the proof-reader, the immune system kicks in. We have immune cells called natural killer cells (**NK cells**) that target cancerous cells and destroy them. But sometimes if your immune system isn't working well that doesn't happen either and the cell starts to divide. The result is the beginning of cancer. So a healthy immune system is crucial.

As well as being immortal, cancer cells produce their energy differently from normal cells. In normal cells, energy is produced in a 3-step process which is very efficient. The first step is called **glycolysis**. This step doesn't use oxygen. It takes glucose and produces pyruvate, lactic acid (which causes your muscles to cramp if you overwork them), and 2 molecules of adenosine triphosphate (**ATP**) (which is what cells use to store energy). The pyruvate then goes through another 2 processes, which need oxygen and can use other fuels, producing about 34 molecules of **ATP** and carbon dioxide.

Cancer cells, on the other hand, use mainly **glycolysis**.[3] This means they're very inefficient, so they need a lot of sugar to produce energy, and they produce lactic acid, which causes the environment around them to become very acidic, which they seem to prefer. In Chapter 2, I'll show you how you can use the fact that cancer cells use mainly glucose to help kill them off. Take a look at Figure 1 below to make the process of energy production described above more clear.

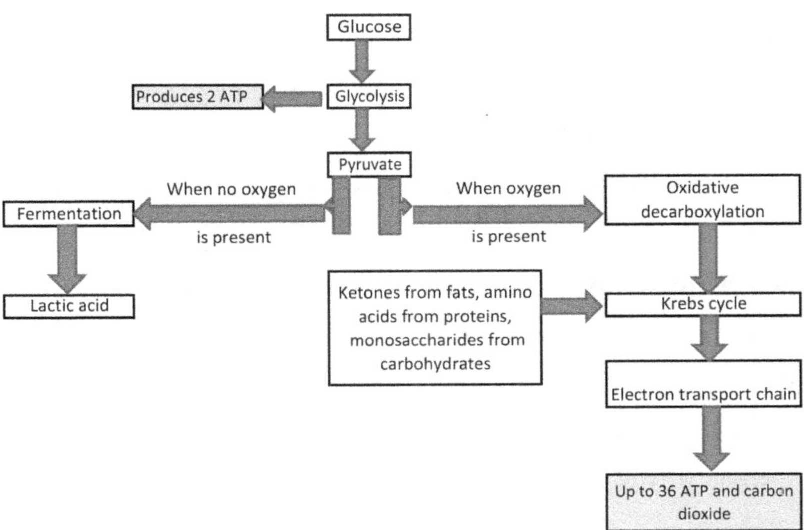

Figure 1: Human energy production

Cancer cells need a blood supply to get enough nutrients to grow. So they form a network of new blood vessels, a process called **angiogenesis**. These blood vessels also form an escape route where some of the cancer cells can break off and circulate to another part of the body, known as **metastasis**. There they can grow more tumours. **Metastasis** can also happen when cancer cells travel through the **lymph**, the fluid that bathes each cell.

Not all cancers produce tumours. The blood-borne cancers (leukaemia, lymphoma and myeloma) are mostly in the bone marrow, which produces the immune cells. The most common treatment is a cocktail of chemo drugs, which target the bone marrow to wipe out a good proportion of the cells there and (hopefully) kill off the cancerous cells as well. This is very different from most chemo regimes, which try to save the bone marrow from being destroyed to protect your immune system. If yours is a blood cancer, it's important not to do anything that protects the bone marrow from being destroyed if the aim of your chemo is to destroy it. I'll highlight this as you go through the book.

That's how cancer starts, but why does it start? What causes a **genetic mutation**? Generally, it's a result of an injury or 'insult' to the body, which could happen because of poor diet, stress, lack of exercise, not enough sleep, or some kind of toxin. I'll go into detail about all of those and show you how to avoid them.

Some viruses, such as Epstein-Barr (which causes glandular fever), human papillomavirus (HPV), and hepatitis B and C can also cause certain cancers. Increasing your natural immunity will help prevent those, and the advice in this book will help you do that.

There's also an increased risk of cancers if you have chronic illnesses, such as diabetes, high blood pressure, increased heart rate, high cholesterol, gouty arthritis, lung disease and chronic kidney disease.[4] All of these cause some sort of ongoing injury to the body.

Being overweight is another risk factor. Fat cells produce hormones like insulin, and growth factors that speed up the rate at which cells divide, increasing the chances of a **mutation** occurring. They also attract immune cells to them, which release chemicals called **cytokines** to 'call for more help', some of which can cause damage. In women after menopause, fat cells also produce oestrogen, which increases the rate of cell division in the breasts and the uterus.[5]

When an injury occurs in the body, we get inflammation. You'll know this from when you cut yourself. The area bleeds, it quickly clots, the skin around it goes red and hot as blood reaches the area and helps healing, and it might swell as white blood cells, fluid and proteins collect there. The healing process occurs with the creation of new cells to replace the damaged ones, and the removal of debris from the damaged cells.

Inflammation is the body's way of defending itself against injury and infection and it's a really important process when you have an acute problem. When the injury keeps happening, though, the inflammation becomes chronic and can dramatically increase cancer risk. In chronic inflammation, the body is constantly churning out new cells. Just like a factory that's gone into overdrive, it's in this state that mistakes can happen and **mutations** can occur. Most of the time the mistakes don't matter. They might be in a part of a **gene** that isn't critical. The more often they happen, though, the more likely a serious **mutation** is to occur, one that can trigger cancer. So treating chronic inflammation is key to stopping cancer from developing or coming back.

References

1. Genomics & Precision Health. Does Breast or Ovarian Cancer Run in Your Family?. Centers for Disease Control and Prevention. https://www.cdc.gov/features/hereditarycancer/. Published 2020. Accessed August 19, 2021.
2. Genomics and Precision Health. What is Epigenetics?. Centers for Disease Control and Prevention. https://www.cdc.gov/genomics/disease/epigenetics.htm. Published 2020. Accessed August 19, 2021.
3. Zheng J. Energy metabolism of cancer: Glycolysis versus oxidative phosphorylation (Review). *Oncol Lett*. 2012;4(6):1151-1157. doi:10.3892/ol.2012.928
4. Tu H, Wen C, Tsai S et al. Cancer risk associated with chronic diseases and disease markers: prospective cohort study. *BMJ*. 2018:k134. doi:10.1136/bmj.k134
5. Cancer Research UK. Does obesity cause cancer?. Cancer Research UK. https://www.cancerresearchuk.org/about-cancer/causes-of-cancer/obesity-weight-and-cancer/does-obesity-cause-cancer. Published 2021. Accessed August 19, 2021.

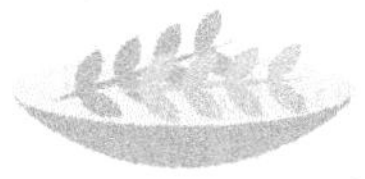

Chapter 2

Tweak your diet

'Let food be thy medicine and medicine be thy food.'
– Hippocrates

Why is diet important?

According to researchers at the University of Texas, between 30% and 35% of cancer deaths are connected with diet.[1] It's an astonishing statistic, and it made me much more optimistic about having a cancer-free future because diet is something we all have total control over.

These figures are confirmed by looking at cancer rates in different countries that have varying diets. You can see changes in cancer rates when, for example, Asian women, who have a low rate of breast cancer in their home country, migrate to the USA, where the rate is high, and change their diet. Their likelihood of contracting breast cancer increases substantially.

The rates vary according to which type of cancer you're talking about. For example, deaths from colon cancer are related to diet in about 70% of cases. But all types are linked to diet to some extent.[1]

The ideal dietary regime if you're fighting cancer or trying to prevent it returning includes the following:

- Eat regularly and enjoy food.
- Where possible, eat organic foods and especially avoid genetically modified foods (GMO).
- Eat plenty of fresh vegetables and some fruit every day. Aim to eat at least one green, one yellow, one red, one orange and one purple vegetable or fruit every day. Hence the saying 'Eat a rainbow a day.'
- Eat no more than 1 or 2 meals of red meat per week.
- Avoid cooking meat at high temperatures, such as barbecuing and frying.
- Include some healthy dairy products (but see my recommendations later in this chapter).
- Eat plenty of healthy fats like avocado, nuts, and fresh (non-rancid) olive and coconut oils.
- Drink plenty of water, tea (especially green tea) and herbal teas, but avoid carbonated drinks, both sugary and artificially sweetened, and alcohol.
- Avoid sugary foods, salt or artificial sweeteners.
- Eat dark chocolate with at least 70% cocoa, avoid milk chocolate and white chocolate.
- Eat fermented foods like yoghurt, sauerkraut, kimchi, kefir and kombucha.
- Avoid eating or drinking anything that interferes with your sleep.
- Avoid using non-stick (Teflon® coated) pans to cook with, and don't store your food in plastic.[2]

Those are the golden rules. Let's look at why each of them is important.

Have regular meals and enjoy them

Mealtimes should be an enjoyable experience, ideally shared with family and friends. This helps you relax, which in turn means better digestion. When under stress, you produce hormones that slow down digestion. In days gone by, if we needed to escape from predators, digestion was put on hold until we were safe again.

If you're having chemo, you may have lost your appetite and you could have difficulty keeping food down. It's important to get as many nutrients as possible because cancer can cause you to lose weight and particularly muscle mass, known as **cachexia**. It's better to eat small meals more often because they're often easier to manage. If you find that hot food makes you nauseous, look for cold foods that you can safely eat, or eat hot food once it's cooled. Sandwiches with fillings such as tinned salmon, nut spreads or hard-boiled eggs, and some carefully washed salad vegetables might work for you.

Eat organic foods and avoid genetically modified foods

Organic foods contain between 18% and 69% higher levels of antioxidants than conventionally grown foods.[3] Antioxidants counteract the effects of free radicals, also known as reactive oxygen species (**ROS**). Our bodies produce **ROS** all the time but when the levels get too high they can cause damage to our cells.

This causes inflammation, which we need to avoid. We produce some antioxidants ourselves but we need a lot from our diet too.

The best-known antioxidants and some of their best sources are shown below.

Antioxidant	Food source
Vitamin A	Apricots, butter, carrots, cheese, egg yolk, fish liver oils, green leafy vegetables, kohlrabi, liver, mint, spinach, orange sweet potatoes
Vitamin C	Blackcurrant, broccoli, Brussels sprouts, cabbage (raw), capsicum, citrus, guava, parsley, pawpaw and papaya, pineapple, potatoes, rosehips, strawberries, sweet potatoes, tomatoes
Vitamin E	Almonds, beef, corn, egg yolk, hazelnuts, other nuts and seeds, wheat germ
Beta-carotene	Broccoli, capsicum, carrots, pawpaw and papaya, spinach, sweet potatoes, tomatoes, yellow and greenish-yellow vegetables
Lutein	Corn, all dark green leafy vegetables, egg yolks
Lycopene	Apricots, guava, pawpaw and papaya, pink grapefruit, tomatoes (cooked) and processed tomato products, such as tomato paste and passata, watermelon
Selenium	Alfalfa, barley, broccoli, brazil nuts (2 per day provide daily requirement. Don't eat more than 6 per day regularly), butter, cashews, crab, celery, eggs, fish, garlic, kidney, liver, mackerel, oysters, peanuts, tuna, wholegrains, yeast, onions, turnip

Organic foods have lower levels of cadmium, a toxic heavy metal, and pesticides, which have been shown to cause **DNA mutations**. Organic meat, milk and dairy products also have higher levels of omega 3 fatty acids.[3] The average Western diet these days has high levels of omega 6 fatty acids, which are pro-inflammatory, whereas omega 3 fatty acids are anti-inflammatory.

Organic foods can be more expensive and difficult to find, although the major supermarkets have begun to stock some. Farmers' markets are usually a good source and they sell local produce, which is usually fresher. Antioxidant levels of some foods can drop significantly if they aren't fresh. If you can't find any stockists locally, you might find online sources that will deliver.

The Environmental Working Group (**EWG**) is a US non-profit organisation whose aim is to educate people to live healthily. They produce a guide to the foods most likely to be contaminated with pesticides. For 2021, these are, starting from the worst:

- strawberries
- spinach
- kale, collard and mustard greens
- nectarines
- apples
- grapes
- cherries
- peaches
- pears
- capsicum and chillies
- celery
- tomatoes.[4]

If you aren't able to buy organic produce, wash these fruit and vegetables in unperfumed Castile soap, as this will help remove any residues on the surface. Alternatively, soak them in a solution of 1 teaspoon of sodium bicarbonate per **litre** of water for about 12 minutes. After washing or soaking them, rinse with fresh water with a few drops of apple cider vinegar. This removes any soap or sodium bicarbonate and kills bacteria and fungi.

Genetically modified foods have been created to be able to withstand herbicides like glyphosate, the main ingredient in Roundup. Glyphosate alone was declared safe for use on foods but Roundup, which is often used by farmers, contains compounds designed to make it 100 times easier to absorb. So the safe level has been well and truly exceeded. There are no human studies showing the effects of Roundup because they wouldn't be approved for ethical reasons, but population studies show a correlation between non-Hodgkin lymphoma and Roundup use (see Chapter 6). Some states in the US have banned its use and on 29 July 2021 Bayer, who took over Monsanto, announced that Roundup would no longer be available in the US for home use. Animal studies show evidence of liver and kidney toxicity, together with effects on blood cells, spleen, adrenals and the heart.[2]

Labelling laws for genetically modified foods are poor, but the major genetically modified crops are canola (rapeseed), corn and soy, so I suggest avoiding these unless they're labelled GMO (genetically modified organism) free. Organic foods are by definition GMO free.

Eat plenty of fresh vegetables and fruit

Eating a wide variety of fresh vegetables and fruit with different colours ensures that you get many of the vitamins and minerals you need. They also contain phytochemicals which have antioxidant properties. These can prevent damage to your **DNA** and counteract some of the toxic effects of your treatment.[5]

Fresh vegetables and fruit are also an important source of fibre. Constipation can be a problem during cancer treatment, and fruit and vegetables can help stop it. The body gets rid of toxins, which include medications and break-down products, via the faeces, so avoiding constipation is important.

All the evidence shows that eating more vegetables and fruit is strongly associated with a protective effect against a range of cancers, including oral, throat, oesophageal, stomach, bowel, pancreatic, lung and endometrial cancers. Vegetables offer greater protection than fruit, and raw vegetables are the most protective. Among the best vegetables are the onion family (onions, garlic, leeks, spring onions etc.), carrots, green leafy vegetables, cruciferous vegetables (broccoli, cabbage and cauliflower), and tomatoes.[6]

Vitamin C is found in vegetables and fruit. The American Institute of Cancer Research (**AICR**) and the World Cancer Research Fund (**WCRF**) found that foods containing high amounts probably protect against oesophageal, oral and throat, lung and stomach cancers, and may also protect against liver, bowel and pancreatic cancers.[2] Vitamin C is a powerful antioxidant, needed for regenerating other antioxidant vitamins like Vitamin E. At normal doses, it also protects **DNA** from **mutations** and prevents the formation of **carcinogens**.

Some fruits like grapefruit and apples contain high amounts of flavonoids, which inhibit formation of **carcinogens** and are antioxidant.[2] Grapefruit can interfere with some medications, so check with your doctor or pharmacist before eating them.

Berries are rich in ellagic acid, an antioxidant which slows cancer cell division and neutralises some **carcinogens**. Raspberries and strawberries are particularly good sources. Strawberries are also rich in flavonoids. The most powerful antioxidants known are anthocyanosides and they are found in purple, blue and red berries and in purple vegetables such as eggplant and beetroot.[2]

Cruciferous vegetables are particularly good for cancer patients. They contain compounds such as indole-3-carbinol and glucosinolates, which have anti-cancer properties.[7] They reduce inflammation[8] and are high in fibre. If you have a hormone-sensitive cancer, such as breast, ovarian, endometrial or prostate cancer, cruciferous vegetables can reduce the hormonal effects, and help with anti-oestrogenic and anti-androgenic therapies.[9, 10]

Cruciferous vegetables can affect your thyroid if you eat large amounts of them raw, but they're safe to eat if you cook them, even if you have thyroid problems.[11] However, boiling for just 5 minutes reduces the anti-cancer effects significantly, so stir frying or lightly steaming/microwaving them for 3–4 minutes is best.[2]

Cruciferous vegetables include:

- bok choy
- broccoli
- brussels sprouts

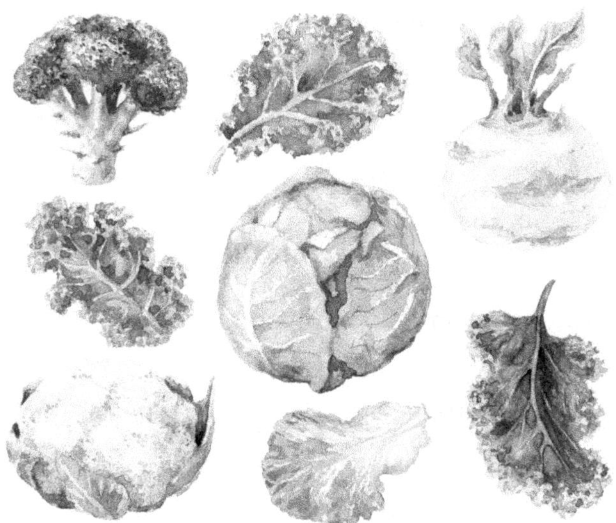

- cabbage
- cauliflower
- kale
- kohlrabi
- maca
- radish
- rocket (arugula)
- swede
- turnip
- watercress.

Tomatoes contain high levels of lycopene, which is powerfully antioxidant. ***In vitro*** research shows it encourages cancer cells' **apoptosis** and stops them growing, stops **metastasis** and **angiogenesis**, and is anti-inflammatory. It's particularly helpful for anyone undergoing prostate cancer treatment.[12] Lycopene levels are higher in cooked tomatoes than raw, and adding some olive oil makes it easier to absorb.[2]

Mushrooms have anti-cancer properties and boost the immune system, have an antioxidant effect, block the effects of oestrogen, encourage **apoptosis** of cancer cells, prevent **metastasis**, and can even stop cancer recurrences. Not all mushrooms have this effect. Shiitake mushrooms do and are easily available.[13] You'll find further information about mushroom extracts in Chapter 8. Beware of eating wild mushrooms: they can be deadly.

Eat red meat no more than twice a week

Eating a lot of red meat has been convincingly linked to many cancers, especially in the bowel, but also breast, lung, endometrium, pancreas, kidney, oesophagus, stomach and bladder cancers, and non-Hodgkin lymphoma. Processed meats such as bacon, ham and deli meats contain nitrites and nitrates that are linked to these cancers particularly and others too.[14]

In 2007, the **WCRF** and **AICR** advised that red meat was a cause of colorectal cancer, and that higher red meat intake was linked to higher cancer rates.[15] The same report showed there was 'convincing evidence' that processed meats cause colorectal cancer and 'limited evidence' that they cause lung, prostate, oesophageal and stomach cancers.[15]

In 2015, the International Agency for Research on Cancer (**IARC**) classified processed meats as '**carcinogenic** to humans' and red meat (including lamb, goat, mutton, veal, pork, beef and horse) was classified as 'probably **carcinogenic** to humans', causing colorectal, prostate and pancreatic cancers.[16] A **meta-analysis** of 800 studies concluded that for each 50 **g** portion of processed meat eaten daily, the risk of colorectal cancer rose by 18%.[16]

Processed meats include any meat, including beef, pork, poultry, offal and blood, that has been cured, salted, fermented, smoked or processed by any means that improves shelf-life. That includes sausages, ham, bacon, corned beef, hot dogs, beef jerky, canned and deli meats, and meat-based foods and sauces.[16]

Nowadays, red meat contains a lot of omega 6 fatty acids. Livestock used to be put out into the fields to graze, whereas now they're generally raised in feedlots, where they're fed grains. Grass-fed meat has higher levels of omega 3s than grain fed meat and is therefore less inflammatory.[17] The grains that livestock are fed are quite often genetically modified too, which means they're potentially very high in glyphosate (Roundup).

All that being said, red meat provides nutrients that are difficult to find in a vegetarian diet:

- Vitamin B12, essential for maintaining nerves, developing red blood cells and normal brain function. Deficiency causes fatigue and weakness, anaemia, problems with concentration, confusion, low white blood cells and many other issues. Deficiency may also be linked to Alzheimer's[18] and heart disease.[19] A long-term deficiency can lead to death. Vitamin B12 is particularly depleted during cancer treatment because of the effects of chemo on the digestive system.[20] Vitamin B12 is only found naturally in animal foods and certain types of seaweed[21], although some vegetarian foods are fortified with it.

- Creatine is a natural substance found in meat. Although we can manufacture some in the liver, vegetarians tend to be low in it. It's needed for energy production.[22] It improves muscle strength and muscle mass, both of which are affected by cancer treatment. It's also connected with brain function.[21]
- Carnosine is a nutrient mainly found in meat. It isn't essential for us because we can make it, but our diets contribute a significant amount and vegetarians have reduced levels. We need it to maintain muscle mass and to improve stamina.[21]
- Haem iron is found in meat alone. Some plant foods contain iron but it's non-haem iron, which isn't easy for our bodies to absorb. Strangely, haem iron also helps the absorption of non-haem iron.[21] Iron is necessary for making haemoglobin in red blood cells.

So red meat is beneficial in the diet, but to get these benefits we only need 2 meals of red meat a week, preferably organic or free range, each portion less than 200 **g** for men and 160 **g** for women. Processed meats should be avoided completely.

Avoid cooking at high temperatures

Cooking at high temperatures, such as toasting, roasting, baking, frying, grilling and barbecuing, produces a range of chemicals classified by the **IARC** as possibly or probably **carcinogen**ic.[23] These chemicals are collectively known as advanced glycation end-products (**AGEs**). They can occur in cooked meat, vegetables and grain foods.

A **systematic review** summarised the evidence for the links between cancer and acrylamides, which are **AGE**s. It found significant evidence for links to endometrial, lung, mouth, ovarian, oesophageal, renal and stomach cancers.[24]

Foods high in protein and fats, primarily meats and especially beef, produce higher levels of **AGE**s after high temperature cooking, but deep-fried vegetables and grains are problematic too.[24]

To reduce the levels of **AGE**s:

- Steaming, poaching, stewing, slow cooking, microwaving and boiling keep the levels of **AGE**s at from 20—50% lower than high temperature cooking methods.[24]
- Marinating beef for an hour in acidic marinades, such as vinegar or lemon juice before roasting reduced the levels of **AGEs** by about 50% in a controlled trial.[24] This would probably help with other meats too.
- When making toast, don't brown it too much. Cut the crusts off, because they brown more quickly. The darker the toast, the higher the level of **AGE**s.[24]
- When cooking at high temperatures, cook food for the shortest time and at the lowest temperature needed to thoroughly cook but not brown too much.
- Higher fat and aged cheeses, such as cheddar and parmesan, are also high in **AGE**s, so eat them sparingly. Cottage cheese, reduced fat mozzarella and low-fat cheddar are better choices.[24]
- High fat spreads, such as cream cheese, mayonnaise, margarine and butter are high in **AGE**s too, so choose lower-fat options.[24]

- Oils and nuts cooked at high temperatures also have high levels of **AGE**s.[24] Stick to natural nuts rather than roasted ones.
- Processed foods cooked with dry heat, such as potato chips, crackers and biscuits are high in **AGE**s[24], so are best avoided.
- Non-fat milk is significantly lower in **AGEs** than whole milk[24], but see the next section on dairy.
- Avoid deep-fried foods, such as French fries. If you cook them yourself, keep the potatoes in a cool, dark place (not the fridge) before you fry, roast or bake them. Soaking and drying reduces the **AGEs** when cooked, or parboil for a few minutes before cutting them into pieces. Oven roast with spray oil rather than frying and don't overcook them. This reduces **AGEs** to the minimum.[25] This method is also significantly lower in calories than frying. Or switch to baked potatoes, which have even fewer **AGEs.**
- Dark roasts of coffee are higher in **AGEs** than lighter ones[25], so consider switching to a lighter roast.

Include some healthy dairy products

Healthy dairy products include natural yoghurt and kefir, both of which are fermented and contain probiotics. Make sure you buy products that contain live cultures: many commercial products are heat-sterilised, which kills the bacteria. Probiotics are covered in Chapter 7. They're important for maintaining healthy gut bacteria, which is crucial for anyone suffering from cancer.

I don't recommend eating a lot of dairy, though. Many doctors consider that dairy products are our major source of calcium, which is important for bones. However, in some cultures, such as China, dairy products aren't eaten at all and they have low rates of osteoporosis, whereas it's a serious problem in the West.

One problem with dairy products is that, although they contain a large amount of calcium, they don't contain the other minerals bones need in the right proportions for the body to use. If you can't use it, calcium is laid down in the arteries and organs instead of the bones.[26] This can cause heart disease and other issues. Better sources of calcium are green, leafy vegetables, almonds, eggs, tinned sardines and salmon (with the bones, which are edible), and bone broth.

Making your own bone broth is simple, especially in a pressure cooker or a slow cooker. Use about 1 **kg** of beef, lamb or chicken bones. Chicken wings, necks and feet are particularly good. Cover with water, add any herbs or spices you like, an onion, a carrot and a celery stick, plus about 2 tablespoons of organic apple cider vinegar. You won't taste the vinegar but it's important because it helps extract the calcium and other minerals from the bones. Cook at high pressure for about 2 hours or more, slow cook for 24 hours, or simmer for about 5–6 hours, then strain it and store in glass jars. Mason jars are ideal. The broth keeps in the fridge for about 3 days, or you can freeze it. It may set once it's cooled. If it does, it means you've extracted a lot of collagen, which strengthens your skin, hair and nails. It's wonderful for helping heal your gut, often badly hit by chemo. You can drink it straight or use it in soups and casseroles, wherever you would use stock.

Milk contains toxins, such as pesticide and herbicide residues from the grass and feed that the cows eat.[27] In some countries, the milk from cows treated with antibiotics reaches the shops. This happens occasionally in Australia, despite measures taken to prevent it.[28] Drinking milk containing antibiotics increases the risk of developing antibiotic resistance.

Dairy products have other unwanted effects on the body. Cows produce milk when they've calved and this is intended to accelerate calf growth. So it contains a lot of growth hormones, which can increase cancer growth. However, consuming low-fat dairy products, but not milk, protects against developing prostate[29], breast[30] and endometrial[31] cancers, and also against the growth of these cancers once they've begun.

Milk itself, though, seriously increases the risk of breast cancer. A recent study followed 52,975 women for 9 years. Some drank milk regularly whilst others drank soy milk. The results showed that those drinking milk, either whole or low-fat, had an increased risk of breast cancer. Those drinking just 60 **ml** per day increased their risk by 30% and those drinking 500—750 **ml** per day increased their risk by an incredible 70—80%. This applied equally to pre-menopausal and post-menopausal women and to all kinds of breast cancer. However, cheese and yoghurt didn't have this effect. Soy products didn't affect breast cancer risk either and they may even be protective.[32]

There's conflicting evidence about the effect of milk on prostate cancer. Some studies find that a high intake of calcium from dairy products increases the risks, whilst others disagree.[33]

So the take-away messages are:

- Avoid full-fat dairy products, such as whole milk, high-fat cheeses and full-fat yoghurt.

- Avoid dairy milk. Use low-fat cheeses such as cottage cheese and low-fat ricotta, and eat low-fat yoghurt.
- Cut down on butter. Margarine, although high in fat, doesn't contain saturated fats like butter. Solid margarines, such as those used in cooking, contain high levels of trans fats, which increase inflammation, particularly in the gut[34] and the cardiovascular system.[35]

Eat plenty of healthy fats

Although highly saturated fats in meat and dairy cause and promote cancer growth, many unsaturated fats, mostly found in oily fish and plant foods, have the opposite effect.

Fats are important in our diet for many reasons:

- They're needed for making the membranes that surround each cell, which are a combination of fat (lipid) and phosphate molecules.
- They help us absorb Vitamins A, D, E and K, which are all fat soluble.
- They're used to produce steroid hormones, which are made from cholesterol. These include cortisol and our sex hormones.
- They contain more energy than carbohydrate and proteins.
- The fat layer under our skin insulates against heat loss and protects our organs.

Although eating carbohydrates enables fat production, essential fatty acids must be included in our diet. The best-known are polyunsaturated omega 3 and omega 6 fatty acids. We need both, ideally in a ratio of 4 parts omega 6s to 1 part omega 3s. However, the average Western diet has a ratio of between 10:1 and 50:1.[36] Omega 6s are pro-inflammatory. Increasing levels of omega 3s reduces the risk of cancer, particularly breast and colorectal cancers.[37]

The best sources of omega 3s are fish oils, found in oily fish like salmon, sardines, herrings and mackerel. The best plant source is flax seeds. Flax oil goes rancid quickly, producing toxic chemicals, so put the seeds in smoothies and grind fresh for cooking. Flax seeds also contain compounds that reduce tumour growth, especially skin cancer and the hormone-sensitive cancers.[38]

Other polyunsaturated fats, like sunflower, rapeseed (canola), corn, soybean and safflower oils are higher in omega 6s. Although we need omega 6s, most people get enough of them, because they're particularly high in most processed foods, which also tend to have high saturated fats.

Canola (rapeseed), corn and soybean oils are all likely to be genetically modified so it's safest to avoid them. Canola contains erucic acid, a fatty acid associated with fibrotic lesions in the heart. Although genetically modified canola oil contains less erucic acid, the safety of eating even small quantities hasn't been established. It also goes through a deodorisation process that converts omega 3s into trans-fats, which are bad for heart health.[2] I recommend you avoid it.

Monounsaturated fats are a healthy option, containing omega 9s. High quantities are found in olive oil, nuts and seeds (especially hemp), olives, pork and avocadoes, and there are some in eggs. If you replace the saturated fats in your diet with monounsaturated fats, you're likely to:

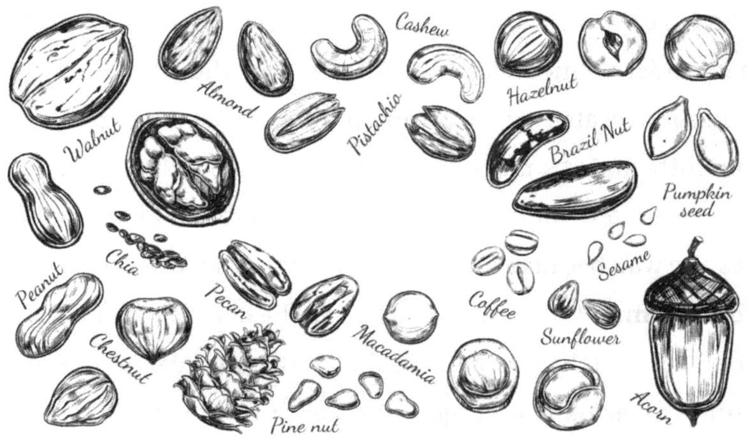

- Reduce your risk of heart disease.
- Maintain or even lose weight.
- Reduce insulin resistance, lowering your risk of diabetes.
- Reduce inflammation.
- Reduce your risk of some cancers, particularly breast cancer.[39]

Ensure that the olive oil you use is extra-virgin, cold-pressed and in a dark-coloured bottle to keep out the light. This ensures you get all the health benefits and that it isn't contaminated by other, possibly genetically modified oils.

Coconut oil has developed a reputation for being unhealthy because it's a saturated fat. Saturated fats have been labelled as promoting heart disease. However, in 2010 a **meta-analysis** of 21 studies covering almost 348,000 people over a 5–23 year period found that there is no significant evidence that saturated fat is linked to heart disease.[40] Another study showed that virgin coconut oil has a beneficial effect on cardiovascular health.[41]

Coconut oil is unlike other saturated fats. All fats consist of fatty acids. Coconut oil is different because many of the fatty acid chains are considered 'medium' in length, rather than the long chains found in saturated fat in animal products. The body processes it differently and it's much easier to break down during digestion. Most saturated fats can't enter the bloodstream through the intestine wall because the molecules are too big. Instead they cross into the **lymph** fluid and are carried to the liver for manufacturing into cholesterol that can be carried in the bloodstream. The medium chain fatty acids from digested coconut oil, however, are small enough to cross directly into the bloodstream and can be used directly by the cells for energy, so they don't turn into cholesterol.[42]

Coconut oil has antibacterial, antiviral, anti-parasitic and antifungal effects, and can help to balance the immune system.[43] It can also be used as a moisturiser for these effects, and as a mouthwash before cleaning your teeth to help remove plaque and fight oral thrush infections, which are common during chemo.[43]

My advice is:

- Eat more oily fish.
- Eat more flaxseeds, other seeds and nuts.
- Avoid polyunsaturated oils like canola, soybean and corn oil.
- Use olive oil or coconut oil in cooking.

Drink plenty but choose the best drinks

Water is vital for good health. It:

- Helps regulate temperature.
- Flushes out waste products via the kidneys, liver and digestive system.

- Keeps body tissues moist, including the nose, mouth and eyes.
- Cushions bones and joints.
- Helps with digestion.

How much you need depends on the weather, exercise levels, and your health, but most of us need 6—8 glasses of water or other healthy drinks each day. Drink more if your urine is a dark colour.

Water is the ideal drink. Try carrying a water bottle, preferably of glass or stainless steel. I recommend using a water filter to remove any contaminants, ideally one that alkalises and remineralises the water. Most filters sold in supermarkets and chainstores only filter out particles. A good filter will remove:

- Chlorine, which damages your gut bacteria.
- Heavy metals, which are poisonous.
- Fluoride. There is some evidence that fluoride is toxic and may cause a number of diseases, including cancer.[44, 45]
- Phthalates (see Chapter 6), which are released from the PVC pipes used in modern plumbing.

Don't like the taste of water? Try adding a few berries, other fruit, cucumber, or herbs such as mint. It really lifts the flavour.

How about coffee? In 1991 the **IARC** classified it as 'possibly **carcinogenic'** but they changed their minds in 2016 and it's now classified as 'unclassifiable as to its **carcinogenicity** to humans'.[46] In fact, a paper published in 'The Lancet', quoted several meta-analyses that found coffee reduces the risk of some cancers. These include endometrial and liver cancers, and a possible reduction in breast cancer.[46] Coffee contains antioxidants but the roasting of coffee beans creates **AGEs**[25], since they're roasted at high temperatures. Very hot drinks, over 65°C, can encourage the growth of tumours, especially in the oesophagus[46], probably because they cause damage as they're being swallowed. So if you enjoy coffee:

- Limit it to 1 or 2 cups per day to reduce your exposure to **AGE**s.
- Choose a lighter roast.
- Drink it at a lower temperature.

Green tea is an excellent choice. Studies on animals show it has anti-cancer properties, preventing cancers of the oesophagus, stomach, liver, lung, mouth, prostate, skin, pancreas, colon and others.[47] Human studies on green tea drinkers also show a reduced risk of cancers of the prostate, lung, colon, ovary and breast.[48] Green tea is rich in antioxidants, particularly epigallocatechin-3-gallate (EGCG), believed to be the main reason for its anti-cancer effects. Black tea contains very small amounts of EGCG but would be unlikely to have therapeutic effects. Concentrations are significantly higher in green tea. Again, don't drink it too hot. Choose organic teas to avoid toxins and brew it for less than 3 minutes to avoid heavy metals. However, green tea can interact with certain drugs, including those used in chemo treatments. Check out this article at https://www.naturallysupportingcancertreatment.com.au/blog/dark-side-green-tea.

Shop-bought fruit juices are high in sugar, which produces an insulin spike when they're consumed. Sugar feeds cancer cells, so they're best avoided. Eating fruit whole rather than juicing is better, because it's easy to drink large quantities of juice. Although juice gives you more antioxidants, the sugar outweighs the benefit. If you eat whole fruit, the fibre content stops you eating too much and also slows down sugar absorption. If you like juices, try blending fruit whole with non-dairy milk.. Better still, blend a mixture of vegetables and use a little fruit to sweeten it. Try to find organic fruit and vegetables to juice. Otherwise you'll drink a lot of pesticides with the good stuff.[2]

Cordials and carbonated drinks aren't good choices. They're high in sugar and don't contain any useful nutrients. Sugar-free drinks contain a lot of additives and are no better for you than their sugary counterparts.[2] Carbonated drinks also contain phosphoric acid, which is highly acidifying. Acidity in the blood encourages cancer growth.

Drinking alcohol is risky. It can cause cancer of the breast, oesophagus, throat, colon, bowel and liver.[49] It also increases prostate cancer risk.[50] It's estimated that 5.8% of all cancer deaths worldwide are related to alcohol consumption[49], and the more you drink the higher the risk.[51]

So should you give up alcohol completely? In Western culture, alcohol plays a large part in our social lives. Cancer shouldn't mean giving up everything you enjoy. If you aren't currently undergoing chemo, it probably isn't going to make a significant difference to your outcome if you have the occasional drink. Just don't make it a regular habit. The **WCRF** and **AICR** report recommends a limit of 2 alcoholic drinks each day for men and one for women.[15] In Chapter 8, I've given some suggestions for herbs that support your liver, which I recommend if you're going to drink alcohol. If you're currently undergoing chemo, though, it would be wise to avoid alcohol during treatment. Your liver will be detoxifying the drugs and doesn't need an additional burden. Some chemo drugs change your sense of smell and taste, so alcohol may taste unpleasant anyway.

Avoid sugary foods, artificial sweeteners and salt

Refined sugar has been linked to inflammation.[52] High blood sugar, usually a result of eating too many sugary foods, reduces the body's immune defences[53], which protect against cancers starting.

The Western diet contains large amounts of sugar, especially in processed foods. This includes most breakfast cereals, packaged foods, sauces, pies, pastries, muffins, cakes, lollies and ice cream. Most bread also contains high levels of sugars. Wholegrain bread is less likely to cause a spike in blood sugar levels. It would be impractical to suggest completely eliminating them from your diet, but try to reduce these foods as much as possible. The best source of sugar in the diet is fruit. It's metabolised more slowly because of the fibre in it, and fruit contains vitamins and phytonutrients that are beneficial.

So are artificial sweeteners the answer? Sadly, although there isn't any direct evidence that they cause cancer, acesulfame K, saccharin, aspartame (Equal), sucralose and stevia have been shown to disrupt gut bacteria. In animal trials, they've been shown to cause weight gain, which should be avoided if you're fighting cancer, especially if you're already on the heavy side.[54]

Aspartame also causes a rise in insulin levels, which can lead to type II diabetes, and worsens atherosclerosis, which can cause heart attacks.[54] Using aspartame regularly has been shown to affect liver detoxification and result in liver damage.[55] Chemo is hard on the liver, so avoiding any further damage is important.

Sugar alcohols, such as erythritol, mannitol, sorbitol and xylitol, often used in sugar-free foods, are no better. They've also been shown to cause changes to gut bacteria.[54]

So what's the answer to the sugar dilemma? Well, ideally, we need sweeteners that are natural but don't cause an insulin spike, which means sugars that have a lower glycaemic index (GI).

For coffee, tea, herbal teas and other drinks, use a little raw honey. Honey is sweeter than sugar, contains some useful nutrients and antioxidants, and has anti-inflammatory and antimicrobial effects (particularly Manuka honey). It also helps the **p53 gene** and some other cancer-fighting mechanisms, so it assists with **apoptosis**. There's some evidence it can also inhibit tumour growth.[56] The glycaemic index (GI), which determines how quickly a food is absorbed and therefore how much blood sugar rises, varies according to the type of honey used and can be anything from about 45–64, compared with 65 for white sugar. The lowest are sourced from a single flower species, with Yellow Box and Stringybark being the lowest in Australia.[57]

For baking, try fresh dates (not dried ones, which have very high levels of sugar like any other dried fruit). Blended, they make a good substitute for sugar in cooking and smoothies. They're also a powerhouse of nutrition. They're high in fibre, so they're absorbed slowly, high in potassium, which is needed to balance sodium, and contain antioxidants, vitamins and minerals. They increase energy, relieve constipation and reduce cholesterol levels.[58]

If you have a sweet tooth, they also make a good snack, but stick with just 1 or 2 and savour them, as they're fairly high in calories. They're also wonderful for snacking when they're frozen.

If you're watching your weight or have diabetes, the best artificial sweetener is stevia. Despite its effects on gut bacteria, it has useful properties:

- It can help to reduce blood sugar — helpful if you're diabetic or have insulin resistance, the precursor to diabetes.[59]
- It helps reduce blood pressure.[59]
- It's antimicrobial, killing bacteria, fungi and viruses.[59]
- Most importantly, it helps kill cancer cells.[59]

There are various brands of stevia available. I recommend liquid stevia, which is available in health food shops. It only contains stevia and a little alcohol to preserve it. Stevia tablets and powders usually contain erythritol, which can leave an aftertaste that many people find unpleasant. Liquid stevia is more economical than the tablets or powdered varieties. Some dispensers must be refrigerated after opening, which isn't very convenient if you're not home, but some do not.

Another, possibly better, alternative is monk fruit. This article compares stevia and monk fruit. https://www.naturallysupportingcancertreatment.com.au/blog/is-monk-fruit-healthier-than-stevia

Eat dark chocolate

You can enjoy a few squares of dark chocolate each day and feel good about it. A cocoa content of 70% plus is best, though, and milk chocolate usually contains about 10% cocoa. White chocolate doesn't contain cocoa at all, only cocoa butter. Dark chocolate usually contains much less sugar than milk or white chocolate too.

Cocoa contains polyphenols, which are antioxidant and affect various stages of cancer development. They're especially helpful for normal **apoptosis** but also help prevent damage to **DNA** that can start cancer growth. Their anti-inflammatory effects reduce damage.[60] They stop **angiogenesis**, and they help stop **metastasis.**[61]

In trials, cocoa protected against colon cancers in animals and there's evidence for the same effect in humans.[60] It reduces insulin resistance, blood pressure, and total and **LDL cholesterol** ('bad cholesterol'), and makes blood less sticky, which is good for heart health. It may be helpful for reducing inflammation in ulcerative colitis and Crohn's disease[61], both of which can be precursors to cancer.

A couple of pieces about half an hour before a meal can reduce your appetite, so it can help with weight loss.

Don't over-indulge but enjoy a few pieces each day.

Eat fermented foods

Fermented foods that aren't pasteurised or heat treated contain live bacteria and yeasts that help diversify our gut microbiome. The good bacteria thrive on vegetable fibre in food. These are important for many reasons, including:

- Producing natural antibiotics that kill off the bacteria responsible for infections and diarrhoea.[62]
- Helping stop cancer-treatment related diarrhoea.[63]

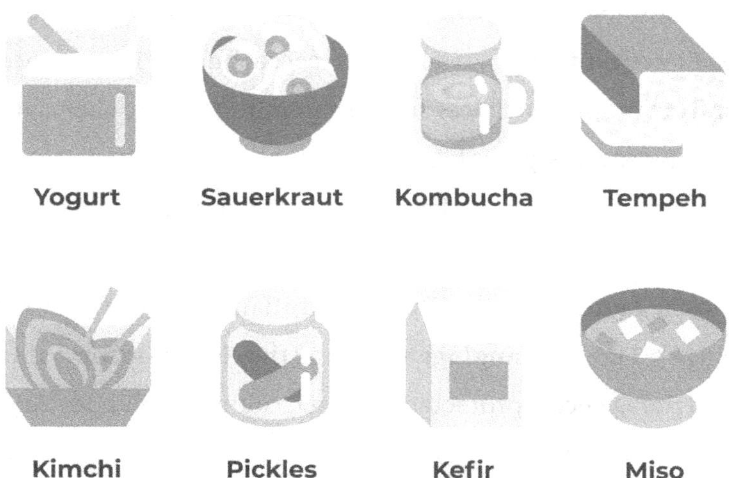

- Strengthening the immune system, especially in the gut. They also affect other body systems, such as the urinary and respiratory systems, salivary and tear glands, the prostate and breast tissue.[2]
- Producing enzymes, such as lactase, which aid digestion, and reducing enzymes that can help promote cancers.[62]
- Producing some vitamins.[62]
- Helping prevent food allergies.[62]
- Assisting in the fight against cancer in many different ways. They produce short chain fatty acids, which make the environment of the colon more acidic. This is associated with a lower incidence of bowel cancer.[62] They're also effective against breast cancer, cervical cancer, liver cancer and fibrosarcoma.[2]

- Some probiotic bacteria increase natural killer (**NK**) cell numbers and effectiveness.[64]
- Repopulating the gut with good bacteria after taking antibiotics.

If your white blood cell count is very low (neutropenic) it may be wise to avoid probiotic foods until your levels rise. A handful of neutropenic patients have contracted infections which have been associated with probiotics.[64]

Fermented foods include:

- Yoghurt, but not those high in added sugars. Plain yoghurt is ideal. Add fruit to sweeten it.
- Kefir, a fermented milk drink. You can buy it or use kefir grains from health food stores to make your own.
- Sauerkraut (fermented cabbage) and kimchi, the Korean equivalent that can be quite spicy.
- Kombucha (fermented tea).
- Miso, made from fermented soybeans, is a paste you can make into soups, use in dressings or on vegetables, or use as a savoury drink. It's also rich in protein.
- Tempeh, also made from fermented soybeans, has a nutty taste and is good in stir fries.
- Soft cheeses made from unpasteurised milk, such as those made from goat's and sheep's milk.

Probiotic bacteria live on prebiotics. These are foods that aren't digested in the small intestine and feed the bacteria in the colon. Eating prebiotics helps promote the growth of good bacteria. Prebiotics are found in the following foods.[65]

Prebiotic	Best food source
Vegetables	All the onion family, Jerusalem artichokes, asparagus, beetroot, fennel, green peas, snow peas, sweetcorn and Savoy cabbage
Legumes	Chickpeas, lentils, red kidney beans, baked beans etc.
Fruit	Custard apples, grapefruit, nectarines, white peaches, persimmon, pomegranate, rambutan, tamarillo, watermelon
Cereals	Rye bread and crackers, barley, pasta, gnocchi, couscous, oats
Nuts	Cashews and pistachios

Don't consume anything sleep-disrupting

Sleep is really important when you're fighting cancer or trying to prevent recurrences (see Chapter 5). If you have sleeping problems, avoid eating or drinking anything that might disrupt it.

The biggest problem is coffee, tea, cola or energy drinks, which contain caffeine. Caffeine breaks down relatively slowly. After 5 hours, we have metabolised about half of it. After 10 hours most people still have about 25% left in their system. Some people metabolise it even more slowly. So a cup in the afternoon could cause sleep issues.

Chocolate also contains some caffeine and another stimulant called theobromine. If you're sensitive to caffeine, eat chocolate earlier in the day.

It's unwise to drink alcohol late at night. Most people feel that it helps with sleep but, although it helps you fall sleep, it disrupts your sleep later. It also reduces rapid eye movement (REM) sleep[66], which is associated with learning. The more you drink, the worse the effects, and even wine can cause some disruption. If you want a drink with dinner, eat earlier and have one glass. Avoid drinking anything, including alcohol, within about 2 hours of bedtime. Otherwise, you may need a night-time bathroom trip.

Eating a large meal late at night disrupts sleep too. Ideally, eat at least 3 hours before bed. That gives the body a chance to digest dinner while you're upright. It also reduces the risk of heartburn.

If you suffer from heartburn, fatty foods are a likely trigger. So avoid them in the evening. Spicy foods can also cause heartburn and tend to delay and disrupt your sleep. This may be because of capsaicin, the chemical in chillies that makes them hot. The theory is that it raises your core temperature, which needs to be lowered before sleep.[67]

Some foods help us to produce the brain chemicals (neurotransmitters) that promote sound sleep. These include:

- Almonds, which contain melatonin. We produce melatonin naturally. The more we produce, the more soundly we sleep. Almonds also contain magnesium. Magnesium helps reduce cortisol, the stress hormone, which can disrupt sleep.[68] A handful of almonds is all you need and they make a good evening snack.
- Kiwifruit contain serotonin, which the body uses to produce melatonin, and they're also full of antioxidants. In a 4 week

trial, participants ate 2 kiwifruit an hour before bedtime. They reduced the time it took participants to get to sleep by 35%, they slept 13% longer, and the quality of their sleep was improved.[69]

- Tart cherry juice is high in melatonin and a number of small studies showed it improves sleep quality.[70-72] It's also rich in vitamins A and C, and anthocyanins and flavonols, both powerful antioxidants.
- Turkey contains high levels of tryptophan, which increases melatonin production. Breast meat contains more than dark meat but both help with sleep. The protein also keeps you satisfied for longer and helps with sleep quality.[73]
- Chamomile tea in the evening may help with sleep. It contains apigenin, which binds to benzodiazepine receptors in the brain (Valium is a benzodiazepine), so it's helpful if your insomnia is caused by anxiety. It also relieves indigestion, another common cause of insomnia. A few laboratory tests on cancer cells show that it may also have some anti-cancer effects.[74]

Take care over what contacts your food

Saucepans

Did you know that non-stick pans contain toxic chemicals? Teflon® coating is made using perfluorooctanoic acid, known as PFOA, which is part of a group of chemicals known as perfluoroalkyl substances (PFASs). When PFOA is heated, the coating degrades and releases dangerous toxins into the air. What's more, when the surfaces get scratched, as they inevitably do if they're used regularly, you eat particles of PFOA. In animal studies, some PFASs caused tumours in the pancreas, liver and testicles, and a human study linked exposure to PFOA with testicular and kidney cancers.[75] There are also links to thyroid disease, ulcerative colitis, high cholesterol and pregnancy-induced high blood pressure[75], and they're associated with obesity.[76]

The leading manufacturers of PFOA products agreed to phase them out by the end of 2015, but the **EWG** found that its replacements are still PFASs, and they're no safer than PFOA.[77]

The safest alternatives are cast iron and stainless steel[76], but neither of them is non-stick. If you want non-stick, ceramic cookware is best, ideally solid ceramic as opposed to ceramic-coated. Although solid ceramic is more expensive it'll last a lifetime. For baking, glass is a good choice. It's inert, doesn't stick or stain, and is easy to clean, but it doesn't come in many different shapes. If you're making muffins or looking for a baking sheet, silicon is a good choice. It can safely be used in the oven up to 220°C, and doesn't react with food or liquids, or give off fumes.

Food wrappers and containers

PFASs are also found in food wrappers such as pizza boxes, microwave popcorn bags, fast food wrappers and grease-resistant wrappers. Very low levels have been found in baking paper too.[78, 79] By avoiding fast foods you avoid consuming most PFASs.

Plastics leach chemicals into your food that disrupt hormones, which is serious if you are fighting or trying to avoid hormone-related cancers. Most people are aware that bisphenol A (**BPA**) in plastics is a hormone disruptor, but **BPA**-free plastics are based on a similar molecular structure and have the same effect. If you're using **BPA**-free plastic containers to cook in the microwave or store food, glass or ceramic dishes are a safe alternative.

Plastics fall into 7 different types and many display an identifying number inside a triangle with curved arrows.

Types of plastics, their uses and their safety

No.	Type	Uses	Safety
1	Polyethylene terephthalate (PET)	Disposable bottles for water, carbonated drinks, cordials and juices, plus jars for items such as peanut butter.	If PET is stored at high temperatures, highly likely in storage areas in summer, it releases antimony, a heavy metal.[80] Antimony trioxide is used in plastic manufacture and is classified as 'possibly **carcinogenic**' by the **IARC**.[81]
2	High density polyethylene (HDPE)	Used for milk cartons, yoghurt containers, sippy cups, breakfast cereal bags lining packets, kitchen utensils, and some reusable containers for food and drinks.	Have a low melting point (125–135°C), so are unsuitable for heating foods in the microwave. Take care when using kitchen utensils made from HDPE.[82]

No.	Type	Uses	Safety
3	Polyvinyl chloride (PVC)	Mainly used for plastic cling wraps. Some manufacturers are switching from **BPA** to PVC to line food cans.[83] Used under the lids of jars to improve the seal and used in modern plumbing pipes.	PVC contains plasticisers such as DEHA or phthalates which can leach into food. Phthalates are hormone disruptors, they reduce testicular function and reduce semen quality, are linked with endometriosis, increases in waist circumference and **BMI**. One phthalate was designated a **carcinogen** in California.[84] PVC is made by joining molecules of vinyl chloride, which has been designated as a **carcinogen** by the **EPA**.[85]
4	Low density polyethylene (LDPE)	Bread wrappers and frozen food bags, takeaway containers, waterproof coating on milk cartons, cling wrap and click lock bags.	Like HDPE it has a low melting point, starting to soften at 80°C, so it's unsuitable for use in the microwave.[82]
5	Polypropylene (PP)	Food storage containers, microwave cookware, margarine and yoghurt containers, bottle caps, drinking straws.	PP has a high melting point (165°C) and a low freezing point (–10°C), and it's stabilised with antioxidants, so it's sold as a 'safe' plastic.[82]

No.	Type	Uses	Safety
6	Polystyrene (PS)	Foam is used for coffee cups and trays for fruit and vegetable packs in the supermarkets. Plastic cutlery and cups for drinking and yoghurt.	PS is made from chains of styrene, which is **carcinogenic** in rats and mice. Population studies in humans who are exposed to styrene regularly show a higher incidence of blood cancers, and possible evidence of oesophageal and pancreatic cancers.[86]
7	A catch-all grouping for any other type of plastic, including polycarbonate	Feeding bottles for babies, drinking cups for infants, sauce bottles, reusable water bottles.	**BPA** is used in the manufacture of polycarbonate, so it will have the same hormone-disrupting effects as **BPA** itself. Polycarbonate has been linked to **carcinogenesis** and to promotion of growth in cancer cells.[87]

Almost all commercially available plastics release oestrogenic chemicals. A study measured the oestrogenic effects of over 500 commercially available plastic products, including many claiming to be **BPA** free. The effects were magnified if the plastics were exposed to microwaving, boiling water or UV light.[88]

My advice is:

- Opt for foods preserved in glass jars instead or, better still, use fresh foods rather than canned.[89]
- To avoid PET, carry a stainless steel or glass water bottle filled

with filtered water. Not only is it healthier and protects the environment but it also saves you money.

- Many people store food, particularly for freezing, in click-lock bags made from polyethylene. Instead, wrap the food in unbleached baking paper coated with silicone before you put food into these bags or any other type of plastic. Unbleached is important: the bleaching process uses chlorine, which creates dioxins when heated. Dioxins are classified by the **IARC** as a 'known human **carcinogen**'.[90] If the food doesn't touch plastic, it can't absorb problem chemicals. Beeswax and silicone wraps are other alternatives.
- Avoid cooking frozen foods in plastic bags, as this increases the likelihood of migration of chemicals.
- Invest in glass feeding bottles and sippy cups for children to avoid exposing them to oestrogenic chemicals.
- Instead of cling wrap, use unbleached baking paper, beeswax wraps or silicone covers.
- Aluminium from foil can be absorbed by food. High levels of aluminium are associated with neurological, bone and blood problems.[91] It also blocks absorption of minerals we need, such as magnesium, iron and calcium.[92] Unbleached baking paper is better.
- Wherever possible, avoid buying anything sold in plastic.

Specialised diets for cancer

Ketogenic diet

To be effective against cancer, this diet should consist of 5% carbohydrate, 20% protein and 75% fat, which should be healthy fats like avocado, olive or coconut oil, nuts and seeds. The diet works because most cancer cells only use glucose for energy. Positron emission tomography (PET) scans, where a radioactive substance is injected that combines with blood sugar, use this. The radioactive combination can be tracked to see where it's most used, which can locate cancer activity.

When carbohydrates are restricted, the body processes the fats into ketones, which cancer cells can't usually use for energy but the rest of your body can, and it puts the body into a state called 'ketosis'. Ketosis isn't the same as ketoacidosis, which is a complication of type I diabetes[93], and it's quite safe.

It's effective at reducing glioblastoma, a type of brain tumour, and 2 or 3 studies show good evidence for its effectiveness in pancreatic, colon, lung and prostate cancers.[94] However, a study on rats showed that the diet caused a pro-tumour effect on a tuberous sclerosis complex (TSC), a **genetic** condition causing benign tumours. A study in mice showed that the diet caused significant growth in a type of melanoma.[94] On the other hand, a review of 29 animal and 24 human studies (although they were small ones) showed some evidence for an anti-tumour effect and none showing it promoted tumour growth.[95]

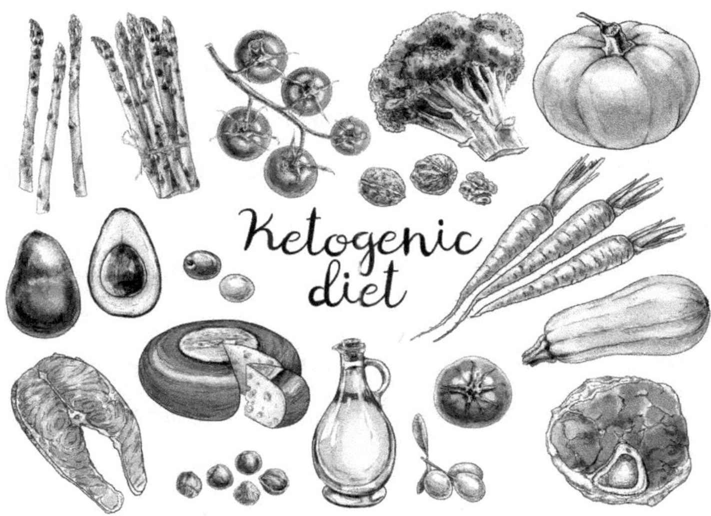

Because of the high fat, this diet isn't suitable for those with liver or gallbladder cancers, or gallstones.

Ideally, this diet should be supervised by a nutritionist to ensure you consume all the nutrients you need. Your markers should be monitored by your oncologist to ensure the diet works on your particular tumour.

Full details of the diet are beyond the scope of this book but if you want more information, a couple of books may help you:

- 'Keto for Cancer' by Miriam Kalamian, a nutritionist and educator, whose book has good reviews from a number of oncologists.
- 'Fight Cancer with a Ketogenic Diet' by Ellen Davis, who holds a Master of Science and is an expert on ketogenic diets. Her website is www.ketogenic-diet-resource.com

Gerson diet

The Gerson diet is a low-salt diet, very high in fresh organic fruit and vegetables (about 9 **kg** per day, which are juiced), which contain high levels of potassium. You take supplements of vitamin B12, pancreatic enzymes, Lugol's iodine, thyroid hormone and potassium, and undergo coffee enemas to detoxify and stimulate metabolism. Meals are vegetarian, using more organic fruit and vegetables, and wholegrains. No salt or spices are used.

The diet was developed in the 1930s as a treatment for tuberculosis and then became an alternative cancer therapy. The idea behind it is that changes the sodium and potassium balance in the body caused by processed foods and toxins in the environment, which promote cancer.

I too would advocate plenty of organic fruit and vegetables because of their high antioxidant levels. However, if you also take potassium supplements you can end up with too little sodium and too much potassium, which is potentially lethal. If you choose this diet, I strongly recommend close monitoring of your sodium and potassium levels by your doctors.

It's been suggested that some tumours may be sensitive to aldosterone, a hormone that would be significantly raised by the Gerson diet. Some research also shows that low sodium, high potassium diets can change damaged cell proteins back to their original undamaged state.[96]

The coffee enemas can cause serious infections, inflammation of the colon, dehydration, constipation and even death. There are several reports of deaths in those using the Gerson diet.[97]

Few scientific studies of the therapy have been carried out:

- One was conducted by the Gerson Research Organization, where the numbers of patients studied was relatively small and results could be biased.[98] It showed that the 5 year survival rate of melanoma patients was significantly improved.
- The other study was more recent and studied just 6 people with various different types of cancers: 1 malignant melanoma, 2 with metastatic breast cancer, 1 non-Hodgkin lymphoma, 1 inoperable cancer of the bile duct, and one astrocytoma (a type of brain tumour). It showed a very significant improvement in survival, but in each case except the bile duct cancer they also received some kind of medical treatment. In the non-Hodgkin lymphoma case, though, the patient only had one cycle of chemo, which wouldn't be enough to cure them on its own. Of the 6 patients, 5 were still alive and were clear of disease when the study ended, with the bile duct cancer patient being the only death.[96]

It could be a helpful additional therapy if it's carefully supervised. However, the medical community is very much opposed to it.

Budwig diet

Dr Johanna Budwig, who developed the Budwig diet, discovered that the blood of thousands of people with degenerative diseases like cancer, diabetes and liver disease was deficient in certain nutrients, particularly linolenic acid, phosphatide and lipoprotein. Her conclusion was that essential fatty acids, phosphatide and sulphur-based proteins were critical to maintaining and building healthy cells. She was violently opposed to the use of hydrogenation to create margarine, which she believed was **carcinogenic**.

The mainstay of the diet is a mixture of flaxseed oil and cottage cheese or quark, known as 'The Spread'. This is rich in sulphur-based amino acids to increase absorption of alpha-linolenic acid (ALA).

The 'Spread' recipe

Mix or blend 1 cup (250 **ml**) of flaxseed oil into a bowl with 450 **g** organic low-fat cottage cheese or quark and 60 **ml** of raw honey, adding enough filtered water or organic low-fat milk to get the mixture to blend together. After 5 minutes, it forms a custard-like consistency with no oily taste (when you rinse out the bowl there shouldn't be an oily 'ring'). You can also use organic yoghurt by blending 30 **g** (1 oz) of yoghurt with 15 **ml** of flaxseed oil and 15 **ml** of honey. The Spread can be used however you like, including (but not limited to) with nuts and seeds as a kind of muesli, as a dressing, or eaten with vegetables or fruit as a meal.

Budwig diet rules

- 'The Spread' should be freshly prepared each day.
- A minimum of 120 **g** of 'The Spread' must be eaten daily, distributed through the day.
- Flaxseed oil must be refrigerated and used quickly, as it goes rancid easily.
- Include freshly squeezed vegetable juices.
- Drink at least 3 cups of warm herbal teas, such as green tea, rosehip or peppermint, daily.

- Include plenty of organic fruit and vegetables, nuts and seeds.
- Add buckwheat, brown rice, quinoa, oat flakes, soya flakes or millet.
- Avoid all meat, especially processed meats, dairy (except 'The Spread'), butter, margarine (including the ones sold as 'healthy'), processed fish (i.e. smoked, canned, salted), all salad oils (including commercial mayonnaise and olive oil), all ready-made meals and processed foods, eggs, sugar of **any** sort (except for a small amount of raw honey), white bread and peanuts, which are legumes, not nuts.
- If you want meat, stick to wild caught organic game meats, such as rabbit, venison etc. Wild caught fish can also be added.
- A little alcohol is permitted.
- Eat your night meal before 6 pm.
- Avoid using any pesticides and chemicals, such as those in household products.

For full details, go to the website www.budwig-diet.co.uk which has the complete list of foods to eat, forbidden foods, suggested meal plans, recipes and more.

The diet is healthy and can be adapted to suit yourself to a large extent. By including small amounts of wild-caught meat and fish you can avoid losing muscle mass.

There are plenty of testimonials (e.g. http://www.budwigdvds.com/budwig-diet-healing-stories.htm) but there have been no formal studies done on the diet. Although there's no scientific evidence for it, it's unlikely to harm you.

Macrobiotic diet

Macrobiotic diets were created by George Ohsawa, a Japanese philosopher, and Michio Kushi, his student. They believed that the balance between Yin and Yang was important. The diet is based on an organic, vegetarian and wholefoods diet, together with clean living.

It consists of 50—60% wholegrain cereals, mainly brown rice, 25—30% organic vegetables with minimal processing, 5—10% soups, especially miso soup, and 5—10% seaweeds and legumes. Limited amounts of white meat, fish and fruit can be eaten. Foods to avoid are sweet potatoes and potatoes, tomatoes, capsicum, chilli, eggplant (aubergine), asparagus, beetroot, spinach, avocado, zucchini (courgette), red meat, mayonnaise, tea and coffee. Dairy is discouraged.

Exercise, fresh air, meditation and the wearing of cotton, preferably organic, is recommended. Television is restricted. Cooking with electric appliances and microwaves is discouraged. Gas and wood-fired cooking is preferred.

Research shows that women following a macrobiotic diet have slightly lower blood levels of oestrogen, which reduces their chances of breast cancer.[99] This is probably because of the phyto-oestrogens in the diet. However, it's a very low calorie diet and is often used for weight loss. If you need to lose some weight, that's fine. If you're currently having treatment and particularly if your cancer is fairly advanced, you may be losing weight already from **cachexia**. This diet would exacerbate that. It also has low levels of **B** group vitamins (particularly B12), calcium and iron, and some people even get scurvy because of low vitamin C. If you choose to use this diet, ensure you take vitamin and mineral supplements to counteract these deficiencies.

For more details of the macrobiotic diet, this website may be useful for background and some recipes: www.ohsawamacrobiotics.com

Calorie restriction

There are 2 types of calorie restriction: fasting, and a reduction in calories that doesn't cause malnutrition. Both have a place in cancer treatments.

Fasting for 4–5 days when you have active cancer causes changes in the body that inhibit the growth of cancer cells without any unwanted side-effects.[100] This is because of the reduction in blood glucose levels.

Calorie restriction of 20–40% can be maintained for long periods, while ensuring you have all the necessary nutrients you need to stay healthy. This has been studied extensively for its effects on tumours, and most cancers show a reduction in tumour growth.[100] However, other research shows it might be less effective in cancers that have a particular **mutation** that enables them to grow independently of insulin and insulin growth factor 1. This includes glioblastomas, some prostate cancer types and one breast cancer type.[101] Your oncologist should be able to tell you whether you have one of these types.

Even a 20% reduction in calories can cause a significant (about 15%) drop in body mass index (**BMI**). If you aren't overweight, this isn't good. Long term, it can also reduce immunity and delay wound healing, which is unwise if you're undergoing chemo, surgery or immune therapy.[100]

Studies on the effects of dietary restrictions on cancer prevention in rhesus monkeys showed that, over 20 years, a 30% reduction in calories resulted in a 50% reduction in tumours.[100]

Another option is 'periodic fasting', defined as a fasting period of 48 hours to 3 weeks followed by normal eating to regain the weight lost. In trials on mice, a fast of 48–60 hours prior to receiving the drug Etoposide increased survival. Fasting for 72 hours before exposure to lethal doses of the drug Doxorubicin, which can damage the heart, protected them.[102] This may not translate to humans.

An alternative is a fasting-mimicking diet of about 4,560 kJ (1,090 Calories) on day 1 and 3,033 kJ (725 Calories) on days 2–5 (roughly 10% protein, 56% fat and 34% carbohydrate with supplements to ensure sufficient vitamins, minerals etc.), followed by normal eating for 25 days. This was tested on 19 people with an equal **control group**, all of whom were healthy. The cycle was repeated 3 times. The diet changed markers for inflammation and cardiovascular disease risk factors, and reduced blood sugar levels. The participants found the diet quite manageable. Many effects continued after completion of the third cycle of fasting, suggesting they may be long-lasting. The authors noted that protein restriction was as important as carbohydrate restriction in reducing cancer growth.[103] This diet can be a viable alternative for the longer term, once treatment is complete, as it means you eat 'normally' most of the time. It offers significant benefits.

A variation of the fasting-mimicking diet with even lower calorie content was tested on breast cancer patients, with the diet followed for 3 days prior to and the day of chemo. Their responses to chemo were significantly improved.[104]

Alkalising diet

Our bodies are generally very good at keeping our acid/alkaline balance. The Western diet is high in animal protein and processed grains, and low in vegetables, making it highly acidic. This can put such a strain on the body that it can't maintain that balance and it ends up in low-grade metabolic acidosis[105], meaning that the blood is acidic.

Acidosis inhibits the immune system[106], reducing the body's ability to detect cancerous cells and allowing cancers to start. Acidity in the fluid surrounding cancer cells also induces **metastasis** and encourages more aggressive cancers.[106] Because most cancers use **glycolysis** for energy production, they produce lactic acid, raising the acidity of their environment.[107]

Acidosis raises cortisol levels, which not only increases stress but also induces insulin resistance. Higher insulin levels are associated with increased risk of cancers of the breast, kidney, endometrium, pancreas and bowel.[105]

Diets with a high acid load are associated with a significant increase in breast cancers, particularly oestrogen-receptor negative and triple-negative cancers. However, alkaline diets were associated with a significantly reduced risk.[108] In 2 studies of about 3,000 early-stage breast cancer survivors, an acid diet increased the likelihood of pre-diabetes[109], and pre-diabetic survivors had a higher risk of recurrence.[110]

A high acid diet is linked with higher risk of contracting glioma.[111]

A study in Japan found no association between an acidic diet and cancer[112], but in areas of the world where the soil contains high concentrations of alkalising minerals there are very low cancer rates.[113] A Swedish study found a modest increase in all-cause mortality in both highly acidic and highly alkaline diets.[114]

I recommend a balanced acid–alkaline diet. This involves having a modest amount of animal protein and grains, balanced with a lot of vegetables and fruit. As a very general guide, for each 100 **g** of animal protein you need about 500 **g** of vegetables or fruit to balance it.

For the nerds among you, this is based on the Potential Renal Acid Load (PRAL), which is calculated using this equation:

$$\text{PRAL (mEq/d)} = (0.49 \times \text{protein (g)}) + (0.037 \times \text{phosphorus (g)}) - (0.021 \times \text{potassium (g)}) - (0.026 \times \text{magnesium (g)}) - (0.013 \times \text{calcium (g)})$$

Acidic foods, such as those containing high protein and phosphorus have a positive PRAL. Alkaline foods, which are those with high potassium, magnesium and calcium, have a negative PRAL. Ideally, your daily food intake should total a PRAL of around zero.

An excellent explanation of PRAL can be found at: https://

thekidneydietitian.org/pral/ and a useful calculator is at: http://www.foodnutritiontable.com/calculate/pral/, although it doesn't cover everything. If you want exact calculations, find the government nutrition data for your country, as minerals in soil vary. For Australia, they're at: https://www.foodstandards.gov.au/science/monitoringnutrients/ausnut/ausnutdatafiles/Pages/foodnutrient.aspx

I've created a spreadsheet of common foods, which you'll find on my website: **www.NaturallySupportingCancerTreatment.com.au.**

If you have kidney disease, you should avoid foods containing high amounts of potassium, even though they have a low PRAL. For most people, though, this diet is an extremely healthy one.

Mediterranean Diet

The Mediterranean diet has become very popular recently. That's because it's associated with a wide range of health benefits. It reduces the incidence of cardiovascular problems, including the risk factors for it, such as being overweight, high blood pressure, insulin resistance and high blood pressure.

Followers of the diet have a lower incidence of diabetes. There's less age-related cognitive decline in those who eat this way, including a lower incidence of Alzheimer's disease.

A recent **meta-analysis** showed that people who stuck to the diet most closely had a lower incidence of a wide range of cancers, including breast, colorectal, liver, lung, bladder, stomach, blood cancer, endometrial, pancreatic, and head and neck, but, surprisingly, not prostate[115]. They also have lower cancer mortality and lower all-cause mortality[115].

The basis of the Mediterranean diet is that the daily intake should be based on:

- 3-9 servings of vegetables.
- 0.5-2 servings of fruit.
- 1-13 servings of wholegrains.
- Up to 8 servings of olives and olive oil.
- Together with beans, nuts, legumes, seeds, herbs and spices.
- There's a recommendation to eat fish and seafood at least twice a week.
- Eat moderate portions of eggs, poultry, cheese and yoghurt daily to weekly.

MEDITERRANEAN DIET PYRAMID

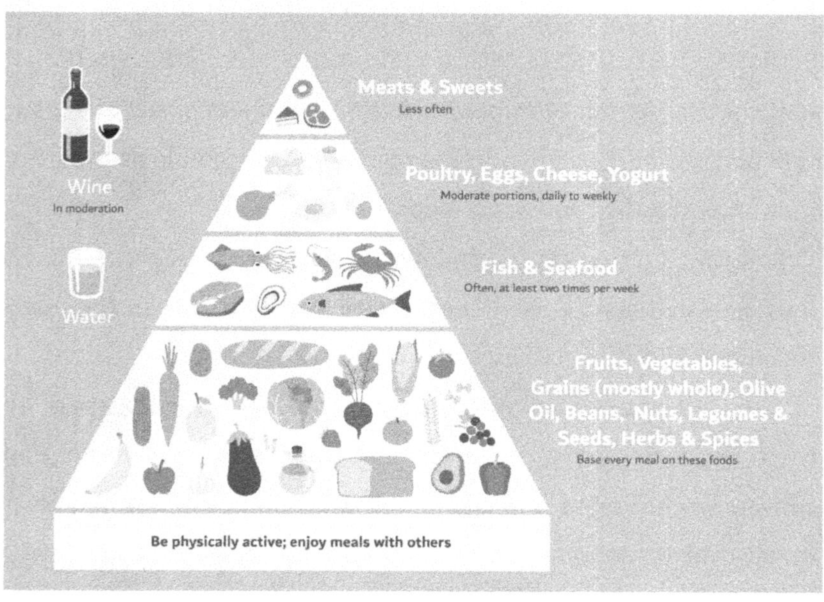

- Eat meat and sweets less often.
- You're encouraged to be physically active and to make each meal a social occasion.

You might have noticed that this list pretty much mirrors what I've said earlier in this chapter.

Mediterranean Keto diet

There is another option that you could consider when weighing up the options on diets for cancer, and that is the Mediterranean Keto diet. It combines the best of both the Mediterranean and Keto diets.

One potential issue with the Mediterranean diet is the high levels of carbohydrates. If you have Type II diabetes or insulin resistance, both of which are a risk factor for cancer, a low-carb diet is a better option, as it can help to improve blood sugar levels[116].

A very high fibre diet, such as the high levels of beans and wholegrains in the Mediterranean diet, can also exacerbate some digestive problems. Many of the high-carb foods are also high in FODMAPS, which can aggravate problems like Irritable Bowel Syndrome (IBS).

Some of the less healthy foods on a typical American Keto diet, such as fatty meats, cheese and cream, are high in saturated fats.

A Mediterranean Keto diet is based on:

- Proteins: any fish (especially oily fish like salmon, mackerel and sardines) and seafood, poultry, eggs, small amounts of lean meat.

- Fats: olive oil, avocado oil, coconut oil, MCT oil, and small amounts of dairy.
- Non-starchy vegetables: these include leafy green vegetables (such as lettuce, spinach, kale, cabbage, rocket (arugula), watercress, Chinese greens such as bok choy, choy sum, wombok (Napa cabbage)), avocado, broccoli, cauliflower, asparagus, celery, fennel, red capsicum (bell pepper), tomatoes, green beans, Brussels sprouts, celery, cucumber, mushrooms, eggplant (aubergine), zucchini (courgette). You can also include small amounts of onion, radish, carrot and beetroot (beets), but anything that grows below ground is usually higher in carbs.
- Small amounts of low carb fruits, such as lemons, strawberries, blueberries and other berries, and apricots.
- Low carb nuts include pecans, Brazil nuts, macadamias, hazelnuts, pine nuts, almonds and peanuts (technically a legume, but low carb). Nut butters made from these are also good, and flours made from grinding nuts (and seeds) make excellent substitutes for wheat flour in baking and to thicken sauces.
- Low carb seeds include sesame seeds, sunflower seeds, hemp seeds, chia seeds, flax seeds and pumpkin seeds.
- Herbs and spices, such as black pepper, chilli pepper, curry powder, paprika and garlic. Garlic salt and onion salt are lower-carb alternatives to fresh garlic and onion.
- Sweeteners, such as monk fruit and stevia.

This may sound restrictive, but it's surprising how much variety you can introduce using these ingredients.

I can help you with both the Mediterranean and the Keto Mediterranean diets. I have a range of digital cookbooks for sale in both genres on my website at https://www.naturally supportingcancertreatment.com.au/mealplanning.

If you would prefer a personalised meal plan prepared for your personal likes and dislikes, including allergies and cultural diets, whether you want to lose weight, gain muscle or maintain your current weight, how long you would like to spend preparing meals etc., go to https://www.naturallysupportingcancertreatment.com.au/mealplanning for more details.

References

1. Anand P, Kunnumakkara A, Sundaram C et al. Cancer is a Preventable Disease that Requires Major Lifestyle Changes. *Pharm Res.* 2008;25(9):2200-2200. doi:10.1007/s11095-008-9690-4
2. O'Brien K, Sali A. *A Clinician's Guide To Integrative Oncology.* Cham, Switzerland: Springer International Publishing; 2017.
3. Barański M, Rempelos L, Iversen P, Leifert C. Effects of organic food consumption on human health; the jury is still out!. *Food Nutr Res.* 2017;61(1):1287333. doi:10.1080/16546628.2017.1287333
4. Environmental Working Group. Dirty Dozen™ Fruits and Vegetables with the Most Pesticides. Ewg.org. https://www.ewg.org/foodnews/dirty-dozen.php. Published 2021. Accessed August 19, 2021.
5. Ferguson L, Chen H, Collins A et al. Genomic instability in human cancer: Molecular insights and opportunities for therapeutic attack and prevention through diet and nutrition. *Semin Cancer Biol.* 2015;35:S5-S24. doi:10.1016/j.semcancer.2015.03.005
6. Steinmetz K, Potter J. Vegetables, Fruit, and Cancer Prevention. *J Am Diet Assoc.* 1996;96(10):1027-1039. doi:10.1016/s0002-8223(96)00273-8
7. Keck A, Finley J. Cruciferous Vegetables: Cancer Protective Mechanisms of Glucosinolate Hydrolysis Products and Selenium. *Integr Cancer Ther.* 2004;3(1):5-12. doi:10.1177/1534735403261831

8. Jiang Y, Wu S, Shu X et al. Cruciferous Vegetable Intake Is Inversely Correlated with Circulating Levels of Proinflammatory Markers in Women. *J Acad Nutr Diet*. 2014;114(5):700-708.e2. doi:10.1016/j.jand.2013.12.019

9. Khurana N, Talwar S, Chandra P et al. Sulforaphane increases the efficacy of anti-androgens by rapidly decreasing androgen receptor levels in prostate cancer cells. *Int J Oncol*. 2016;49(4):1609-1619. doi:10.3892/ijo.2016.3641

10. Meng Q, Yuan F, Goldberg I, Rosen E, Auborn K, Fan S. Indole-3-Carbinol Is a Negative Regulator of Estrogen Receptor-α Signaling in Human Tumor Cells. *J Nutr*. 2000;130(12):2927-2931. doi:10.1093/jn/130.12.2927

11. Bajaj J, Salwan P, Salwan S. Various Possible Toxicants Involved in Thyroid Dysfunction: A Review. *Journal of Clinical and Diagnostic Research*. 2016;10(1):FE01-FE02. doi:10.7860/jcdr/2016/15195.7092

12. Kucuk O, Sarkar F, Sakr W et al. Phase II Randomized Clinical Trial of Lycopene Supplementation before Radical Prostatectomy. *Cancer Epidemiology, Biomarkers & Prevention*. 2001;10(8):861-868. https://cebp.aacrjournals.org/content/10/8/861. Accessed August 19, 2021.

13. Patel S, Goyal A. Recent developments in mushrooms as anti-cancer therapeutics: a review. *3 Biotech*. 2011;2(1):1-15. doi:10.1007/s13205-011-0036-2

14. Lippi G, Mattiuzzi C, Cervellin G. Meat consumption and cancer risk: a critical review of published meta-analyses. *Crit Rev Oncol Hematol*. 2016;97:1-14. doi:10.1016/j.critrevonc.2015.11.008

15. Glade M. Food, nutrition, and the prevention of cancer: a global perspective. American Institute for Cancer Research/World Cancer Research Fund, American Institute for Cancer Research, 1997. *Nutrition*. 1999;15(6):523-526. doi:10.1016/s0899-9007(99)00021-0

16. Terrasse V, Gaudin N. IARC Monographs evaluate consumption of red meat and processed meat. International Agency for Research on Cancer. https://www.iarc.who.int/wp-content/uploads/2018/07/pr240_E.pdf. Published 2015. Accessed August 19, 2021.

17. Daley C, Abbott A, Doyle P, Nader G, Larson S. A review of fatty acid profiles and antioxidant content in grass-fed and grain-fed beef. *Nutr J*. 2010;9(1):1475-2891-10. doi:10.1186/1475-2891-9-10

18. Wang H. Vitamin B12, folate, and Alzheimer's disease. *Drug Dev Res*. 2002;56(2):111-122. doi:10.1002/ddr.10066

19. Woo K, Kwok T, Celermajer D. Vegan Diet, Subnormal Vitamin B-12 Status and Cardiovascular Health. *Nutrients*. 2014;6(8):3259-3273. doi:10.3390/nu6083259

20. Osiecki H. *The Nutrient Bible*. 9th ed. Eagle Farm: Bio Concepts Publishing.

21. Arnarson A. 7 Nutrients You Can't Get from Plants. Healthline. https://www.healthline.com/nutrition/7-nutrients-you-cant-get-from-plants. Published 2021. Accessed August 19, 2021.

22. Mayo Clinic. Creatine. Mayo Clinic. https://www.mayoclinic.org/drugs-supplements-creatine/art-20347591. Published 2021. Accessed August 19, 2021.

23. Jägerstad M, Skog K. Genotoxicity of heat-processed foods. *Mutation Research/Fundamental and Molecular Mechanisms of Mutagenesis*. 2005;574(1-2):156-172. doi:10.1016/j.mrfmmm.2005.01.030

24. Virk-Baker M, Nagy T, Barnes S, Groopman J. Dietary Acrylamide and Human Cancer: A Systematic Review of Literature. *Nutr Cancer.* 2014;66(5):774-790. doi:10.1080/01635581.2014.916323

25. Sanders H. How to Avoid Acrylamide in Food. Health Ambition. https://www.healthambition.com/acrylamide-in-food-how-to-avoid-it/. Accessed August 19, 2021.

26. Thompson R, Barnes K. *The Calcium Lie II.* Brevard, N.C.: Take Charge Books; 2013.

27. Liener I. Toxins in Cow's Milk and Human Milk. *J Nutr Environ Med.* 2002;12(3):175-186. doi:10.1080/13590840210000006830

28. Vassallo R. Preventing antibiotic residues in milk | Agriculture and Food. WA Department of Primary Industries and Regional Development. https://www.agric.wa.gov.au/dairy-cattle/preventing-antibiotic-residues-milk. Published 2014. Accessed August 19, 2021.

29. Peisch S, Van Blarigan E, Chan J, Stampfer M, Kenfield S. Prostate cancer progression and mortality: a review of diet and lifestyle factors. *World J Urol.* 2016;35(6):867-874. doi:10.1007/s00345-016-1914-3

30. Zang J, Shen M, Du S, Chen T, Zou S. The Association between Dairy Intake and Breast Cancer in Western and Asian Populations: A Systematic Review and Meta-Analysis. *J Breast Cancer.* 2015;18(4):313. doi:10.4048/jbc.2015.18.4.313

31. Li X, Zhao J, Li P, Gao Y. Dairy Products Intake and Endometrial Cancer Risk: A Meta-Analysis of Observational Studies. *Nutrients.* 2017;10(1):25. doi:10.3390/nu10010025

32. Fraser G, Jaceldo-Siegl K, Orlich M, Mashchak A, Sirirat R, Knutsen S. Dairy, soy, and risk of breast cancer: those confounded milks. *Int J Epidemiol.* 2020;49(5):1526-1537. doi:10.1093/ije/dyaa007

33. Baron J, Beach M, Wallace K et al. Risk of Prostate Cancer in a Randomized Clinical Trial of Calcium Supplementation. *Cancer Epidemiology Biomarkers & Prevention.* 2005;14(3):586-589. doi:10.1158/1055-9965.EPI-04-0319

34. Okada Y, Tsuzuki Y, Ueda T et al. Trans fatty acids in diets act as a precipitating factor for gut inflammation?. *J Gastroenterol Hepatol.* 2013;28(54):29-32. doi:10.1111/jgh.12270

35. Micha R, Mozaffarian D. Trans fatty acids: Effects on cardiometabolic health and implications for policy. *Prostaglandins, Leukotrienes and Essential Fatty Acids.* 2008;79(3-5):147-152. doi:10.1016/j.plefa.2008.09.008

36. Robertson R. Omega-3-6-9 Fatty Acids: A Complete Overview. Healthline. https://www.healthline.com/nutrition/omega-3-6-9-overview. Published 2020. Accessed August 19, 2021.

37. Simopoulos A. The Importance of the Omega-6/Omega-3 Fatty Acid Ratio in Cardiovascular Disease and Other Chronic Diseases. *Experimental Biology and Medicine.* 2008;233(6):674-688. doi:10.3181/0711-mr-311

38. Touré A, Xueming X. Flaxseed Lignans: Source, Biosynthesis, Metabolism, Antioxidant Activity, Bio-Active Components, and Health Benefits. *Compr Rev Food Sci Food Saf.* 2010;9(3):261-269. doi:10.1111/j.1541-4337.2009.00105.x

39. Robertson R. What Are the Benefits of Monounsaturated Fats?. Healthline. https://www.healthline.com/nutrition/monounsaturated-fats. Published 2017. Accessed August 19, 2021.

40. Siri-Tarino P, Sun Q, Hu F, Krauss R. Meta-analysis of prospective cohort studies evaluating the association of saturated fat with cardiovascular disease. *Am J Clin Nutr.* 2010;91(3):535-546. doi:10.3945/ajcn.2009.27725

41. Nevin K, Rajamohan T. Beneficial effects of virgin coconut oil on lipid parameters and in vitro LDL oxidation. *Clin Biochem.* 2004;37(9):830-835. doi:10.1016/j.clinbiochem.2004.04.010

42. Boateng L, Ansong R, Owusu W, Steiner-Asiedu M. Coconut oil and palm oil's role in nutrition, health and national development: A review. *Ghana Med J.* 2016;50(3):189-196. doi:10.4314/gmj.v50i3.11

43. DebMandal M, Mandal S. Coconut (Cocos nucifera L.: Arecaceae): In health promotion and disease prevention. *Asian Pac J Trop Med.* 2011;4(3):241-247. doi:10.1016/s1995-7645(11)60078-3

44. Lee L. Fluoride - A Modern Toxic Waste. Vianovalife.com. http://www.vianovalife.com/wp-content/uploads/2016/09/Fluoride-A-Modern-Toxic-Waste-Product.pdf. Published 2005. Accessed August 20, 2021.

45. Peckham S, Awofeso N. Water Fluoridation: A Critical Review of the Physiological Effects of Ingested Fluoride as a Public Health Intervention. *The Scientific World Journal.* 2014;2014:1-10. doi:10.1155/2014/293019

46. Loomis D, Guyton K, Grosse Y et al. Carcinogenicity of drinking coffee, mate, and very hot beverages. *The Lancet Oncology.* 2016;17(7):877-878. doi:10.1016/s1470-2045(16)30239-x

47. Lambert J, Yang C. Mechanisms of Cancer Prevention by Tea Constituents. *J Nutr.* 2003;133(10):3262S-3267S. doi:10.1093/jn/133.10.3262s

48. National Cancer Institute. Tea and Cancer Prevention. National Cancer Institute. https://www.cancer.gov/about-cancer/causes-prevention/risk/diet/tea-fact-sheet. Published 2010. Accessed August 20, 2021.

49. Connor J. Alcohol consumption as a cause of cancer. *Addiction.* 2016;112(2):222-228. doi:10.1111/add.13477

50. Zhao J, Stockwell T, Roemer A, Chikritzhs T. Is alcohol consumption a risk factor for prostate cancer? A systematic review and meta-analysis. *BMC Cancer.* 2016;16(1). doi:10.1186/s12885-016-2891-z

51. Bagnardi V, Rota M, Botteri E et al. Alcohol consumption and site-specific cancer risk: a comprehensive dose–response meta-analysis. *Br J Cancer.* 2014;112(3):580-593. doi:10.1038/bjc.2014.579

52. Aeberli I, Gerber P, Hochuli M et al. Low to moderate sugar-sweetened beverage consumption impairs glucose and lipid metabolism and promotes inflammation in healthy young men: a randomized controlled trial. *Am J Clin Nutr.* 2011;94(2):479-485. doi:10.3945/ajcn.111.013540

53. Turina M, Fry D, Polk H. Acute hyperglycemia and the innate immune system: Clinical, cellular, and molecular aspects. *Crit Care Med.* 2005;33(7):1624-1633. doi:10.1097/01.ccm.0000170106.61978.d8

54. Suez J, Korem T, Zilberman-Schapira G, Segal E, Elinav E. Non-caloric artificial sweeteners and the microbiome: findings and challenges. *Gut Microbes.* 2015;6(2):149-155. doi:10.1080/19490976.2015.1017700

55. Finamor I, Pérez S, Bressan C et al. Chronic aspartame intake causes changes in the trans-sulphuration pathway, glutathione depletion and liver damage in mice. *Redox Biol*. 2017;11:701-707. doi:10.1016/j.redox.2017.01.019

56. Samarghandian S, Farkhondeh T, Samini F. Honey and Health: A Review of Recent Clinical Research. *Pharmacognosy Res*. 2017;9(2):121-127. doi:10.4103/0974-8490.204647

57. Arcot J, Brand Miller J. *A Preliminary Assessment Of The Glycemic Index Of Honey*. Barton, A.C.T.: Rural Industries Research and Development Corporation; 2005.

58. Axe J. 11 Best Sugar Substitutes (the Healthiest Natural Sweeteners). Dr Axe. https://draxe.com/nutrition/sugar-substitutes/. Published 2020. Accessed August 20, 2021.

59. Marcinek K, Krejpcio Z. Stevia rebaudiana Bertoni: health promoting properties and therapeutic applications. *Journal für Verbraucherschutz und Lebensmittelsicherheit*. 2015;11(1):3-8. doi:10.1007/s00003-015-0968-2

60. Martín M, Goya L, Ramos S. Preventive Effects of Cocoa and Cocoa Antioxidants in Colon Cancer. *Diseases*. 2016;4(1):6. doi:10.3390/diseases4010006

61. Andújar I, Recio M, Giner R, Ríos J. Cocoa Polyphenols and Their Potential Benefits for Human Health. *Oxid Med Cell Longev*. 2012;2012:1-23. doi:10.1155/2012/906252

62. Donaldson M. Nutrition and cancer: A review of the evidence for an anti-cancer diet. *Nutr J*. 2004;3(1). doi:10.1186/1475-2891-3-19

63. Redman M, Ward E, Phillips R. The efficacy and safety of probiotics in people with cancer: a systematic review. *Annals of Oncology*. 2014;25(10):1919-1929. doi:10.1093/annonc/mdu106

64. Ho Y, Lu Y, Chang H et al. Daily Intake of Probiotics with High IFN-γ/IL-10 Ratio Increases the Cytotoxicity of Human Natural Killer Cells: A Personalized Probiotic Approach. *J Immunol Res*. 2014;2014:721505. doi:10.1155/2014/721505

65. Department of Gastroenterology. Prebiotic diet - FAQs. Monash University. https://www.monash.edu/medicine/ccs/gastroenterology/prebiotic/faq#3. Published 2020. Accessed August 20, 2021.

66. Ebrahim I, Shapiro C, Williams A, Fenwick P. Alcohol and Sleep I: Effects on Normal Sleep. *Alcoholism: Clinical and Experimental Research*. 2013;37(4):539`-549. doi:10.1111/acer.12006

67. Edwards S, Montgomery I, Colquhoun E, Jordan J, Clark M. Spicy meal disturbs sleep: an effect of thermoregulation?. *International Journal of Psychophysiology*. 1992;13(2):97-100. doi:10.1016/0167-8760(92)90048-G

68. Elliott B. 9 Foods and Drinks to Promote Better Sleep. Healthline. https://www.healthline.com/nutrition/9-foods-to-help-you-sleep. Published 2020. Accessed August 20, 2021.

69. Lin H, Tsai P, Fang S, Liu J. Effect of kiwifruit consumption on sleep quality in adults with sleep problems. *Asia Pacific Journal of Clnicial Nutrition*. 2011;20(2):169-174. https://pubmed.ncbi.nlm.nih.gov/21669584/. Accessed August 20, 2021.

70. Garrido M, Gonzalez-Gomez D, Lozano M, Barriga C, Paredes S, Moratinos A. A Jerte Valley cherry product provides beneficial effects on sleep quality. Influence on aging. *J Nutr Health Aging*. 2013;17(6):553-560. doi:10.1007/s12603-013-0029-4

71. Howatson G, Bell P, Tallent J, Middleton B, McHugh M, Ellis J. Effect of tart cherry juice (Prunus cerasus) on melatonin levels and enhanced sleep quality. *Eur J Nutr*. 2012;51(8):909-916. doi:10.1007/s00394-011-0263-7

72. Losso J, Finley J, Karki N et al. Pilot Study of the Tart Cherry Juice for the Treatment of Insomnia and Investigation of Mechanisms. *Am J Ther.* 2018;25(2):e194-e201. doi:10.1097/mjt.0000000000000584

73. Halson S. Sleep in Elite Athletes and Nutritional Interventions to Enhance Sleep. *Sports Medicine.* 2014;44(S1):13-23. doi:10.1007/s40279-014-0147-0

74. Srivastava J, Shankar E, Gupta S. Chamomile: A herbal medicine of the past with a bright future (Review). *Mol Med Rep.* 2010;3(6):895-901. doi:10.3892/mmr.2010.377

75. Nicole W. PFOA and Cancer in a Highly Exposed Community: New Findings from the C8 Science Panel. *Environ Health Perspect.* 2013;121(11-12):A340-A340. doi:10.1289/ehp.121-a340

76. EWG. EWG Guide to PFCs. Environmental Working Group. https://static.ewg.org/reports/2015/poisoned_legacy/EWG_Guide_to_PFCs.pdf?_ga=2.33158590.1259416286.1524461200-392654626.1519713981. Accessed August 20, 2021.

77. Amarelo M. The Toxic Truth About A New Generation of Nonstick and Waterproof Chemicals. Environmental Working Group. https://www.ewg.org/release/toxic-truth-about-new-generation-nonstick-and-waterproof-chemicals#.Wt1xVC5ub4Y. Published 2015. Accessed August 20, 2021.

78. Mercola J. Hundreds of Scientists Issue Warning About Chemical Dangers of Non-Stick Cookware and Water-Repellant Items. Organic Consumers Association. https://www.organicconsumers.org/news/hundreds-scientists-issue-warning-about-chemical-dangers-non-stick-cookware-and-water-repellant. Published 2015. Accessed August 20, 2021.

79. Kotthoff M, Müller J, Jürling H, Schlummer M, Fiedler D. Perfluoroalkyl and polyfluoroalkyl substances in consumer products. *Environmental Science and Pollution Research.* 2015;22(19):14546-14559. doi:10.1007/s11356-015-4202-7

80. Westerhoff P, Prapaipong P, Shock E, Hillaireau A. Antimony leaching from polyethylene terephthalate (PET) plastic used for bottled drinking water. *Water Res.* 2008;42(3):551-556. doi:10.1016/j.watres.2007.07.048

81. Sundar S, Chakravarty J. Antimony Toxicity. *Int J Environ Res Public Health.* 2010;7(12):4267-4277. doi:10.3390/ijerph7124267

82. Hansen E. Hazardous substances in plastic materials. COWI. https://www.byggemiljo.no/wp-content/uploads/2014/10/72_ta3017.pdf. Published 2021. Accessed August 20, 2021.

83. Groh K. BPA and PVC in U.S. food can coatings | Food Packaging Forum. Food Packaging Forum. https://www.foodpackagingforum.org/news/bpa-and-pvc-in-u-s-food-can-coatings. Published 2017. Accessed August 20, 2021.

84. Serrano S, Braun J, Trasande L, Dills R, Sathyanarayana S. Phthalates and diet: a review of the food monitoring and epidemiology data. *Environmental Health.* 2014;13(1). doi:10.1186/1476-069x-13-43

85. Agency for Toxic Substances and Disease Registry. Toxicological Profile for Vinyl Chloride. Environmental Protection Agency. https://nepis.epa.gov/Exe/ZyPDF.cgi/9101SL6G.PDF?Dockey=9101SL6G.PDF. Published 1989. Accessed August 20, 2021.

86. Huff J, Infante P. Styrene exposure and risk of cancer. *Mutagenesis.* 2011;26(5):583-584. doi:10.1093/mutage/ger033

87. Prins G. Endocrine disruptors and prostate cancer risk. *Endocrine Related Cancer.* 2008;15(3):649-656. doi:10.1677/erc-08-0043

88. Yang C, Yaniger S, Jordan V, Klein D, Bittner G. Most Plastic Products Release Estrogenic Chemicals: A Potential Health Problem That Can Be Solved. *Environ Health Perspect.* 2011;119(7):989-996. doi:10.1289/ehp.1003220

89. Brotons J, Olea-Serrano M, Villalobos M, Pedraza V, Olea N. Xenoestrogens released from lacquer coatings in food cans. *Environ Health Perspect.* 1995;103(6):608-612. doi:10.1289/ehp.95103608

90. World Health Organization. Dioxins and their effects on human health. World Health Organization. http://www.who.int/en/news-room/fact-sheets/detail/dioxins-and-their-effects-on-human-health. Published 2016. Accessed August 20, 2021.

91. Alfrey A. Aluminum Toxicity in Humans. *Trace Elements in Clinical Medicine.* 1990:459-464. doi:10.1007/978-4-431-68120-5_59

92. Bernardo J. Aluminium Toxicity. Medscape. https://emedicine.medscape.com/article/165315-overview?pa=gq7VNGLoC3vLhSuDYjBtc+HiEaNMhw/eNTHlJsmVHcz2eShODbPlMJaHW1ykpQhxs7CF3wx2Tu1U792SxywYLg==. Published 2021. Accessed August 20, 2021.

93. Butler N. Ketosis vs. Ketoacidosis: What's the Difference?. Healthline. https://www.healthline.com/health/ketosis-vs-ketoacidosis. Published 2019. Accessed August 20, 2021.

94. Weber D, Aminazdeh-Gohari S, Kofler B. Ketogenic diet in cancer therapy. *Aging (Albany NY).* 2018;10(2):164-165. doi:10.18632/aging.101382

95. Klement R. Beneficial effects of ketogenic diets for cancer patients: a realist review with focus on evidence and confirmation. *Medical Oncology.* 2017;34(132 (2017). doi:10.1007/s12032-017-0991-5

96. Molassiotis A, Peat P. Surviving Against All Odds: Analysis of 6 Case Studies of Patients With Cancer Who Followed the Gerson Therapy. *Integr Cancer Ther.* 2007;6(1):80-88. doi:10.1177/1534735406298258

97. PDQ® Integrative, Alternative, and Complementary Therapies Editorial Board. Gerson Therapy (PDQ®)–Patient Version. National Cancer Institute. https://www.cancer.gov/about-cancer/treatment/cam/patient/gerson-pdq. Published 2015. Accessed August 20, 2021.

98. Hildenbrand G, Hildenbrand L, Bradford K, Cavin S. Five-year survival rates of melanoma patients treated by diet therapy after the manner of Gerson: a retrospective review. *Altern Ther Health Med.* 1995;1(4):29-37. https://pubmed.ncbi.nlm.nih.gov/9359807/. Accessed August 20, 2021.

99. Kushi L, Cunningham J, Hebert J, Lerman R, Bandera E, Teas J. The Macrobiotic Diet in Cancer. *J Nutr.* 2001;131(11):3056S-3064S. doi:10.1093/jn/131.11.3056s

100. Lee C, Longo V. Fasting vs dietary restriction in cellular protection and cancer treatment: from model organisms to patients. *Oncogene.* 2011;30(30):3305-3316. doi:10.1038/onc.2011.91

101. Kalaany N, Sabatini D. Tumours with PI3K activation are resistant to dietary restriction. *Nature.* 2009;458(7239):725-731. doi:10.1038/nature07782

102. Brandhorst S, Longo V. Fasting and Caloric Restriction in Cancer Prevention and Treatment. *Metabolism in Cancer.* 2016;207:241-266. doi:10.1007/978-3-319-42118-6_12

103. Brandhorst S, Choi I, Wei M et al. A Periodic Diet that Mimics Fasting Promotes Multi-System Regeneration, Enhanced Cognitive Performance, and Healthspan. *Cell Metab.* 2015;22(1):86-99. doi:10.1016/j.cmet.2015.05.012

104. de Groot S, Lugtenberg R, Cohen D et al. Fasting mimicking diet as an adjunct toneoadjuvant chemotherapy for breast cancer in the multicentre randomized phase 2 DIRECT trial. *Nat Commun.* 2020;11(1):3083. doi:10.1038/s41467-020-16138-3

105. Robey I. Examining the relationship between diet-induced acidosis and cancer. *Nutr Metab (Lond).* 2012;9(1):72. doi:10.1186/1743-7075-9-72

106. Ibrahim-Hashim A, Estrella V. Acidosis and cancer: from mechanism to neutralization. *Cancer and Metastasis Reviews.* 2019;38(1-2):149-155. doi:10.1007/s10555-019-09787-4

107. Pillai S, Damaghi M, Marunaka Y, Spugnini E, Fais S, Gillies R. Causes, consequences, and therapy of tumors acidosis. *Cancer and Metastasis Reviews.* 2019;38(1-2):205-222. doi:10.1007/s10555-019-09792-7

108. Park Y, Steck S, Fung T et al. Higher diet-dependent acid load is associated with risk of breast cancer: Findings from the sister study. *Int J Cancer.* 2018;144(8):1834-1843. doi:10.1002/ijc.31889

109. Wu T, Seaver P, Lemus H, Hollenbach K, Wang E, Pierce J. Associations between Dietary Acid Load and Biomarkers of Inflammation and Hyperglycemia in Breast Cancer Survivors. *Nutrients.* 2019;11(8):1913. doi:10.3390/nu11081913

110. Wu T, Hsu F, Wang S, Luong D, Pierce J. Hemoglobin A1c Levels Modify Associations between Dietary Acid Load and Breast Cancer Recurrence. *Nutrients.* 2020;12(2):578. doi:10.3390/nu12020578

111. Mousavi S, Milajerdi A, Sshayanfar M, Esmaillzadeh A. Relationship between Dietary Acid Load and Glioma: A Case-Control Study. *Qom University of Medical Sciences Journal.* 2019;13(1):11-20. doi:10.29252/qums.13.1.11

112. Akter S, Nanri A, Mizoue T et al. Dietary acid load and mortality among Japanese men and women: the Japan Public Health Center–based Prospective Study. *Am J Clin Nutr.* 2017;106(1):146-154. doi:10.3945/ajcn.117.152876

113. Alessandra L. Manipulating pH in Cancer Treatment: Alkalizing Drugs and Alkaline Diet. *Journal of Complementary Medicine & Alternative Healthcare.* 2017;2(1):555580. doi:10.19080/jcmah.2017.02.555580

114. Xu H, Åkesson A, Orsini N, Håkansson N, Wolk A, Carrero J. Modest U-Shaped Association between Dietary Acid Load and Risk of All-Cause and Cardiovascular Mortality in Adults. *J Nutr.* 2016;146(8):1580-1585. doi:10.3945/jn.116.231019

115. Guasch-Ferré M, Willett WC. The Mediterranean diet and Health: A Comprehensive Overview. *Journal of Internal Medicine.* 2021;290(3):549-566. doi:10.1111/joim.13333

116. Dening J, Mohebbi M, Abbott G, George ES, Ball K, Islam SMS. A web-based low carbohydrate diet intervention significantly improves glycaemic control in adults with type 2 diabetes: Results of the T2DIET study randomised controlled trial. *Nutrition & Diabetes.* 2023;13(12). doi:10.1038/s41387-023-00240-8

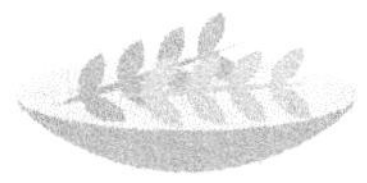

Chapter 3

Reduce your stress

'If you ask what is the single most important key to longevity, I would have to say it is avoiding worry, stress and tension.And if you didn't ask me, I'd still have to say it.'

– George Burns

What happens when you're stressed?

The medical definition of stress is 'an emotional, mental or physical factor that causes mental or bodily tension'. It's a survival mechanism. When our ancestors were being chased by a predator or in a dangerous situation, it helped them escape.

When our bodies are stressed, the first thing that happens is a rush of hormones, including adrenalin (also known as epinephrine) or noradrenalin (also known as norepinephrine), both produced by our adrenal glands. The effect is immediate and prepares you for quick actions. These include:

- an increase in heart rate and breathing, providing the muscles and the brain with more oxygen
- dilation of blood vessels in the muscles, and constriction

of them in body systems that aren't necessary during times of danger, such as the kidneys, and the digestive and reproductive systems

- triggered by the kidneys' blood supply being reduced, the release of hormones that move fluid from the urine back into the blood, pushing up blood pressure
- the release of glucose and fats from temporary storage sites in the body, ready to fuel the muscles.

Once the glucose and fats from temporary storage sites are used up, cortisol is released. The actions of cortisol are to:

- stimulate the breakdown of fat, to provide energy for most of the body except the brain, which can only use glucose as fuel
- help the breakdown of protein in the muscles to provide glucose for the brain
- slow down the uptake of glucose by most of the body, to maximise energy for the brain
- control the immune and inflammatory responses that could be caused by an injury.

Whenever the situation that triggered the stress response is gone, the hormones stop being produced and the body goes back to its natural relaxed state. The trouble is that, these days, stress tends to come as a result of a deadline at work, a fight with a loved one, sitting in a traffic jam, or something similar, and it can become a chronic situation rather than a temporary response.

If you have chronic stress, a few things happen that can cause illness:

- The increase in blood volume can cause hypertension – high blood pressure. That in turn damages the linings of the arteries, which can trigger atherosclerosis and heart disease, possibly resulting in a heart attack or stroke.
- Reduction of blood to the digestive system causes problems digesting food. That can result in nutrient deficiencies because you aren't absorbing them properly, which can lead to a myriad of problems, including cancers. The bacteria in the gut can be affected. In Chapter 7 we discuss probiotics, but there is a link between disrupted gut bacteria and some cancers.
- Reduction of blood to the reproductive system can cause erectile dysfunction in men.
- Reduction of blood to the kidneys affects how well they can remove toxins. Chapter 6 covers the effects of toxins. They include a higher risk of some cancers.
- Higher blood sugar levels can result in diabetes. This can also damage the blood vessels, which increases your risk of heart disease and stroke, kidney disease, nerve damage and damage to your vision. Diabetes can also affect immunity, which prevents the body from fighting the beginnings of cancer effectively.
- Stress can affect memory too, usually badly, although interestingly sometimes it can improve it. Think of when you've crammed for an exam. Long-term, though, it can change the structure of the brain for the worse.[1]

A study of a large number of British civil servants found those in low-level jobs with a high level of stress, low control and little support from their supervisors and co-workers had lower life expectancies.[2]

A cancer diagnosis is a stressful event. Reading this book should help you feel that you have some control over the situation, empowering you and lowering your stress levels.

The importance of social support

Cancer can disrupt almost every aspect of your life: family relationships, work and daily activities. You may feel a high degree of uncertainty about what is happening, the potential side-effects of treatment, how it might affect you physically, your prognosis, and a fear of impending death. One of the best ways of de-stressing is to talk about your feelings.

Cancer patients who have a good support system tend to live longer.[3] Support may come in various ways:

- Family and friends can help with emotional support, comfort, love and security.
- Support groups are available to help with emotional support. It can be helpful to talk to someone who has been in your situation.
- Nurses can help. In my experience, oncology nurses are wonderful at talking about feelings. They can also advise about side-effects and the physical outcomes of treatment.
- Doctors can provide you with information about the disease, the treatment you will need and your prognosis.
- Social workers are usually available in hospitals to advise on the practical side of things: equipment or modifications at

home that can help you, financial assistance that might be available, counselling services and so on.

It's important for your health that you take advantage of this support. I've found most people will rally around you when you're sick. I know some people feel that they would rather be alone, but it's really crucial that you unload your stress on people who are there to help.

Meditation

The word 'meditation' tends to conjure up pictures of Eastern yogis sitting cross-legged on the ground contemplating their navels. This kind of meditation originated in the East and some people continue to practise it this way. Most people in the West aren't comfortable with the idea of religious meditation but don't let it put you off.

I want to discuss mindfulness meditation. When you're mindful, you pay close attention to one thing at a time, very often your breathing or how your body feels. When your mind wanders, as it inevitably will, you simply return to whatever you were focussing on without beating yourself up. The main point is not to judge or label what's happening but simply to observe. You begin to notice your thoughts but not engage with them, rather than acting emotionally to them. You're no longer on autopilot.

The benefits of mindfulness meditation are huge. As you focus, you relax and your breathing tends to slow. This engages your vagus nerve, a nerve that runs from the brain stem (your 'primitive' brain that controls basic survival, like breathing) down to your abdomen, travelling via many major organs, including your heart and lungs. The vagus nerve notes your slow breathing and interprets it as meaning you aren't in any danger, and then it tells your brain. The brain passes control to the parasympathetic nervous system, which controls the 'rest and digest' response rather than 'fight or flight'.

Mindfulness meditation practice changes the brain itself by:

- shrinking the amygdala, the 'fear centre' of the brain
- increasing the size of the prefrontal cortex, which controls decision-making, concentration and awareness
- weakening the connections between the amygdala and the rest of the brain
- increasing connections between the prefrontal cortex and other parts of the brain associated with awareness.[4]

On top of that, mindfulness meditation can:

- reduce blood pressure
- improve outcomes for those with heart disease
- reduce sensitivity to chronic pain
- improve sleep
- reduce gastrointestinal difficulties
- reduce anxiety
- alleviate depression
- improve well-being.[5]

In a trial, cancer patients tested the effectiveness of mindfulness meditation over 7 weekly 90-minute sessions, followed by homework. The sessions included information as well as practice. The average daily practice at home was 32 minutes. After 7 weeks the participants had reduced fatigue, reduced mood disturbance and lower stress-related symptoms than the **control group**.[6]

Five **meta-analyses** studied the use of mindfulness-based meditation on cancer patients. These showed a significant reduction in stress, fatigue, mood fluctuations, and sleep disturbances, and an improvement in the patients' quality of life.[7]

Mindfulness meditation, and possibly other kinds of meditation too, is helpful for most people. Keeping the practice going is difficult for many people. To help, set a time of day when you're able to consistently meditate. That might be first thing in the morning or bedtime. The secret is to make it as much a part of your day as brushing your teeth.

There are some useful apps available on both phone or desktop. I recommend Headspace and Calm. Both explain how to meditate as well as guiding you through the process.

Meditation doesn't have to be done sitting down. Getting out into nature and really focusing on what you're experiencing, using all your senses, is an effective form of mindfulness. Really look at everything around you, notice all the different greens of the plants and all the different flora and fauna. Inhale deeply and relish the different smells. Listen to the birds, the crackle of leaves and twigs under your feet, and the sound of leaves rustling in the breeze. Touch the trees and plants. The Japanese call it 'forest bathing'. The psychological effects of communing with nature are an effective form of stress relief, and the higher your stress levels the greater the effects.[8] It also increases the levels and activity of natural killer (**NK**) cells, so it helps fight cancer.[9]

A word of warning: if you've been diagnosed with chronic depression or another mental illness, meditation may exacerbate the problem. It's really rare, but it does happen. If you haven't meditated before but would like to try, I suggest you talk to an experienced meditation teacher to see whether meditation is right for you.

Yoga

Yoga is an ancient tradition originating in India. The origins of yoga included a spiritual element, but in the West most yoga classes only involve stretching movements, controlled breathing and relaxation techniques. Focus on the poses can become a form of mindfulness meditation.

There are a number of different types of yoga, including the following:

- Hatha yoga is where you slowly get into various poses which you hold for a few breaths. It's ideal for beginners, as it's usually quite gentle.
- Restorative yoga is a slow-moving practice and poses are held for longer, so it's ideal for unwinding. Yoga props like blocks, blankets and bolsters are used to help you stay in the poses.
- Yin yoga involves holding poses for a few minutes at a time. It's designed to allow your body to loosen and targets the deeper tissues. Yoga props are used. It's more of a meditative practice, and is perfect if you want to unwind and stretch. It isn't recommended for anyone with a connective tissue disorder, or those who are already super flexible, as it's possible to overdo some poses.

- Iyengar yoga uses props, such as straps, blankets, ropes or blocks, and poses are held for a period of time. There's focus on getting body alignment just right, so this may suit you if you like detail and appreciate the importance of balance exercises.
- Ashtanga yoga comprises 6 series of specific sequences of movements that flow together, with focus on breathing. The sequences are always performed in the same order, so this will suit you if you're a perfectionist.
- Vinyasa yoga is more dynamic, linking movement and breathing together in dance-like movements. The pace can be quite quick, so you need high energy levels. If you're currently having treatment, check with your doctor before attempting this.

- Bikram yoga is performed in a room heated to 40°C (105°F) and with 40% humidity. In a 90 minute sequence, you perform a series of 26 vigorous poses and 2 breathing exercises. The warmth and humidity allow your joints to loosen, but they can also make it more tiring. If you're currently undergoing treatment, check with your doctor and the yoga instructor before taking a bikram yoga class.
- Hot yoga is similar to bikram yoga, as it's done in a heated room. But the teacher chooses the poses rather than being limited to the same routine. Again, it's vigorous, so check with your doctor and the instructor if you're undergoing treatment.
- Kundalini yoga involves chanting, meditating and singing, as well as breath work and repetitive physical exercises. If you're looking for a spiritual practice as well as a physical one, this may suit you.[10]

In 2015, people with chronic illnesses participated in a study to discover whether practising yoga was helpful in reducing anxiety and depression levels. It found that the longer people practised yoga the more benefit they got. The amount of time they spent each day, for 4 days a week, was related to a lowering in anxiety, but not depression.[11]

Research on breast cancer patients showed the beneficial results of yoga, at least in the short term, on depression, fatigue, anxiety, quality of life, perceived stress and well-being. It also showed positive effects on pain reduction and lymphoedema, swelling caused by an accumulation of lymphatic fluid that often occurs after removal of **lymph** nodes.[7]

T'ai Chi and Qi Gong

T'ai Chi and Qi Gong are derived from Chinese martial arts. They combine gentle movements with deep breathing and awareness. There's significant evidence for an improvement in a number of physical conditions, psychological symptoms, sleep disorders and quality of life measurements with their practice. They may also help reduce pain. The studies aren't considered high quality, but the conclusion was that T'ai Chi and Qi Gong are helpful additions to cancer care.[7]

Another study found conclusive evidence that T'ai Chi has a positive effect on psychological health and also on balance[12], which can be damaged by chemo treatment.

Clinical hypnosis

Anton Mesmer introduced hypnosis in the 18th century and there's been extensive research into the subject. It's defined as 'a state of highly focused attention and concentration, often connected with relaxation and heightened susceptibility, where many people are more open to helpful suggestions'. Not everyone can be hypnotised and you won't do anything under hypnosis, or as a result of it, that you wouldn't be willing to do normally. You must be comfortable with the practitioner and be willing to be hypnotised. Best results come from a qualified clinical hypnotist and several sessions are usually needed for good effects. Some self-hypnosis recordings are also very good and are less expensive.

Research shows it helps reduce anxiety both in the general population and in cancer patients.[13]

Massage therapy

Massage involves the use of rhythmic stroking, pressure and kneading of the body. There are various types of massage. For combating stress, I suggest Swedish massage, also known as relaxation massage.

Most people find it pleasurable and relaxing, so it's not surprising that various trials show it benefits cancer patients' stress levels, reducing their anxiety.[14] In a large study of cancer patients on a massage program, it resulted in a 50% reduction in stress/anxiety, depression, nausea, fatigue and pain.[15]

Contact your local massage association to find a therapist who specialises in working with cancer patients, as there can be issues that need to be considered. These include:

- coagulation problems, complicated by internal haemorrhage and bruising
- low platelet count (platelets help with clotting)
- bone metastases, especially if complicated by fractures
- anti-coagulant medications, such as heparin, warfarin (Coumadin) and aspirin
- radiation dermatitis or open wounds
- catheters.

It was once thought massage could encourage **metastasis**, but that's been shown to be a myth.[16]

The effects of massage are relatively short-lived, so you may need to indulge in a weekly massage to maintain the effects.

Acupuncture

Acupuncture has been used in China and other Asian countries for centuries. It involves insertion of very fine needles into very specific locations, which vary according to what's being treated. In Chinese medicine, practitioners believe the needles stimulate movement of Qi, an energy force that regulates health, and enable its balancing. This restores the body's overall health. In the West, Qi is considered to be a metaphor for the body's metabolism. The needles are inserted close to nerves and, depending on their insertion point, they can stimulate endorphins (the body's painkillers), help the body heal, or stimulate the brain area controlling emotions, including anxiety.[17]

In 2003, the **WHO** produced a report recognising acupuncture's effectiveness for many different conditions.[18]

A skilled practitioner shouldn't cause pain. You may not even feel the needles penetrating your skin. Look for someone who's properly qualified and registered with the Chinese Medicine Board of Australia or the equivalent in your country.

It's difficult to find robust studies of acupuncture trials for a number of reasons:

- A good study should be double-blinded (neither the researcher nor the participant should know whether they're receiving real treatment or **placebo**). Obviously the researcher in acupuncture studies always knows, although it's possible to administer sham treatment that the participant won't recognise. This avoids a **placebo** effect by the participant affecting the outcome.
- Bias is often perceived in acupuncture research. Many studies

with positive results for acupuncture are conducted in Asia, whereas many with negative results come from elsewhere. It's feasible that practitioners are more experienced in Asia, but it's impossible to tell whether the research is sound.

- Acupuncture is individualised, so the location of the needles is, by definition, going to differ, which makes replication very difficult.

However, evidence from animal studies shows that acupuncture prior to exposure to cold significantly reduced the production of stress hormones compared with the **control group**.[19]

Pat your pet

Many studies on the use of animals in hospitals show they reduce patients' stress levels. Naturally, you can also enjoy the benefits of pets at home, stroking your cat or dog, or even watching fish in an aquarium.

A **systematic review** identified quite a few studies showing the benefits of animal therapy. They showed that therapy animals in hospitals improve quality of life for cancer patients and others with chronic illnesses. Other studies showed just having a friendly animal around reduced stress and anxiety in the patients, and their families and friends. Blood pressure and heart rate were reduced. Effects were particularly good in young patients, where animal therapy distracts them from their treatment, helps them relax, gives unconditional support, helps them stay motivated and optimistic, and brings joy.[20]

As a bonus, in several studies therapy dogs were associated with reduced pain in both children and adults.[20]

If you're immunocompromised, it's important to ensure that any animals you contact are checked for disease by a vet and that the animal is clean. You should wash your hands, or at least use hand sanitiser, after handling a pet.

Write all your worries down

Keeping a journal or a diary is easy to do and costs next to nothing except time. Many of us kept a diary or journal when we were younger and found it helpful for sorting out our emotions. It's a useful tool for managing stress, anxiety and depression.

Writing down how you're feeling helps in a number of ways, including:

- prioritising your concerns, fears and problems
- tracking your symptoms and maybe helping identify any triggers
- giving an opportunity to spot any negative thought patterns
- providing an outlet for when you don't feel you have the social support you need
- helping to understand yourself better
- using a creative outlet to open up the right-sided, more creative, brain and helps you come up with innovative solutions (most of us problem-solve using our left, analytical brains).

A group of blood cancer patients was asked to complete a 20 minute writing task, an assessment following the task and a follow-up 3 weeks later. After 3 weeks, about half found their thoughts about their condition were more positive.[21]

The effects of journaling are even better if you make it a regular practice. Brandeis University's Department of Community Service gives the following advice:

- Set aside time in your schedule to write.
- Do it somewhere you feel comfortable.
- Use a special 'journal writing' pen (you could also use a PC, iPad or tablet if that's more comfortable).
- Write about whatever comes to mind.
- Don't worry about asking questions and not answering them. Just asking them can start your brain thinking and the answers will come to you later.
- Say exactly what you're thinking. You don't have to worry about what anyone else thinks.
- Write about what you feel **and** think, so that both your heart and brain are engaged.
- Look back at your journal periodically to see what's changed.
- Don't force yourself to write more or less than you want to.[22]

Keep your feet on the ground

You know how good you feel at the beach or when you walk on grass? Do you sleep better after walking barefoot? That's what's known as 'grounding' or 'earthing'.

The concept started when Clinton Ober, a cable TV executive, noticed that when cables are earthed, signal interference is eliminated. He wondered whether humans, who rely on electrical impulses for nerve signal transmission, would be affected by being connected to earth. Together with Stephen Sinatra, a cardiologist, bioenergetic psychotherapist, certified nutritionist and anti-ageing specialist, and Martin Zucker, a well-known writer on alternative health, he wrote a book called 'Earthing: The Most Important Health Discovery Yet?'.

The surface of the earth carries a negative charge and the atmosphere has a positive charge. When we walk barefoot, we absorb the negative charge and this has significant effects on our physiology. Grounding has been shown to reduce pain, stress and inflammation, improve sleep, energy and blood flow and generally improve quality of life.[23]

You can buy mats to sleep on with an earthing connection. Grounding during sleep has been shown to realign your natural cortisol levels, so if you're stressed it helps you to relax. It also improves sleep, and reduces stress and pain.[24]

Another study used medical infra-red imaging, which measures body heat, to demonstrate the effectiveness of grounding on inflammation. Inflammation causes heat. Grounding reduced the amount of heat produced in an injury, showing inflammation was lowered.[25]

Grounding speeds up healing, which is helpful if you've undergone surgery. It also improves heart rate variability, which is a measure of stress, and reduces loss of calcium and phosphorus at least in the short term, suggesting it may help reduce osteoporosis risk. Blood is less likely to clot, making it helpful for those with heart problems.[26]

Most of these studies were quite small, which makes the evidence less reliable. But given that walking barefoot doesn't cost anything, is easy and pleasurable, what do you have to lose?

For stronger effects, you can buy grounding pads to sit or sleep on, underlays for your bed, pillows, sheets and throws.

Find something to laugh at

It may sound strange to suggest that you could find anything funny when you're going through cancer treatment, but if you can find ways to giggle, it does help keep your spirits higher. I found laughter an invaluable tool in my own cancer journey and I took every opportunity to see the funny side of life whenever I could. I recommend you do the same. When you think about some of the indignities you go through with cancer treatment, it's not difficult to find them funny.

One story in particular comes to mind and still amuses me. I have a good friend who would have been in her early 80s when I was diagnosed. She visited me in hospital just before my first round of chemo started. The conversation went like this:

Friend: So will you lose your hair when you have the chemo?

Me: They say I almost certainly will. I can't help feeling that the Universe is playing tricks on me because I've always wanted my hair to look perfect. And more than once I've wished that everyone didn't have hair to save all the hassle.

Friend: So when you lose it, is it just from on your head, or do you lose it from everywhere else on your body?

Me: I think it's all over.

Friend: What, even down below?

Me: I think so. Look on the bright side, a lot of people pay good money for a Brazilian.

Friend: What's a Brazilian?

Me: When you wax the whole area down there.

Friend: (Horrified look on her face) You mean people actually **pay** to do that??

I almost fell off the bed laughing and the nurses wondered what was going on. True story!

If you're finding it difficult to laugh, I have a few suggestions. There are heaps of hilarious YouTube videos (search for the Try Not To Laugh series, which is excellent), or you could watch funny films. If cash is tight, most libraries have DVD collections that you can borrow for free. Look for collections of jokes, cartoons or books written by comedians. Join a Laughter Club, either in person if there's one locally, or online. Even just smiling lifts your mood and you'll be brightening someone else's day at the same time, which can give you a warm and fuzzy feeling.

The research backs me up. Breast cancer patients undergoing radiotherapy given 4 sessions of Therapeutic Laughter Program therapy felt it reduced depression, anxiety and stress, even after just one session.[27] In another study, cortisol levels were lowered after watching a funny video.[28] This doesn't just show a physiological reason for stress reduction. It also suggests an effect on the immune system, because cortisol suppresses the immune system.

The power of prayer

If you're religious you may or may not find prayer helpful. The research is mixed and seems to depend on whether you're looking for help or angry because you thought your religious beliefs would protect you against cancer. For example, a small study in Brazil, where religious beliefs are strong, found listening to an audio recording of a prayer reduced their anxiety and stress levels.[29] But a systematic review concluded the evidence wasn't convincing either for or against the power of prayer.[30]

A **systematic review** was conducted on 23 randomised controlled trials of distant healing, including prayer, mental healing, Therapeutic Touch, and spiritual healing, such as Reiki. Some significant treatment outcomes were shown in 13 people, 9 showed no effects and one showed a negative treatment result. The researchers concluded that the subject was worth further exploration.[31]

I don't have a strong religious belief, although I believe in a Higher Power. However, my sister-in-law, who has strong Christian beliefs, added my name to 3 different prayer groups when I was in hospital. I have to say I felt fantastic that complete strangers were praying for me. After I'd recovered, some of those people specifically wanted to meet me, so it wasn't just lip service. I really felt it raised my spirits when I was low, and I believe that has a significant effect on how the body heals.

Change your thinking

I'm talking about cognitive behaviour therapy (CBT), a branch of psychotherapy. The underlying premise of CBT is that sometimes our thinking becomes inaccurate, unhealthy or unhelpful in some situations. CBT interventions use a number of techniques, including cognitive, emotion-focused and behavioural ones. It's practised by psychiatrists who are well-trained in this area and has proved really helpful for cancer patients.

The results of CBT on 790 cancer patients were compared with 702 cancer patients who didn't receive CBT. CBT was found to reduce anxiety and depression, at least in the short term, and quality of life was improved in both the short and long term.[32]

Get a mental picture

Close your eyes. Imagine yourself on a beach on a tropical island. Feel the sun and a gentle breeze on your skin, and the soft sand under you. See the blueness of the ocean and the sky. Hear the sound of the palm trees rustling in the breeze. Smell the salty air.

I'm betting that feels good and your anxiety levels have dropped. That's visualisation or guided imagery, showing the power of the mind over your body.

Guided imagery can help with controlling anxiety and depression in cancer patients, even those undergoing chemotherapy. Breast and prostate cancer patients who were given guided imagery and progressive muscle relaxation felt better, and their stress hormone levels were improved.[33]

Visualisation can do so much more than this, though. A respected psychologist who specialises in evidence-based medicine suggests the following experiment to test it:

- Tie a small heavy object, such as a bolt or a lead weight, to a piece of string about 30 cm long.
- Hold the end of the string so that the object hangs straight down like a pendulum.
- Now sit at a table, rest your elbow on the table and dangle the string so that the object is about one cm above the table. Sit up straight and hold the string about 15 cm away from your nose.
- Blink and breathe naturally and imagine the object on the end of the string start to make small circles.
- Keeping your eyes open, imagine the circles getting bigger. In most cases, it does just that.

This isn't magic. The brain sends tiny signals to the muscles in your fingers, which contract and cause the pendulum to move.[34]

It isn't just your muscles that can be affected by the power of visualisation but also your immune system, increasing the number of white blood cells to fight infection and even cancer cells. Imagine that your white blood cells are armies of little soldiers fighting for you. Call up all the reserves as well and see them knocking out the cancer cells or the bacteria, viruses or fungi causing an infection. The more you practise visualising this, the more effective it is.[34]

I used this technique when I had my first round of chemo. My white blood count was rock bottom and I got a partial blockage in my small intestine. It was excruciatingly painful. The doctors would normally have operated to relieve it but it was too dangerous because of the risk of infection. So they inserted a naso-gastric tube to relieve the pressure, which it did to some extent, and hoped nature would take its course. After about 2 days of this, with no sleep and in a lot of pain, I thought I'd try visualising my intestine relaxing enough to let the blockage move. I focused for about 10 minutes on this. Suddenly, there was a gurgling sound and the blockage shifted. Mind power really is that strong.

I have Raynaud's Syndrome, an autoimmune condition that causes the capillaries in my fingers to clamp shut when I'm cold or stressed. The fingertips go white and then blue, then very red when the blood returns. When I get an attack, I focus on opening those capillaries and within a few minutes I can see the blood coming back into them.

I believe we all have the power to do this. I'm certainly not unique. So when your body is struggling with something, try visualising the problem area and correcting it.

References

1. Yaribeygi H, Panahi Y, Sahraei H, Johnston T, Sahebkar A. The impact of stress on body function: A review. *EXCLI J*. 2017;16:1057-1072. doi:10.17179/excli2017-480
2. Brower V. Mind–body research moves towards the mainstream. *EMBO Rep*. 2006;7(4):358-361. doi:10.1038/sj.embor.7400671
3. Usta Y. Importance of Social Support in Cancer Patients. *Asian Pacific Journal of Cancer Prevention*. 2012;13(8):3569-3572. doi:10.7314/apjcp.2012.13.8.3569
4. Ireland T. What Does Mindfulness Meditation Do to Your Brain?. Scientific American Blog Ne2rk. https://blogs.scientificamerican.com/guest-blog/what-does-mindfulness-meditation-do-to-your-brain/. Published 2014. Accessed August 20, 2021.
5. Helpguide. Benefits of Mindfulness. HelpGuide. https://www.helpguide.org/harvard/benefits-of-mindfulness.htm. Accessed August 20, 2021.
6. Speca M, Carlson L, Goodey E, Angen M. A Randomized, Wait-List Controlled Clinical Trial: The Effect of a Mindfulness Meditation-Based Stress Reduction Program on Mood and Symptoms of Stress in Cancer Outpatients. *Psychosom Med*. 2000;62(5):613-622. doi:10.1097/00006842-200009000-00004
7. Bhatnagar S, Satija A. Complementary therapies for symptom management in cancer patients. *Indian J Palliat Care*. 2017;23(4):468. doi:10.4103/ijpc.ijpc_100_17
8. Morita E, Fukuda S, Nagano J et al. Psychological effects of forest environments on healthy adults: Shinrin-yoku (forest-air bathing, walking) as a possible method of stress reduction. *Public Health*. 2007;121(1):54-63. doi:10.1016/j.puhe.2006.05.024
9. Li Q, Morimoto K, Nakadai A et al. Forest Bathing Enhances Human Natural Killer Activity and Expression of Anti-Cancer Proteins. *Int J Immunopathol Pharmacol*. 2007;20(2_suppl):3-8. doi:10.1177/03946320070200s202
10. Yu C. The Beginner's Guide to Every Type of Yoga Out There. Daily Burn. https://dailyburn.com/life/fitness/yoga-for-beginners-kundalini-yin-bikram/. Published 2017. Accessed August 20, 2021.
11. Telles S, Pathak S, Kumar A, Mishra P, Balkrishna A. Influence of intensity and duration of yoga on anxiety and depression scores associated with chronic illness. *Ann Med Health Sci Res*. 2015;5(4):260-265. doi:10.4103/2141-9248.160182
12. Lee M, Ernst E. Systematic reviews of t'ai chi: an overview. *Br J Sports Med*. 2012;46:713-718. doi:10.1136/bjsm.2010.080622
13. Mayden K. Mind-Body Therapies: Evidence and Implications in Advanced Oncology Practice. *J Adv Pract Oncol*. 2012;3(6):357-373. doi:10.6004/jadpro.2012.3.6.2
14. Greenlee H, DuPont-Reyes M, Balneaves L et al. Clinical practice guidelines on the evidence-based use of integrative therapies during and after breast cancer treatment. *CA Cancer J Clin*. 2017;67(3):194-232. doi:10.3322/caac.21397
15. Cassileth B, Vickers A. Massage therapy for symptom control: outcome study at a major cancer center. *J Pain Symptom Manage*. 2004;28(3):244-249. doi:10.1016/j.jpainsymman.2003.12.016

16. MacDonald G. Massage therapy in cancer care: an overview of the past, present, and future. *Altern Ther Health Med*. 2014;20(Supplement 2):12-5. https://pubmed.ncbi.nlm.nih.gov/25362212/. Accessed August 20, 2021.

17. Hohman M. Why Acupuncture Works for Anxiety Relief - Everyday Health. Everyday Health. https://www.everydayhealth.com/news/why-acupuncture-works-anxiety-relief/. Published 2014. Accessed August 20, 2021.

18. Amaro J. Acupuncture: review and analysis of controlled clinical trials. International Academy of Medical Acupuncture. https://iama.edu/wp-content/uploads/2019/10/WHO-LIST-OF-CONDITIONS.pdf. Published 2003. Accessed August 20, 2021.

19. Eshkevari L, Permaul E, Mulroney S. Acupuncture blocks cold stress-induced increases in the hypothalamus–pituitary–adrenal axis in the rat. *Journal of Endocrinology*. 2013;217(1):95-104. doi:10.1530/joe-12-0404

20. McCullough A, Ruehrdanz A, Jenkins M et al. Measuring the Effects of an Animal-Assisted Intervention for Pediatric Oncology Patients and Their Parents: A Multisite Randomized Controlled Trial. *Journal of Pediatric Oncology Nursing*. 2018;35(3):159-177. doi:10.1177/1043454217748586

21. Morgan N, Graves K, Poggi E, Cheson B. Implementing an Expressive Writing Study in a Cancer Clinic. *Oncologist*. 2008;13(2):196-204. doi:10.1634/theoncologist.2007-0147

22. Department of Community Service. Journal Writing Tips. Brandeis University. https://www.brandeis.edu/community-service/volunteers/resources/helpful-information/journaling-tips.html. Accessed August 20, 2021.

23. Menigoz W, Latz T, Ely R, Kamei C, Melvin G, Sinatra D. Integrative and lifestyle medicine strategies should include Earthing (grounding): Review of research evidence and clinical observations. *EXPLORE*. 2020;16(3):152-160. doi:10.1016/j.explore.2019.10.005

24. Ghaly M, Teplitz D. The Biologic Effects of Grounding the Human Body During Sleep as Measured by Cortisol Levels and Subjective Reporting of Sleep, Pain, and Stress. *The Journal of Alternative and Complementary Medicine*. 2004;10(5):767-776. doi:10.1089/acm.2004.10.767

25. Oschman J. Can Electrons Act as Antioxidants? A Review and Commentary. *The Journal of Alternative and Complementary Medicine*. 2007;13(9):955-967. doi:10.1089/acm.2007.7048

26. Chevalier G, Sinatra S, Oschman J, Sokal K, Sokal P. Earthing: Health Implications of Reconnecting the Human Body to the Earth's Surface Electrons. *J Environ Public Health*. 2012;2012:1-8. doi:10.1155/2012/291541

27. Kim S, Kim Y, Kim H. Laughter and Stress Relief in Cancer Patients: A Pilot Study. *Evidence-Based Complementary and Alternative Medicine*. 2015;2015:1-6. doi:10.1155/2015/864739

28. Bennett M, Lengacher C. Humor and Laughter May Influence Health: III. Laughter and Health Outcomes. *Evidence-Based Complementary and Alternative Medicine*. 2008;5(1):37-40. doi:10.1093/ecam/nem041

29. Carvalho C, Chaves E, Iunes D, Simão T, Grasselli C, Braga C. Effectiveness of prayer in reducing anxiety in cancer patients. *Revista da Escola de Enfermagem da USP*. 2014;48(4):684-690. doi:10.1590/s0080-623420140000400016

30. Andrade C, Radhakrishnan R. Prayer and healing: A medical and scientific perspective on randomized controlled trials. *Indian J Psychiatry.* 2009;51(4):247. doi:10.4103/0019-5545.58288

31. Astin J, Harkness E, Ernst E. The Efficacy of "Distant Healing". *Ann Intern Med.* 2000;132(11):903-910. doi:10.7326/0003-4819-132-11-200006060-00009

32. Osborn R, Demoncada A, Feuerstein M. Psychosocial Interventions for Depression, Anxiety, and Quality of Life in Cancer Survivors: Meta-Analyses. *The International Journal of Psychiatry in Medicine.* 2006;36(1):13-34. doi:10.2190/eufn-rv1k-y3tr-fk0l

33. Charalambous A, Giannakopoulou M, Bozas E, Paikousis L. A Randomized Controlled Trial for the Effectiveness of Progressive Muscle Relaxation and Guided Imagery as Anxiety Reducing Interventions in Breast and Prostate Cancer Patients Undergoing Chemotherapy. *Evidence-Based Complementary and Alternative Medicine.* 2015;2015(27086):1-10. doi:10.1155/2015/270876

34. Lazarus C. Can Visualization Techniques Treat Serious Diseases?. Psychology Today. https://www.psychologytoday.com/au/blog/think-well/201601/can-visualization-techniques-treat-serious-diseases. Published 2016. Accessed August 20, 2021.

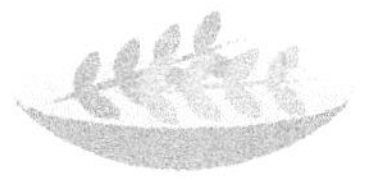

Chapter 4

Move your body

'Lack of activity destroys the good condition of every human being, while movement and methodical physical exercise save it and preserve it.'

— **Plato (427–347 BC)**

I didn't name this chapter 'Exercise' because I groan inwardly every time someone reminds me that I should exercise. But please bear with me and I'll explain why movement really is a matter of life and death for us, and I'll help you find ways to make it pleasurable instead of a burden.

Physical activity is something that humans really need. It helps us in so many ways, including by:

- improving anxiety
- reducing fatigue
- boosting mood
- raising self-esteem
- developing cardiovascular fitness
- increasing muscle strength

- avoiding obesity
- enhancing immunity
- strengthening bones
- improving brain health
- removing toxins.

If exercise was a pill it would be the most prescribed pill on the market.

One of the reasons exercise is so important involves the lymphatic system. This is one of the body's systems for removing toxins from the body. It carries a clear fluid called **lymph** to all the body's cells. It works a bit like the plumbing in your house, by draining away all the rubbish produced by the cells, tissues and organs in your body as they go about their daily work. It also produces white blood cells that defend against disease, and absorbs fats and fat-soluble vitamins from the digestive system, carrying them to the cells. The catch is that, unlike the way that blood circulates, there's no pump for the lymphatic system. It relies totally on physical movements of the skeletal muscles and breathing to pump **lymph** around the body. If you don't move, the lymphatic system can't do its job properly and that has serious consequences.

Epidemiological studies show that the better your cardiovascular fitness, the lower your risk of dying from cancer. Intermediate levels of cardiovascular fitness reduced the risk by 20%, while high levels reduced it by 45%. Even when obesity was factored in, the same reductions were true.[1]

A **systematic review** examined 100 studies involving thousands of participants to determine the effects of exercise on cancer mortality and recurrence, and its influences on the side-effects suffered by the participants. The studies covered a wide range of different types of cancers. It concluded that exercise helped 28—44% of cancer patients overcome cancer, and resulted in 21—35% fewer recurrences of cancers.[2]

Also:

- One of the studies showed breast symptoms were reduced by half when breast cancer participants walked 10,000 steps daily.
- Another showed results were better with high intensity than low intensity exercise.
- Cognitive health was improved in 5 trials with breast and prostate cancer patients.
- In 22 **meta-analyses,** which covered a range of cancers, including people undergoing chemo, there was less fatigue.
- Quality of life was enhanced for most cancer patients.
- Anxiety, depression and mental health were examined in 12 **meta-analyses**: one on prostate cancer patients, 8 with a variety of diagnoses, and 3 on breast cancer patients. Ten showed a significant improvement in at least one area with exercise. Of the 2 that didn't show an improvement, one was a small **meta-analysis** that only looked at 2 trials, and the other specifically looked at depression among prostate cancer patients.[2]

The mechanisms by which exercise reduces cancer risk, mortality, recurrence and side-effects aren't completely understood, but are thought to include:

- Switching on and off the **genes** that affect cancer initiation and progression, in a positive way.
- Reducing blood pressure and risk of diabetes, heart disease, obesity and osteoporosis, all of which can affect cancer survival.
- Findings that more active patients are generally diagnosed with less aggressive cancers.
- Increasing tolerance to higher doses of treatment.
- Reducing side-effects, enabling treatment to be completed.
- Improving healing after surgery.
- Potentially increasing the transport of systemic drugs to the cancer cells.
- Positively affecting immunity, oxidative stress, inflammation, sex hormones and metabolic hormones, all of which are believed to cause cancer progression.[2]

Types of exercise

There are 4 main types of exercise:

- Aerobic exercise. This is exercise that raises the heart rate and breathing but that can be maintained for a reasonable period. You should be able to talk while you're doing aerobic exercise. It's sometimes referred to as 'cardio' exercise and includes walking, swimming, hiking, aerobics classes, cross-country skiing, dancing, kickboxing, and many more. It's important for improving cardiovascular health.
- Anaerobic exercise. In anaerobic exercise, such as in sprinting and lifting heavy weights, you run out of breath very quickly. Aerobic exercise carried out at high intensity can become

anaerobic as you run out of breath. Think of walking up a steep hill quickly. Anaerobic exercise helps build fitness and endurance, can build muscle, and improves weight loss.

- Strength or resistance training. This involves using weight, either your body or external weights, to progressively overload the muscles and strengthen them. As your muscles get stronger, your bones do too, so it's important for osteoporosis prevention. It also helps with maintaining balance, as many muscles are needed to keep you upright.
- Flexibility training. This increases or maintains the range of motion of your joints by increasing the length of your tendons, muscles and ligaments. Good flexibility also helps with balance, prevents injuries and back pain.

All these have their place in a good exercise program. It's important to check with your medical practitioner before starting any exercise regime, particularly if you're currently undergoing cancer treatment. Exercise physiologists are experts in designing exercise programmes to suit a person's physical capabilities and preferences. I suggest that you ask your doctor for a referral to one.

The 'Australian Physical Activity and Sedentary Behaviour Guidelines', issued by the Commonwealth Department of Health, suggest that adults aged 18–64 should carry out either:

- 150–300 minutes of moderate exercise a week, or
- 75–150 minutes of vigorous exercise a week, or
- a combination of the 2, spread over most days of the week.

They should also carry out muscle strengthening exercises at least 2 days per week.[3]

As a guide, one minute of vigorous activity equals 2 minutes of moderate activity.[4] You may be thinking that exercise isn't appropriate if you're undergoing chemo and/or radiotherapy at the moment. You may be anaemic and exercise may make you breathless. However, movement of any kind will help to raise your mood and get the blood circulating. If you feel a bit fragile, try stints of, maybe, 10 minutes at a time, 3 times a day.

Let's look at what might be achievable and try to find something you'll enjoy doing, so that it doesn't feel like a chore.

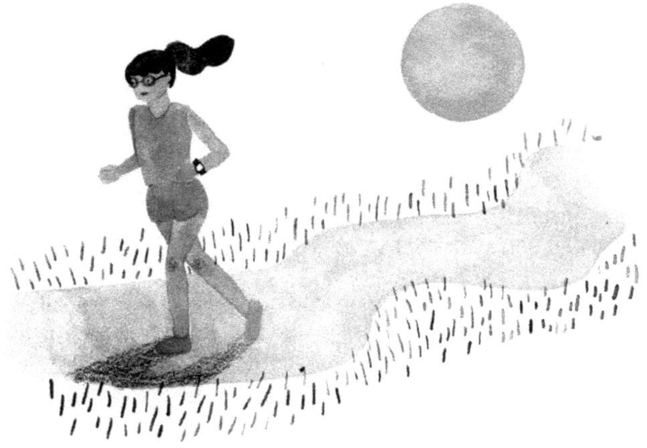

Walking

If you have a dog, this is a no-brainer. Even if you don't go far, you can exercise your dog and get some fresh air, which is usually enjoyable. As mentioned in Chapter 3, walking in nature is a good way to de-stress. You could also throw a ball for your dog. The act of bending down to pick up the ball and throwing it will exercise a few muscles. Walking costs nothing and most people enjoy getting outside.

Even without a dog, a short stroll around the neighbourhood gives an opportunity to talk to your neighbours. Social interaction is as important to your wellbeing as moving your body.

You might consider joining a walking group if you are able to manage a longer walk. This way, you can combine socialising with exercise. In Australia, the Heart Foundation has a free walking network that connects you with other people in your area.[5] This gives you a support network as well as a social group. You stay motivated to go walking because you're part of a group and you aren't alone if you become ill. Being in a group makes you more visible to other road users and makes you feel more secure. They even have a Walker Recognition Scheme, where you get incentives, certificates and discounts on Heart Foundation merchandise when you reach certain milestones. A Walker Handbook is available when you sign up, giving useful information about warming up and cooling down before and after walking, and other practical advice.

Dancing

For many people, dancing is an enjoyable pastime rather than exercise. However, all types of dance involve movement, and you might enjoy it while you get some exercise.

Dancing is as effective as cycling, swimming, jogging or running on a treadmill. Its benefits include toning and building muscle, increasing endurance, increasing flexibility, improving spatial awareness and balance, as well as an increased sense of wellbeing. It can help with weight loss, burning between 800 kJ (191 Calories) and over 2,000 kJ (478 Calories) an hour. You could also improve your cardiovascular fitness with vigorous dancing. The swaying movements of many dance steps help strengthen the weight-bearing bones in your legs, helping to ward off osteoporosis. Some dance steps also improve range of motion in the lower back and hips, improving posture and increasing muscle tone, and helping avoid lower back problems. Learning new dance steps builds new neural connections, so it helps avoid mental decline.[6] And you get all of these benefits while having fun.

Sports

Do you enjoy sports? If you do, find yourself a tennis partner or join a netball or cricket team. If you live near the beach, you could play beach volleyball. Badminton, bowls, 10 pin bowling, golf and croquet are other ideas. The list is endless. Just make it something you find fun and that you feel is manageable for you at the moment. Most sports are also social activities, giving you the stress-busting benefits of mixing with like-minded people as well.

If you prefer something more solitary, consider swimming. If you don't live near the beach, there's usually a swimming pool nearby. Aqua aerobics could be fun for you. These activities are gentler on your joints, which is important if your bones aren't strong or if you have arthritis.

Cycling

If you enjoy exploring the countryside, cycling may appeal to you. It's also a great way to get from A to B and is environmentally friendly to boot. You get the benefits of fresh air (assuming you don't live in a busy city) and sunshine, which boosts your vitamin D levels. We'll cover the importance of vitamin D in Chapter 7. Another bonus is a saving on travel costs.

Playing with children

You may not think of it as exercise, but the games children play are very often pretty active. Think of hopscotch, tag, blind man's buff, kite flying, hula hooping, and all those other games children enjoy. A Frisbee can keep you laughing for ages. What about a pillow fight with them (or your partner)? They'd love to play with you and I'm sure you'd have fun too.

Take up yoga or T'ai Chi

We discussed these in Chapter 3 but, as well as being good stress-busters, they are good exercise and help with flexibility and balance.

Learn martial arts

If you're reasonably fit, martial arts can be a wonderful way of getting exercise, mixing with other people, and learning to defend yourself. Get clearance from your doctor first.

Buy some exercise DVDs

If you prefer to exercise at home, you can buy exercise DVDs covering every type of exercise class you can imagine and every fitness level. Alternatively, look on YouTube for classes.

Grab a surf board, body board or a windsurfer

If you love the beach, try surfing or body boarding for good exercise and great fun. You can windsurf on any body of water and it's an exhilarating way to build some activity into your life.

Work out with light weights

This is the way to get your strength training in. You can buy dumbbells weighing 1–2 kg fairly inexpensively and they don't take up much room. This website has some good exercises using weights: https://www.livestrong.com/article/389963-best-exercises-to-do-with-small-weights-at-home/

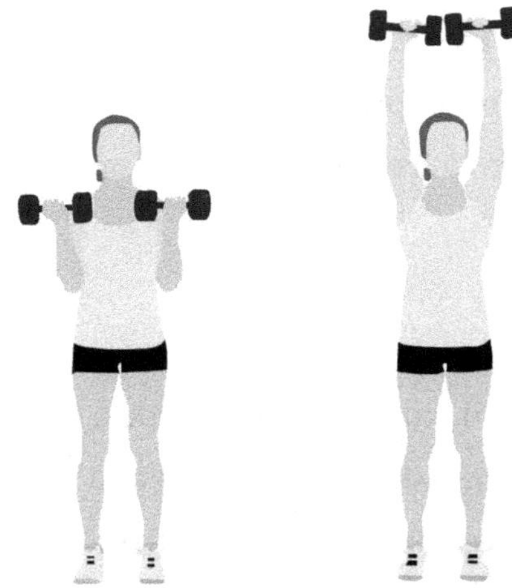

Catch up on your TV viewing

While you're watching your favourite programmes, get on an exercise bike and see how far you can travel while the show is on. If you have a more sophisticated machine, set it for different hill patterns to add interest.

Run or walk for a good cause

Look out for charity runs or sponsored walks and raise money for your favourite charities while you get some exercise. Working for a good cause is a great motivator.

Learn something new

While you're on the treadmill or exercise bike, watch a TED talk or download some good podcasts. It's amazing how much more you can achieve when you take your mind off the muscle fatigue.

Sit and Be Fit

Sit and Be Fit is a low-impact workout developed by a Registered Nurse. It's aired on television in the US but it's also available on a low-cost subscription for streaming on a PC. Find it at: https://www.sitandbefit.org/product/streaming-club/

Have a good belly laugh

Laughter is a really good workout as well as a stress buster. It causes the muscles in your abdomen to expand and contract and helps tone your abs. Not only that, it also gets your heart pumping and improves your mood. If you're chairbound, put on comedy films or watch YouTube videos. You could also join a Laughter Club, run all over the world and also online. Check out: https://www.laughteronlineuniversity.com/laughter-yoga-clubs/.

Make housework fun

It has to be done, so why not make housework into a game? Put on your favourite upbeat music track and see how much you can get done while it's playing. Or go out into the garden and pull up some weeds, mow the lawn, do some pruning and commune with nature. Clear out a cupboard or 2, tidy your shed, or do some spring cleaning. Housework involves plenty of movement and this way you can kill 2 birds with one stone: get your exercise and do your chores at the same time.

Summary

Hopefully that has got your imagination working. The general idea is to find an activity that you really enjoy doing. That way you'll be happy to do it on a regular basis and for much longer than slogging in a gym (unless you enjoy that). The results are well worth it.

References

1. Schmid D, Leitzmann M. Cardiorespiratory fitness as predictor of cancer mortality: a systematic review and meta-analysis. *Annals of Oncology*. 2015;26(2):272-278. doi:10.1093/annonc/mdu250
2. Cormie P, Zopf E, Zhang X, Schmitz K. The Impact of Exercise on Cancer Mortality, Recurrence, and Treatment-Related Adverse Effects. *Epidemiol Rev*. 2017;39(1):71-92. doi:10.1093/epirev/mxx007
3. Australian Government Department of Health. Physical activity and exercise guidelines for all Australians. Australian Government Department of Health. https://www.health.gov.au/health-topics/physical-activity-and-exercise/physical-activity-and-exercise-guidelines-for-all-australians. Published 2021. Accessed August 23, 2021.
4. Harvard Medical Service. Healthy Mind, Healthy Body: Benefits of Exercise. Harvard Medical Service. https://hms.harvard.edu/sites/default/files/assets/Sites/Longwood_Seminars/Exercise3.14.pdf. Published 2014. Accessed August 23, 2021.
5. Heart Foundation Walking. Find a walking Group in Australia | Heart Foundation Walking. Heart Foundation Walking. http://walking.heartfoundation.org.au/walking. Published 2021. Accessed August 23, 2021.
6. Alpert P. The Health Benefits of Dance. *Home Health Care Manag Pract*. 2010;23(2):155-157. doi:10.1177/1084822310384689

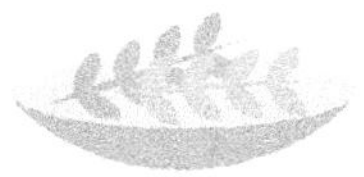

Chapter 5:

The importance of sleep

'The best bridge between despair and hope is a good night's sleep.'
— **Anonymous**

What is sleep?

When we sleep we're unconscious and the brain is more responsive to what's happening internally rather than externally. The cycles of sleep and wakefulness, and the gradual change in responsiveness from external to internal are the features that distinguish sleep from other states of unconsciousness.[1]

Sleep is something of a mystery, but it seems to be controlled by nerve cells in the brain stem, our primitive brain. The nerve cells send signals that seem to switch off the neurotransmitters norepinephrine and serotonin, which keep some areas in the brain active when we're awake. A chemical called adenosine builds up in our blood while we're awake and makes us sleepy when it reaches a certain level. It's slowly broken down whilst we sleep.[2]

Our circadian rhythms also play a part in regulating sleep. When light reaches the retina, a signal is sent to the brain, which relays it to the pineal gland. The pineal gland controls production of melatonin, and light switches production off. Melatonin builds up when it's dark and this makes us tired.[2] Although the 'central' clock is in the brain, recent research has found that we also have body clocks in other organs, such as the stomach and intestines, ovaries, liver, heart, lungs, pancreas and kidneys. These other clocks are less sensitive to light and more affected by other cues, like meal times.[3]

We have a cycle of sleep stages, from 1 to 4 plus REM (rapid eye movement) sleep:

- Stage one is very light sleep, when you can be woken very easily. Muscle activity slows and you have slow eye movements.
- Stage 2 is characterised by slower brain waves with occasional episodes of fast waves, and eye movements stop.
- In Stage 3, very slow delta waves start to occur, interspersed with faster, smaller waves.
- In Stage 4, almost all brain waves are delta waves. Stages 3 and 4 are considered deep sleep. If you're woken from deep sleep, you tend to be very disorientated and groggy.
- REM sleep is when you dream. Our eyes move quickly, our breathing becomes shallow, quick and irregular, and blood pressure and heart rate rise.[2]

Sleep needs vary. Babies need an average of 16 hours, whilst adolescents need about 9 hours. Most adults need 7–8 hours of sleep, with anything less than 5 or over 9 being considered short or long.[2]

Animal studies show we need sleep to survive. For example, rats normally live for 2–3 years. If they don't get REM sleep, survival drops to about 5 weeks. If they don't sleep at all they only live for about 3 weeks.[2]

During sleep, our bodies perform a range of processes important for our health and wellbeing:

- Our heart and blood vessels are repaired and healed, lowering risk of heart disease, stroke, diabetes and kidney disease, and reducing blood pressure.
- Leptin and ghrelin, hormones that affect hunger, are balanced. When you're sleep-deprived, ghrelin levels rise making you hungrier, increasing your chances of overeating and obesity.
- Too little sleep results in higher blood sugar levels, raising the risk of diabetes.
- Healthy growth needs sleep. This is particularly important for children and teenagers, but also affects adults' ability to build muscle, and repair cells and tissues.
- Sleep supports a healthy immune system. Without enough sleep, your body struggles to fight off infections.
- It helps with learning, problem solving, focusing attention, decision making and creativity. That's why driving and working suffer if you haven't had enough sleep.
- It keeps your emotions stable by regulating neurotransmitters. Lack of sleep often results in depression and anxiety.[4]

The links between sleep and cancer

Various studies have shown a link between the risk of developing a number of different cancers and abnormal sleep patterns. For example:

- The Women's Health Initiative study of post-menopausal women found a moderate increase in colon cancer incidence in those who slept more than 9 hours or fewer than 5 hours a night.[5]
- Liver cancer cases tripled in overweight women who slept more than 9 hours a night, and doubled in those of normal weight with similar sleep patterns. Those who slept fewer than 5 hours a night were unaffected.[6]
- The incidence of thyroid cancer was significantly increased in women who suffered insomnia and weren't overweight.[7]

An increasing number of studies link sleep disturbance with cancer incidence. In 2007, the International Agency for Research on Cancer (**IARC**) declared shift work involving a disruption of circadian rhythms to be a probable **carcinogen**. Women who worked night shifts had a 50% higher risk of developing breast cancer compared with those who hadn't worked night shifts. The same applied to shift-working men and prostate cancer.[8]

The research isn't consistent, though. A recent study followed nearly 103,000 women for 10 years who'd worked shifts over the 10 years prior to the beginning of the study. They looked at the associations with the age when they started shift work, whether it was before or after first pregnancy, and how long it had been since they worked shifts. They found no association between shift work and breast cancer in any of these cases.[9] However, in June 2019 the **IARC** evaluated the latest research and concluded that there was limited evidence that night shift work caused prostate, breast and colorectal cancer. They classified night shift work as 'probably **carcinogenic** to humans'. They agreed that the links weren't strong. The link is most pronounced when people work shifts for long periods. Their decision was based on animal studies, as well as human, which show a link between cancer and an alteration in the sleep—wake cycle.[10]

The effects of poor sleep also affect cancer mortality. Poor sleep in breast cancer patients has been linked to cancer growth.[11] Suggested reasons for poor sleep's effects on cancer progression include the following:

- The effects of poor quality sleep on the immune system. Cortisol rhythms are affected by sleep deprivation, and cortisol regulates Natural Killer **(NK)** cells, which protect against cancer.
- Cortisol disruption leads to obesity and poor insulin sensitivity, both of which are factors for cancer risk and growth.
- Melatonin production in the body is reduced. Melatonin slows oestrogen production, so less melatonin causes oestrogen levels to rise and stimulate growth of hormone-sensitive cancer cells.[12]

Sleep apnoea, a disorder of interrupted breathing during sleep, also shows strong links with cancer risk and growth. In the Wisconsin Sleep Cohort study, 1500 healthy participants were monitored for 18 years. Of those with sleep apnoea, 7.9% developed cancer of some type compared with 1.9% of those without apnoea. This is partly because of its effects on sleep and might also be related to the links between obesity and apnoea. You're much more likely to have apnoea if you're overweight. It's also connected with the intermittent lack of oxygen, which animal studies show is associated with increased tumour growth. Broken sleep had the same effect.[13]

The rates of insomnia in people with various cancers going through chemo are about 3 times higher than the general population.[14] In non-metastatic breast cancer patients, 42% reported having problems sleeping 18 months after surgery.[15] It's not surprising: the shock of a cancer diagnosis lingers in many people. Also the side-effects of many treatments, including chemo, surgery, radiation and hormone-blocking drugs, often cause sleep problems. Pain is always worse when you're tired and causes insomnia too, setting up a vicious circle.

The solutions

Train your body clock

Go to bed and wake up at the same time each day (including weekends). Your body clock becomes used to the pattern. After a while you'll find you get sleepy at the same time each night and wake up before your alarm rings.

If you're tired, go to bed. If you aren't tired, don't lie there awake because you'll just get frustrated.

If you've lain awake for half an hour, get up and read something (preferably something not too exciting) until you feel sleepy.

Try to get some sunshine early in the morning. It slows the production of melatonin, the sleep hormone, and tells your body it's time to start the day.

Make sure the bedroom is comfortable

You need a Goldilocks mattress: one that isn't too hard or too soft. An unsupportive mattress or a lumpy one is a sure-fire route to a bad night.

A temperature somewhere from 15—19°C, relatively cool, is ideal. Our body cores have a natural temperature rhythm, with the highest temperature in the early afternoon and the lowest at about 5 am. The body starts to cool about an hour and a half before bedtime, which helps trigger sleepiness. If your bedroom is too hot, the core can't cool as easily.

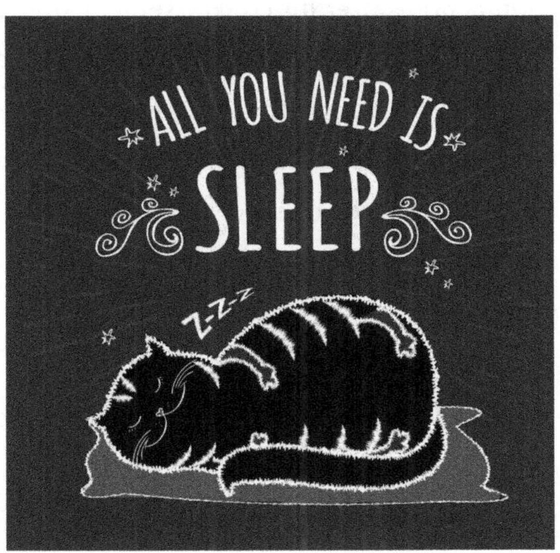

Block out as much light as you can. Sleep without any lights on, if possible. Block out lights from the alarm clock or other digital equipment. Blockout curtains can help, or buy an eye shade. This helps boost melatonin.

If noise is a problem that can't be resolved (barking dogs, noisy neighbours, a partner who snores etc.) get some good earplugs. Listening to relaxing music helps, or use a fan or humidifier to gently hum you to sleep.

Avoid using the bedroom for anything other than sleeping and intimacy. A television in the bedroom means your brain associates the bedroom with staying awake rather than sleep.

Avoid stimulants

Many people who don't sleep well still drink coffee. In most people, the liver processes caffeine in 4–6 hours, so the usual recommendation is none after lunch. For some people it can take significantly longer, which could mean you're still processing coffee at bedtime if you have one in the morning. It's **genetic** and doesn't mean there's a problem with your liver. If you're one of these unfortunate people, you could consider giving up or at least cutting down on coffee. For some people, even tea is problematic, especially strong tea. Energy drinks are high in caffeine and sugar too. If sleep is elusive, these won't help the problem.

Chocolate contains theobromine, a chemical very similar to caffeine. It's also a stimulant, although not as stimulating as caffeine. If you're having trouble sleeping, try eating it (dark chocolate, of course) at lunchtime instead of in the evening.

If you're a smoker, you may think cigarettes relax you. Actually, they're a stimulant. They cause your blood pressure and heart rate to rise, which can keep you awake. If you're a heavy smoker, withdrawal symptoms during the night can wake you. This could be another reason to give them up. If not, at least try to avoid smoking in the evening.

Do you like a nightcap? It does help you doze off but it also disrupts your sleep patterns, preventing deeper, restorative sleep. It stops REM sleep, so you're likely to wake up feeling as though you haven't slept well. It depresses the nervous system and causes your muscles to relax. That includes your throat muscles, so it could cause you to snore or have sleep apnoea. You're likely to wake up during the night to make a trip to the bathroom too because alcohol is a diuretic, not to mention the risk of a hangover in the morning.

Relax your mind and body

You might want to try meditation to relax you and encourage sleep. There are plenty of apps out there designed for this, mostly available free, for both Android and iPhone devices.

Progressive muscle relaxation can be very effective for falling asleep. Start at your feet and tighten the muscles as hard as you can, then relax them completely. Move up to your calves and do the same. Work your way up until you reach your scalp. Do this very slowly and mindfully, focusing on each muscle group. The exercise should take about 20 minutes but don't worry if you're already asleep by then.

If you find yourself worrying at bedtime, try allocating time earlier in the day to focus on all your worries. Once that time is over, put your worries aside until the following day. Remind yourself at bedtime that your worry time is over for the day.

Avoid anything mentally stimulating at bedtime. An adventure book could keep you awake. Relax with something soothing before sleep.

Exercise

Exercising during the day will help you sleep better at night, but do it at least a couple of hours before retiring. Exercise quickens your heart rate and increases your temperature, both of which keep you awake.

Dim your lights in the evening

Turn off any overhead lights in the evening and use table lamps instead to avoid flooding your eyes with blue light. Bright light fools your brain into thinking it's daylight and messes up your circadian rhythms.

If you use LED globes rather than incandescent ones, remember these give off a lot of blue light. It all depends on whether you choose 'Warm white' or 'Cool white' light bulbs. Cool white ones emit blue light, whereas Warm white are yellow, like traditional incandescent bulbs. If you're having sleeping difficulties, I recommend switching to Warm white ones.

Turn off your screens

The blue light produced by electronic screens is interpreted by the brain as sunlight, stopping melatonin production. Avoid using a flat screen TV, computer, tablet or smartphone for at least an hour before sleep to avoid this.

If you're addicted to screens, there are a few solutions:

- Blue screen filters effectively block most blue light.
- Some apps adjust the colour of screens on digital devices to filter out the blue tones. Many are free. My favourite is f.lux for the computer, and Apple and Android devices.
- Blue light filtering glasses are ideal, as they cover all blue light around you, including LED bulbs.

Limit daytime naps

It's tempting to have a nap if you're tired. If you must, set an alarm to wake you in 20–30 minutes. Any longer and you'll go into deep sleep, which can upset your body clock, leaving you wide awake when you get to bed.

Eat your way to sleep

Some foods can help with sleep, usually because they contain high levels of melatonin, tryptophan or magnesium.

Good food sources of melatonin include:

- Eggs.
- Fish.
- Wholegrain cereals, such as brown, black or red rice, wholegrain wheat, barley and oats. Don't overload on carbohydrate-rich foods just before bed, though, as they can keep you awake.
- Nuts and seeds, particularly almonds and pistachios. A handful makes a good evening snack but they're high in fat, so don't overindulge or you'll put on weight.

- Tart cherries and their juice.[16]

Tryptophan is needed to make niacin, which is used for serotonin production. Serotonin in turn produces melatonin. Tryptophan doesn't easily cross the blood brain barrier. It needs a small amount (about 30 **g**) of carbohydrates to carry it across.[17] So try a small amount of these tryptophan-rich foods with some wholegrain crackers or a slice of wholegrain bread as an evening snack:

- hummus
- eggs
- turkey or chicken
- low-fat cottage cheese.

Magnesium helps to relax muscles, which encourages sleep. Good sources are:

- Legumes, so hummus is a good choice again.
- Nuts, particularly cashews and almonds.
- Seeds such as chia, pumpkin and flax.
- Buckwheat, quinoa, oats, barley and wholegrain wheat.
- Salmon and mackerel.
- Bananas.
- Leafy greens, such as kale and spinach. Kale chips make a great evening snack.[18]

Essential oils

Essential oils are concentrated chemicals produced by plants for their protection. They smell wonderful and many have well-documented effects on the body. Several can help with sleep.

Essential oils can be used by inhalation and **topically**, including for massage. For those undergoing chemo, I'd suggest that you consult an aromatherapist who is familiar with anti-cancer drugs, their interactions and contraindications. For example, don't inhale peppermint oil if your chemo drug is 5-fluorouracil or if you have heart problems. If you're undergoing radiotherapy, I don't recommend using any essential oils for 2 days before radiotherapy, as many make skin photosensitive or irritate the skin regardless of light exposure.[19]

The body recognises essential oils as foreign and the liver removes them from your system. While you're receiving chemo, your liver is already coping with detoxifying the drugs and it's wise not to overload it. Inhalation is effective and puts less strain on the liver.

To inhale them, you can use either of the following:

- An inhaler, or aromastick. These tubes contain a cotton pad, onto which you put the oils. The tubes have a hole in the top through which you sniff the oils, similar to the inhalers available for a stuffy nose.
- A diffuser. There are various types of diffusers. Some use heat, which can change the properties of the oils and affect their healing characteristics. Others use evaporation, with a fan blowing through a filter containing the oils. These evaporate the various chemicals in the oils at different rates, which can also influence how well they work. I suggest using an ultrasonic diffuser. These create a fine mist using water and electronic frequencies. They're easily obtainable and won't break the bank.

Essential oils are available from most good health food stores. There are also a few multi-level marketing companies selling essential oils. Compare brands before committing yourself. If you plan to use them **topically**, ensure that they're skin safe. Many cheaper brands are only intended for diffusing.

It's thought that the chemicals in the oils dissolve in the nose and stimulate the olfactory (smell) receptors, which send a signal to the brain's olfactory centre. This is very close to the area that processes emotions and memories, which explains why smells can trigger memories and make you feel a certain way. Our emotions are governed by hormones and neurotransmitters, some of which can affect our sleep.

There's evidence that some oils are effective for sleep. In a cancer centre in the UK, aromasticks were given to 65 cancer patients who were having trouble sleeping. Of those, 64% showed an improvement after using them. The oils used were in 2 blends of the following:

- lavender (*Lavandula angustifolia*)
- bergamot (*Citrus bergamia*)
- sandalwood (*Santalum austrocaladonicum*)
- frankincense (*Boswellia carterii*)
- mandarin (*Citrus reticulata*).[20]

A **systematic review** found that essential oils had a positive effect on people with mild sleep disturbances. Lavender oil was the most studied.[21]

There is also some evidence for cedar (*Cedrus spp.*). Japanese researchers conducted a small trial, diffusing cedar oil when people were taking a daytime nap after a night's sleep. They found the participants fell asleep more quickly.[22]

Lemongrass essential oil (*Cymbopogan citratus*) also has some research behind it, showing it relieves anxiety and helps with falling asleep.[23]

Another study looked at the effects of the following oils on the sleep patterns of dementia patients: lavender (*Lavandula angustifolia*), a blend of lavender and sweet orange (*Citrus sinensis*), and another blend of Japanese cypress (*Chamaecyparis obtuse endl),* cypress (*Cupressus sempervirens*), Virginian cedarwood (*Juniperus virginiana*) and pine (*Pinus sylvestris*) These blends helped with sleep maintenance problems and awakening early.[24]

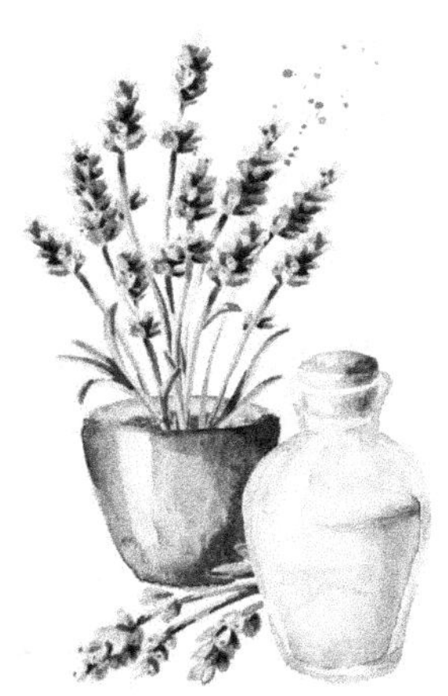

Intensive care patients inhaled a blend of lavender, Roman chamomile (*Chamaemelum nobile*) and neroli (*Citrus aurantium*) before and after undergoing an angioplasty with a stent being inserted. The mixture helped with anxiety and improved sleep quality.[25]

A comprehensive list of oils helpful for insomnia also included the following:

- angelica (*Angelica archangelica rad.*)
- ylang ylang (*Cananga odorata*)
- labdanum (*Cistus ladaniferus*)

- bergamot (*Citrus bergamia*)
- lemon (*Citrus limon*)
- mandarin (*Citrus reticulata*)
- cumin (*Cuminum cyminum*)
- juniper berry (*Juniperus communis fruct.*) (don't use if you have liver or kidney disease)
- may chang (*Litsea cubeba*)
- lemon balm (*Melissa officinalis*)
- myrtle (*Myrtus communis*)
- basil (*Ocimum basilicum*)
- sweet marjoram (*Origanum majorana*)
- ravensara (*Ravensara aromatica*)
- sweet thyme (*Thymus vulgaris ct. geraniol, ct. linalool*) (This is oestrogenic, so don't use it if you have a hormone sensitive cancer, don't use it **topically** on broken skin, and don't use it if you have thyroid disorders.)
- valerian (*Valeriana officinalis*).[26]

Cognitive behavioural therapy

Cognitive behavioural therapy for insomnia (CBT-I) is a psychology-based treatment offered by psychologists trained in treating insomnia and sleep disorders. It focuses on 5 main areas:

1. Cognitive therapy, which challenges the beliefs about sleep that insomniacs might have developed, such as thinking that a minimum of *x* hours sleep is needed to function.
2. Sleep hygiene, covered above.
3. Relaxation training, to learn strategies that can help if you

wake during the night and can't get back to sleep because you're anxious.

4. Stimulus control, which looks at sleep habits and identifies behaviour that might be affecting sleep.
5. Sleep restriction, which forces your body clock to adjust to the times you want to sleep. For example, if you're going to bed early and waking up during the night, you might be told to delay bedtime, making you tired so that you'll sleep longer.[27]

A **systematic review** and **meta-analysis** of CBT-I for 752 cancer patients showed an improvement of 15.5% in their sleep quality. They took an average of 22 minutes less to get to sleep and if they woke during the night their waking time was reduced by an average of 30 minutes. When they were followed up 6 months later, the results had persisted.[28]

Herbal medicines

You might be able to find combinations of these in your local health food stores or online. However, a naturopath or herbalist is able to individually prescribe for your particular needs, can supply superior quality, individual safety and will ensure dosages are correct.

Herbal remedies can be very helpful for some people, but everyone responds differently, so if one doesn't work try another. They're very often found in combination, which seems to increase their effectiveness.

If you're currently undergoing any sort of treatment, please check with your health practitioner before taking any herbs or supplements, as they can interact with drugs. You shouldn't drink alcohol with any of these herbs because they depress the central nervous system (CNS). Alcohol also depresses the CNS, so in combination it can be dangerous. Don't drive or operate machinery if you've taken any sleep medication, including herbs. Stop taking them at least 2 weeks before surgery, as they could increase the effects of anaesthetics.

Valerian (*Valerian officinalis*) and hops (*Humulus lupulus*)

Probably the best-known herb for sleep, valerian has a mild sedative effect. The most recent **systematic review** found most of the studies showed an effect on sleep quality, although some of them were poorly conducted.[29]

A **meta-analysis** summarised 18 studies and concluded that valerian is effective for improvement of insomnia.[30]

There's evidence that a valerian and hops combination work better together than valerian alone[31, 32] but check the contraindications for hops below.

Interactions, contraindications and side-effects

Unlike sleeping pills, valerian doesn't affect driving or operating machinery. Adverse reactions are very rare.[33]

There's no evidence that valerian interferes with chemo drugs[34] but check with your health practitioner.

Valerian may increase the effects of some drugs that are metabolised via a detoxification method called glucuronidation, so check with your pharmacist if you are taking any kind of medication.[35]

Valerian can increase the effects of opioid drugs[36], so avoid using it with these.

Avoid using valerian with tranquillizers or anti-convulsant medications.[37] It may also increase the sedative effects of alcohol.[35]

Hops have an effect similar to oestrogen and can make medications containing oestrogen less effective. Do not use hops if you have, or have had, a hormone-sensitive cancer.[38]

Hops can also interact with a number of medicines. If you're on medication, consult a health practitioner, who can check whether hops are safe for you.[38]

Don't use hops if you suffer from depression.[38]

Dosage

- 600 **mg** of valerian each night[33], and (provided it's not contraindicated)
- 120 **mg** of hops each night.[32]

Kava (*Piper methysticum*)

Kava has been used in the South Pacific since the 18th century to treat insomnia and anxiety. It increases gamma aminobutyric acid **(GABA)**, a neurotransmitter which calms the body. It also inhibits monoamine oxidase B (MAOB).[39] MAO inhibitors (MAOIs) are used to treat depression.

In 2003 (updated in 2010), a Cochrane report, considered to be the gold standard for reviews, conducted a **meta-analysis** on the effects of kava for anxiety. They found it was significantly better than **placebo.**[40]

Another study of the effects of kava on sleep disruption caused by anxiety found there was a significant positive effect on sleep quality and well-being.[41]

Interactions, contraindications and side-effects

There has been a lot of discussion about kava and liver toxicity. This happens very rarely: 0.3 cases per million daily doses. It has been shown to be safer than:

- benzodiazepines, including Valium and Ativan, which vary between 0.9 and 2.12 cases per million daily doses, or
- non-steroidal anti-inflammatory drugs (**NSAID**s), such as aspirin, where it occurs in 3—5% of cases.

In 2005, a review up to 2003 of all the cases of liver damage caused by kava reported worldwide totalled 83 cases. Of these, 3 were found to be possible or definite duplicates. Only a few of the others were shown to be directly attributable to kava. This happens with most drugs and is generally thought to be idiosyncratic.[42]

To minimise risk, look for a preparation made from an aqueous extract (prepared in water) rather than an alcoholic extract, which could contribute to liver problems. It's been suggested that aflatoxins (from fungi) in kava could be responsible for liver problems[43], so ensure you use kava from a reputable source. Please note the following:

- If you're currently undergoing chemo, I don't recommend using kava until treatment is complete and avoid it if your liver enzymes are raised.
- Don't use with tranquillisers or alcohol.[37]

- Don't take with medication that affects dopamine levels, either by increasing or decreasing them.[37]
- Avoid with MAOI drugs.[37]
- Kava could cause liver problems if you use a proton pump inhibitor, such as Nexium, Zoton or Somac.[37]
- Blood thinners, such as warfarin, could interact with kava.[37]

Dosage

Kava should always be taken under the supervision of a trained herbalist or naturopath.

Lemon balm (*Melissa officinalis*)

Lemon balm has been used for centuries to treat anxiety and insomnia. It's also antibacterial, anti-inflammatory and antioxidant. It makes a pleasant tea and is easy to grow, so you could consider planting some. You can also add it to cooking for a gentle lemon flavour.

It works by slowing down breakdown of **GABA**, so more circulates in the body.

In a trial on burns patients, who often suffer from depression, anxiety and insomnia, they were given lemon balm tea or black tea. After 20 days, the lemon balm tea drinkers showed significantly lower levels of anxiety, depression and insomnia than the black tea drinkers.[44]

A combination of lemon balm and valerian was used with children who suffered from insomnia and restlessness. Of those, nearly 81% reduced their insomnia from 'moderate/severe' to 'mild' or 'absent'. Restlessness was reduced in more than 70% of cases.[45]

In an open-label study (where the subjects knew what they were taking), after 15 days almost all those taking a lemon balm extract responded positively. Insomnia was resolved in 85% and anxiety disappeared in 70% of cases.[46]

As well as helping with anxiety and sleep, lemon balm can reduce bloating and wind, and reduce muscle spasms.

Interactions, contraindications and side-effects

Lemon balm can interfere with thyroid medications, although this has only been demonstrated in animals, using freeze-dried extracts[47], but avoid lemon balm if you are taking medication for Graves' disease (hyperthyroidism) or after thyroidectomy.

If you have glaucoma, avoid taking large doses of lemon balm, as it can interfere with glaucoma medication.[47]

It could lower blood sugar levels, so if you have diabetes monitor them carefully.[48]

In large doses, it can cause nausea, vomiting, abdominal pain, increased appetite, wheezing and dizziness.[48]

Dosage

If you are drinking lemon balm as a tea, have a cup several times a day. If you're making your own from fresh herb, use 1.5–4.5 **g** per day.[49]

A standardised preparation containing 80 **mg** of lemon balm and 160 **mg** of valerian, taken 2–3 times per day was shown to be safe, including in children.[49]

Passionflower (*Passiflora incarnata*)

Passionflower originates from Peru and has been used as a traditional sleep aid for many years. It works by increasing **GABA** levels, so it's also helpful for anxiety problems. Its effects are similar to benzodiazepines but without the addiction problems.

Passionflower tea has a significantly positive effect on sleep quality.[50]

Interactions, contraindications and side-effects

Don't use passionflower if you're using anti-convulsants, such as phenytoin.[51]

Avoid use with tricyclic antidepressants.[51]

If you're taking MAO inhibitors, passionflower can increase their effects and side-effects, which could be dangerous.[51]

Passionflower might increase blood clotting time, so avoid with blood thinners, such as warfarin.[51]

It may cause the uterus to contract, so don't use it if you're pregnant.[52, 53]

In high doses, it can cause confusion, dizziness, fainting, affect muscle coordination and inflame blood vessels.[52] It may affect the central nervous system, so stop using it 2 weeks before surgery.[52]

Dosage

Either: a cup of passionflower tea before bedtime[50],

Or in tablet form, 1.5–2.5 **g** per day.[54]

Melatonin

If none of the ideas above work for you, maybe you aren't producing enough melatonin. Some medications, such as beta blockers, suppress the body's production of melatonin. If so, you can use melatonin in tablet form. This is only available on prescription in Australia, but you can buy it over the counter in some other countries.

Melatonin helps with getting to sleep and with frequent waking, particularly if you use slow-release tablets. There's no danger of addiction. Melatonin is also an antioxidant, helping to mop up free radicals[55], and it has anti-cancer effects.[37]

Studies on insomnia sufferers show that melatonin significantly improves their ability to fall asleep.[56] Melatonin is metabolised by the body in about 30–50 minutes, so another study looked at prolonged-release melatonin. It found this form of melatonin helped the subjects get to sleep **and** stay asleep, as well as improving quality of life and morning alertness, suggesting that sleep was more restorative. Melatonin didn't increase risk of falls or cause amnesia, as traditional sleeping tablets can.[56]

Interactions, contraindications and side-effects

Melatonin stimulates the immune system, so it shouldn't be taken by anyone with active blood cancer or active graft vs host disease (GVHD).[57]

Avoid melatonin if you have an autoimmune disease, such as lupus, rheumatoid arthritis, Sjögrens syndrome, psoriasis or severe allergies.[57]

Melatonin could theoretically reduce the effects of corticosteroids, such as dexamethasone or prednisone.[37]

Melatonin can inhibit ovulation, so avoid it if you're trying to conceive.[37]

Melatonin suppresses insulin production, so it's best avoided if you have diabetes or are glucose intolerant.[58]

About 30% of the population have a **genetic mutation** that increases sensitivity to melatonin. To avoid this sensitivity, start with low doses of melatonin (0.3—0.5 **mg**) and avoid eating soon after you've taken it.[58]

Melatonin may exacerbate seasonal affective disorder (SAD), which is usually treated with phototherapy. Melatonin works against this and so it could increase depression in SAD.[59]

There's a theoretical risk of bleeding if you take melatonin with anticoagulants, such as warfarin.[37]

If you're taking methoxamine, clonidine or other drugs designed to increase blood pressure, melatonin might reduce their effectiveness. Advise your doctor and ask to be monitored carefully.[37]

Melatonin supplements could increase inflammation in those suffering from nocturnal asthma.[37]

Melatonin crosses the placenta and its effects on a foetus aren't known, so it's best avoided in pregnancy.[37]

Melatonin has some anti-oestrogenic action, so it could reduce the effectiveness of hormone replacement therapy (HRT) drugs or the contraceptive pill.[37]

Too much melatonin can cause the following side-effects:

- headaches
- dizziness
- nausea
- diarrhoea
- anxiety or irritability
- joint pain
- nightmares or extremely vivid dreams.[60]

Cyclosporine can cause kidney damage, which melatonin can safely and effectively reduce.[37]

Triptorelin is a hormone sometimes used for hormone-sensitive cancers in men and pre-menopausal women. Melatonin increases its effectiveness.[37]

If you're on calcium channel blockers such as verapamil, for hyperparathyroidism, melatonin can safely help reduce insomnia related to it.[37]

Melatonin makes tamoxifen more effective and reduces its side-effects.[37].

At higher doses, melatonin increases the effectiveness of Interleukin-2, a drug sometimes used in chemo, and reduces or prevents the side-effects associated with it.[37]

If you're taking non-steroidal anti-inflammatory drugs (**NSAID**s), including aspirin, melatonin can help with the sleep disturbances you may have and won't interfere with the drug's action.[37]

Dosage

0.3–6.0 **mg** per night, half an hour before bedtime for sleep issues.[37] To avoid unpleasant side-effects, start on a low dose and increase it until your sleep problems disappear.

Most studies have used 10–20 **mg** per day, but up to 40 **mg** per day is appropriate for cancer therapy.[37]

References

1. Bollu P. Normal Sleep, Sleep Physiology, and Sleep Deprivation: Normal Sleep in Adults, Infants, and the Elderly, Sleep Physiology, Circadian Rhythms That Influence Sleep. Medscape. https://emedicine.medscape.com/article/1188226-overview#a1. Published 2019. Accessed August 23, 2021.
2. American Sleep Association. What is Sleep & Why is It Important for Health? | American Sleep Association. American Sleep Association. https://www.sleepassociation.org/about-sleep/what-is-sleep/. Accessed August 23, 2021.
3. Sigurdardottir L, Valdimarsdottir U, Fall K et al. Circadian Disruption, Sleep Loss, and Prostate Cancer Risk: A Systematic Review of Epidemiologic Studies: Table 1. *Cancer Epidemiology Biomarkers & Prevention*. 2012;21(7):1002-1011. doi:10.1158/1055-9965.epi-12-0116
4. National Heart, Lung and Blood Institute. Sleep Deprivation and Deficiency | NHLBI, NIH. National Heart, Lung and Blood Institute. https://www.nhlbi.nih.gov/health-topics/sleep-deprivation-and-deficiency. Accessed August 23, 2021.
5. Jiao L, Duan Z, Sangi-Haghpeykar H, Hale L, White D, El-Serag H. Sleep duration and incidence of colorectal cancer in postmenopausal women. *Br J Cancer*. 2013;108(1):213-221. doi:10.1038/bjc.2012.561
6. Royse K, El-Serag H, Chen L et al. Sleep Duration and Risk of Liver Cancer in Postmenopausal Women: The Women's Health Initiative Study. *J Womens Health*. 2017;26(12):1270-1277. doi:10.1089/jwh.2017.6412
7. Luo J, Sands M, Wactawski-Wende J, Song Y, Margolis K. Sleep Disturbance and Incidence of Thyroid Cancer in Postmenopausal Women The Women's Health Initiative. *Am J Epidemiol*. 2013;177(1):42-49. doi:10.1093/aje/kws193
8. Erren T, Falaturi P, Morfeld P, Knauth P, Reiter R, Piekarski C. Shift Work and Cancer. *Deutsches Aerzteblatt Online*. 2010;107(38):657-662. doi:10.3238/arztebl.2010.0657
9. Jones M, Schoemaker M, McFadden E, Wright L, Johns L, Swerdlow A. Night shift work and risk of breast cancer in women: the Generations Study cohort. *Br J Cancer*. 2019;121(2):172-179. doi:10.1038/s41416-019-0485-7
10. Ward E, Germolec D, Kogevinas M et al. Carcinogenicity of night shift work. *The Lancet Oncology*. 2019;20(8):1058-1059. doi:10.1016/s1470-2045(19)30455-3
11. Trudel-Fitzgerald C, Zhou E, Poole E et al. Sleep and survival among women with breast cancer: 30 years of follow-up within the Nurses' Health Study. *Br J Cancer*. 2017;116(9):1239-1246. doi:10.1038/bjc.2017.8510.1038/bjc.2017.85
12. Stanford University Medical Center. Stanford Research Builds Link Between Sleep, Cancer Progression. Science Daily. https://www.sciencedaily.com/releases/2003/10/031001060734.htm. Published 2003. Accessed August 23, 2021.

13. Owens R, Gold K, Gozal D et al. Sleep and Breathing ... and Cancer?. *Cancer Prevention Research*. 2016;9(11):821-827. doi:10.1158/1940-6207.capr-16-0092

14. Palesh O, Roscoe J, Mustian K et al. Prevalence, Demographics, and Psychological Associations of Sleep Disruption in Patients With Cancer: University of Rochester Cancer Center–Community Clinical Oncology Program. *Journal of Clinical Oncology*. 2010;28(2):292-298. doi:10.1200/jco.2009.22.5011

15. Palesh O, Aldridge-Gerry A, Ulusakarya A, Ortiz-Tudela E, Capuron L, Innominato P. Sleep Disruption in Breast Cancer Patients and Survivors. *Journal of the National Comprehensive Cancer Ne2rk*. 2013;11(12):1523-1530. doi:10.6004/jnccn.2013.0179

16. Meng X, Li Y, Li S et al. Dietary Sources and Bioactivities of Melatonin. *Nutrients*. 2017;9(4):367. doi:10.3390/nu9040367

17. Zamosky L. The Truth About Tryptophan. WebMD. https://www.webmd.com/food-recipes/features/the-truth-about-tryptophan. Published 2009. Accessed August 23, 2021.

18. Spritzler F. 10 Magnesium-Rich Foods That Are Super Healthy. Healthline. https://www.healthline.com/nutrition/10-foods-high-in-magnesium. Published 2018. Accessed August 23, 2021.

19. Cutler N. What You Need to Know About Essential Oils and Cancer Treatment. Institute for Integrative Healthcare. https://www.integrativehealthcare.org/mt/essential-oils-and-cancer-treatment/. Published 2009. Accessed August 23, 2021.

20. Dyer J, Cleary L, McNeill S, Ragsdale-Lowe M, Osland C. The use of aromasticks to help with sleep problems: A patient experience survey. *Complement Ther Clin Pract*. 2016;22:51-58. doi:10.1016/j.ctcp.2015.12.006

21. Lillehei A, Halcon L. A Systematic Review of the Effect of Inhaled Essential Oils on Sleep. *The Journal of Alternative and Complementary Medicine*. 2014;20(6):441-451. doi:10.1089/acm.2013.0311

22. Sano A, Sei H, Seno H, Morita Y, Moritoki H. Influence of cedar essence on spontaneous activity and sleep of rats and human daytime nap. *Psychiatry Clin Neurosci*. 2008;52(2):133-135. doi:10.1111/j.1440-1819.1998.tb00991.x

23. Costa C, Kohn D, de Lima V, Gargano A, Flório J, Costa M. The **GABA**ergic system contributes to the anxiolytic-like effect of essential oil from Cymbopogon citratus (lemongrass). *J Ethnopharmacol*. 2011;137(1):828-836. doi:10.1016/j.jep.2011.07.003

24. Takeda A, Watanuki E, Koyama S. Effects of Inhalation Aromatherapy on Symptoms of Sleep Disturbance in the Elderly with Dementia. *Evidence-Based Complementary and Alternative Medicine*. 2017;2017:1-7. doi:10.1155/2017/1902807

25. Cho M, Min E, Hur M, Lee M. Effects of Aromatherapy on the Anxiety, Vital Signs, and Sleep Quality of Percutaneous Coronary Intervention Patients in Intensive Care Units. *Evidence-Based Complementary and Alternative Medicine*. 2013;2013:1-6. doi:10.1155/2013/381381

26. Ali B, Al-Wabel N, Shams S, Ahamad A, Khan S, Anwar F. Essential oils used in aromatherapy: A systemic review. *Asian Pac J Trop Biomed*. 2015;5(8):601-611. doi:10.1016/j.apjtb.2015.05.007

27. Cunnington D. Cognitive behavioural therapy for insomnia. SleepHub. http://sleephub.com.au/cognitive-behavioural-therapy-for-insomnia/. Published 2016. Accessed August 23, 2021.

28. Johnson J, Rash J, Campbell T et al. A systematic review and meta-analysis of randomized controlled trials of cognitive behavior therapy for insomnia (CBT-I) in cancer survivors. *Sleep Med Rev.* 2016;27:20-28. doi:10.1016/j.smrv.2015.07.001

29. Salter S, Brownie S. Treating primary insomnia, The efficacy of valerian and hops. *Aust Fam Physician.* 2010;39(6):433-437. https://pubmed.ncbi.nlm.nih.gov/20628685/. Accessed August 23, 2021.

30. Fernández-San-Martín M, Masa-Font R, Palacios-Soler L, Sancho-Gómez P, Calbó-Caldentey C, Flores-Mateo G. Effectiveness of Valerian on insomnia: A meta-analysis of randomized placebo-controlled trials. *Sleep Med.* 2010;11(6):505-511. doi:10.1016/j.sleep.2009.12.009

31. Morin C, Koetter U, Bastien C, Ware J, Wooten V. Valerian-Hops Combination and Diphenhydramine for Treating Insomnia: A Randomized Placebo-Controlled Clinical Trial. *Sleep.* 2005;28(11):1465-1471. doi:10.1093/sleep/28.11.1465

32. Koetter U, Schrader E, Käufeler R, Brattström A. A randomized, double blind, placebo-controlled, prospective clinical study to demonstrate clinical efficacy of a fixed valerian hops extract combination (Ze 91019) in patients suffering from non-organic sleep disorder. *Phytotherapy Research.* 2007;21(9):847-851. doi:10.1002/ptr.2167

33. Kelber O, Nieber K, Kraft K. Valerian: No Evidence for Clinically Relevant Interactions. *Evidence-Based Complementary and Alternative Medicine.* 2014;2014:879396. doi:10.1155/2014/879396

34. Block K, Gyllenhaal C, Mead M. Safety and Efficacy of Herbal Sedatives in Cancer Care. *Integr Cancer Ther.* 2004;3(2):128-148. doi:10.1177/1534735404265003

35. Natural Medicines Database. Natural Medicines Database. Natural Medicines Database. https://naturalmedicines.therapeuticresearch.com/#. Published 2021. Accessed August 23, 2021.

36. Abebe W. Herbal medication: potential for adverse interactions with analgesic drugs. *J Clin Pharm Ther.* 2002;27(6):391-401. doi:10.1046/j.1365-2710.2002.00444.x

37. Stargrove m, Treasure J, Mckee D. *Herb, Drug And Nutrient Interactions.* St Louis, Mo: Mosby/Elsevier; 2008.

38. eMedicineHealth. Hops: Uses, Side Effects, Dose, Health Benefits, Precautions & Warnings. eMedicineHealth. https://www.emedicinehealth.com/hops/vitamins-supplements.htm. Published 2021. Accessed August 23, 2021.

39. Bone K, Mills S. *Principles And Practice Of Phytotherapy.* Edinburgh: Churchill Livingstone; 2013.

40. Pittler M, Ernst E. Kava extract versus placebo for treating anxiety. *Cochrane Database of Systematic Reviews.* 2003;1:1465-1485. doi:10.1002/14651858.cd003383

41. Lehrl S. Clinical efficacy of kava extract WS® 1490 in sleep disturbances associated with anxiety disorders Results of a multicenter, randomized, placebo-controlled, double-blind clinical trial. *J Affect Disord.* 2004;78(2):101-110. doi:10.1016/s0165-0327(02)00238-0

42. Mills S, Bone K. *The Essential Guide To Herbal Safety.* St. Louis, Mo.: Elsevier Churchill Livingstone; 2005.

43. Teschke R, Sarris J, Schweitzer I. Kava hepatotoxicity in traditional and modern use: the presumed Pacific kava paradox hypothesis revisited. *Br J Clin Pharmacol*. 2012;73(2):170-174. doi:10.1111/j.1365-2125.2011.04070.x

44. Chehroudi S, Fatemi M, Saberi M, Salehi S, Akbari H, Samimi R. Effects of Melissa officinalis L. on Reducing Stress, Alleviating Anxiety Disorders, Depression, and Insomnia, and Increasing Total Antioxidants in Burn Patients. *Trauma Mon*. 2016;Inpress(Inpress). doi:10.5812/traumamon.33630

45. Müller S, Klement S. A combination of valerian and lemon balm is effective in the treatment of restlessness and dyssomnia in children. *Phytomedicine*. 2006;13(6):383-387. doi:10.1016/j.phymed.2006.01.013

46. Cases J, Ibarra A, Feuillère N, Roller M, Sukkar S. Pilot trial of Melissa officinalis L. leaf extract in the treatment of volunteers suffering from mild-to-moderate anxiety disorders and sleep disturbances. *Med J Nutrition Metab*. 2011;4(3):211-218. doi:10.1007/s12349-010-0045-4

47. Ulbricht C, Brendler T, Gruenwald J et al. Lemon balm (Melissa officinalis L.): an evidence-based systematic review by the Natural Standard Research Collaboration. *J Herb Pharmacother*. 2005;5(4):71-114. https://pubmed.ncbi.nlm.nih.gov/16635970/. Accessed August 23, 2021.

48. WebMD. Lemon Balm: Overview, Uses, Side Effects, Precautions, Interactions, Dosing and Reviews. WebMD. https://www.webmd.com/vitamins/ai/ingredientmono-437/lemon-balm. Published 2020. Accessed August 23, 2021.

49. Drugs.com. Lemon Balm Uses, Benefits & Dosage - Drugs.com Herbal Database. Drugs.com. https://www.drugs.com/npp/lemon-balm.html. Published 2021. Accessed August 23, 2021.

50. Ngan A, Conduit R. A Double-blind, Placebo-controlled Investigation of the Effects of Passiflora incarnata (Passionflower) Herbal Tea on Subjective Sleep Quality. *Phytotherapy Research*. 2011;25(8):1153-1159. doi:10.1002/ptr.3400

51. Mount Sinai. Passionflower Information | Mount Sinai - New York. Mount Sinai. https://www.mountsinai.org/health-library/herb/passionflower. Published 2021. Accessed August 23, 2021.

52. WebMD. Passionflower: Overview, Uses, Side Effects, Precautions, Interactions, Dosing and Reviews. Webmd.com. https://www.webmd.com/vitamins/ai/ingredientmono-871/passionflower. Published 2021. Accessed August 23, 2021.

53. Rokhtabnak F, Ghodraty M, Kholdebarin A et al. Comparing the Effect of Preoperative Administration of Melatonin and Passiflora incarnata on Postoperative Cognitive Disorders in Adult Patients Undergoing Elective Surgery. *Anesth Pain Med*. 2016;7(1):e41238. doi:10.5812/aapm.41238

54. Bone K. *The Ultimate Herbal Compendium*. Warwick: Phytotherapy Press; 2007.

55. Xie Z, Chen F, Li W et al. A review of sleep disorders and melatonin. *Neurol Res*. 2017;39(6):559-565. doi:10.1080/01616412.2017.1315864

56. Zisapel N. New perspectives on the role of melatonin in human sleep, circadian rhythms and their regulation. *Br J Pharmacol*. 2018;175(16):3190-3199. doi:10.1111/bph.14116

57. Cox L. What Is Melatonin?. Live Science. https://www.livescience.com/42066-melatonin-supplement-facts.html. Published 2013. Accessed August 23, 2021.

58. Robards G. Research Reveals a Surprising Link Between Melatonin and Type 2 Diabetes. humanOS. https://blog.humanos.me/research-reveals-an-odd-connection-between-melatonin-and-type-2-diabetes/. Published 2016. Accessed August 23, 2021.

59. Rosenthal N, Sack D, Jacobsen F et al. Melatonin in seasonal affective disorder and phototherapy. *J Neural Transm Suppl*. 1986;21:257-267. https://pubmed.ncbi.nlm.nih.gov/3462335/. Accessed August 23, 2021.

60. Carter A. Melatonin Overdose. Healthline. https://www.healthline.com/health/melatonin-overdose. Published 2019. Accessed August 23, 2021.

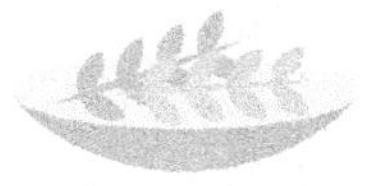

Chapter 6

Stop poisoning yourself

'Deadly poisons are concealed
under sweet honey.'
– Ovid

You probably think that you're not poisoning yourself, but the sad truth is that we're exposed to an enormous number of toxic substances these days. Chapter 2 deals with the toxins you eat. Other areas you need to consider to help your body and maximise your odds of survival are:

- personal care products
- cleaning products
- home furnishings
- garden chemicals
- how you use technology.

All of these things can stress the body, causing inflammatory changes that can result in cancer or prevent your body healing. In many cases, you won't need to spend a lot to avoid the toxins. For some, there are alternatives that do just as good a job and cost significantly less. Some you can't avoid, as they really are everywhere, but using the advice here you might be able to reduce their risk.

First we'll discuss the problem chemicals that are linked to cancer, but bear in mind that many others can cause irritation. Irritation can lead to inflammatory changes, which in turn can trigger cancers.[1] Secondly we'll look at the products that contain these problem chemicals and offer alternatives.

You're only likely to come across certain chemicals if you work with them. Those aren't covered here. Your employer should tell you about any your work involves and advise on how to reduce your risk.

To check out other chemicals in the products you use, check the database Skin Deep that is produced by the Environmental Working Group (**EWG**) at: https://www.ewg.org/skindeep/. Another useful Australian resource for sourcing safe, environmentally friendly products of all sorts is the website of Good Environmental Choice Australia (GECA) at: www.geca.eco.

Aluminium and its salts

Aluminium, together with its salts, is classified as a toxic metal. It's known to be genotoxic: it damages **DNA** molecules, which can cause **mutations** and lead to cancer development.[2]

Arsenic

Arsenic is a heavy metal that's toxic to humans. It comes in both inorganic and organic forms, and inorganic arsenic and its compounds are classified as '**carcinogenic** to humans' by the **IARC**. They can cause cancers of the bladder, lung and skin. They're also linked to cancers of the liver, prostate gland and kidney. Two organic arsenic compounds have also been classified by **IARC** as 'possibly **carcinogenic** to humans': dimethylarsinic acid (DMA, also known as cacodylic acid) and monomethylarsinic acid (MMA).[3] Arsenic doesn't cause **DNA mutations** directly, but it affects the **DNA** repair mechanism that constantly happens.[4] Arsenic consumption from food was covered in Chapter 2, but there are other sources of it, which are covered in this chapter.

Asbestos

Asbestos was known to be **carcinogenic** since the beginning of the 20th century, causing lung cancer, mesothelioma, laryngeal and ovarian cancers. The **WHO**, **IARC** and the Environmental Protection Agency (**EPA**) have all classified it as a known **carcinogen.**[5] Although it hasn't been commonly used in developed countries since the 1980s, its use in developing countries is increasing.[5] Even in developed countries, older properties may have asbestos insulating their roof space, and lining the walls in wet areas, like the bathroom and laundry. If you're going into a roof space or renovating your wet areas, you should take extreme precautions, such as using gloves, face mask and protective clothing, to ensure minimal exposure. This applies particularly if you are younger, as asbestos-related diseases generally take about 30 years to develop. Provided that the asbestos in wet areas and other sheeting is undisturbed, it normally poses little risk, though.

Benzene

We usually think of benzene in connection with vehicle emissions and burning coal, but it's also found in dyes and solvents for plastics, resins and waxes. Benzene can cause headaches, drowsiness, dizziness, irritations of the throat, eyes and skin, anaemia, birth defects, and an increase in leukaemia incidence. The **EPA** classifies benzene as a 'known human **carcinogen** for all routes of exposure'.[6]

Boric acid, borax and borates

Boric acid and its salts are used for their antimicrobial properties and pH (acid/base) buffering, but they're easily absorbed through the skin. They're hormone disruptors, particularly for men. Men involved in boric acid production have low sperm counts and low libido. High doses in animals cause damage to the testicles.[7] In Australia, the European Union and Canada, products containing boric acid or borates must display a notice saying they aren't suitable for children under 3, or for use on broken or irritated skin.

Butylated hydroxyanisole (BHA)

BHA is used as a preservative but the National Toxicology Program and the California Environmental Protection Agency have classified it as a 'possible human **carcinogen**' and the **WHO** and **IARC** state that there is limited evidence of **carcinogenicity.**[84] It's also classified as a human endocrine disruptor by the European Commission on Endocrine Disruption.

Cadmium

Cadmium is a heavy metal that can potentially cause cancer. The IARC classified it as a Group one human carcinogen in 2005, following a systematic review[8] showing an association with renal cancer. It's a potent non-steroidal oestrogen, causing an increase in the weight of the uterus and the size of the mammary glands in rats.[8] Rats injected with cadmium chloride developed prostate cancer and high doses resulted in testicular cancers.[8] It's thought cadmium is related to the high incidence of lung cancer in smokers.[8]

Chlorine bleach

Chlorine bleach is made from sodium hypochlorite with extra sodium hydroxide to make it more alkaline and therefore a more effective cleaner. The sodium hypochlorite is what is responsible for its bleaching and antibacterial effects.

Bleach is a skin irritant and very dangerous if swallowed, but when it's mixed with other chemicals it becomes highly toxic. For example, adding anything acidic to it releases chlorine gas, which is very dangerous, causing build-up of fluid in the lungs that can lead to respiratory failure and death. Ammonia too, is highly dangerous if mixed with bleach, as it releases chloramines, which can have similar effects.

On its own, bleach isn't classified by the **IARC** as **carcinogenic** to humans, as there's insufficient evidence.[9] When mixed with fragrances or surfactants, though, it produces volatile organic compounds (**VOCs**), particularly chloroform and carbon tetrachloride.[10] The **EPA** classifies chloroform as a probable human **carcinogen.**[11] The **IARC** classifies carbon tetrachloride as a possible human **carcinogen** and the **EPA** classifies it as a probable human **carcinogen.**[12]

Coal tar

Coal tar and its ingredients, including diaminobenzene, aminophenol and phenylenediamine, are derived from coal processing. They're classified as **carcinogenic** in humans by the **IARC** and the **NTP.** They're still used in Australia and some other countries in shampoos for dandruff and psoriasis, and in dark hair dyes. They contain a warning that they shouldn't be used in children under 2 and that prolonged use should be avoided. I recommend avoiding them. There are safer options available.

Dihydroxyacetone (DHA)

Dihydroxyacetone (sometimes shortened to DHA but not to be confused with the essential fatty acid docosahexaenoic acid in fish oils) is used in self-tanning lotions. It is a sugar that reacts with proteins in the skin, temporarily turning it brown. This reaction produces advanced glycation end-products (**AGEs**). Applied **topically** at levels of 5% and above, it increases sunlight damage for 24 hours. Until recently, it was thought that dihydroxyacetone only affected the outer, dead layer of skin. But the US Food and Drug Administration (**FDA**) has released a report suggesting that it's absorbed into the skin itself. In living cells, **AGEs** can damage **DNA**, causing **mutations** and potentially cancers.[13]

Ethanolamines

This family of chemicals includes monoethanolamine (**MEA**), diethanolamine (**DEA**) and triethanolamine (**TEA**), amongst others. They're strongly alkaline and are used in personal care products to adjust pH, and as emulsifiers. They can react with certain preservatives to produce various nitrosamines, which the **IARC** classifies as either possible or probable **carcinogens**. The European Commission has banned **DEA**.[14] The **EWG** considers the evidence of contamination is fair for **TEA** with nitrosamines.[15]

Flame retardants

There are a number of different types of flame retardants, some of which aren't used in new products because they have been found to be **carcinogenic**. Sadly those people who still have older products remain exposed to them and the effects persist for a long time. Some of the replacement products are also **carcinogenic**. They can also damage your nervous and reproductive systems. If you have high levels of them in your household dust, you'll also have high levels in your urine, showing they're absorbed by the body. It also suggests our homes are the main source of exposure.

Fire fighters are subjected to high levels from their protective clothing. According to the President of the San Francisco Firefighters Cancer Prevention Foundation, fire retardants aren't even very effective at protecting people or property from fire.[16]

A recent study found exposure to fire retardants is associated with a higher incidence and severity of a type of thyroid cancer[17], but another small study found no association.[18] Prolonged exposure to polybrominated diphenyl ethers (PBDE), a type of flame retardant which has been phased out in recent years but is still widespread, can act as a trigger for thyroid cancer.[19] So the jury is still out on some fire retardants, but the older types, many of which are still found in homes today, may be dangerous to your health.

Formaldehyde

Formaldehyde and products that release it are generally used as preservatives and antiseptics. It's a fairly common chemical and low levels are often found in the air, both indoors and outdoors. It's been classified as a known **carcinogen** by the **NTP** and the **IARC**, as a probable human **carcinogen** by the **EPA**, and researchers at the US National Cancer Institute (**NCI**) have concluded that it causes leukaemia, especially myeloid leukaemia, in humans.[20]

Formaldehyde is known by other names including:

- formic aldehyde
- formalin
- methanal
- methanediol
- methylene glycol
- methyl aldehyde
- methylene oxide.

Some preservatives that can release formaldehyde include:

- 2-bromo-2-nitropropane-1,3-diol
- 5-bromo-5-nitro-1,3-dioxane
- benzylhemiformal

- 1,3-dimethylol-5,5-dimethylhydantoin (or DMDM hydantoin)
- imidazolidinyl urea
- diazolidinyl urea
- quaternium-15
- sodium hydroxymethylglycinate.

It's widely used in the manufacture of particleboard. The half-life of formaldehyde from particleboard is about a year, but long-term studies have shown that there's significant outgassing from it for at least 5 years, possibly longer.[21]

Lauryl and laureth sulphates

Lauryl and laureth sulphates, and cocamide **DEA** are used as foaming agents and cleansers because they're emulsifiers. But they're all known for irritating the skin. In some countries, including Australia, you'll see labels saying that a product is SLS free. That's sodium lauryl sulphate. But ammonium lauryl sulphate is just as bad. To make them less irritating, manufacturers often use ethylene oxide to create sodium (or ammonium) laureth sulphate. The compound 1,4-dioxane is produced in the process, which penetrates the skin quite easily. This compound is classified as a 'probable human **carcinogen**' by the **IARC** and 'reasonably anticipated to be a human **carcinogen**' by the **NTP**.[22] Other common ingredients that may be contaminated by 1,4-dioxane include:

- polyethylene glycol (PEG) compounds
- chemicals including the word 'ceteareth'
- chemicals including the word 'oleth'
- chemicals including the word 'xynol'.

Of the products in the Skin Deep database, 22% could be contaminated with 1,4-dioxane.

Mineral oils

Mineral oils are derived from petroleum. In laboratory testing petroleum derivatives were found to disrupt hormones.[23] They also accumulate in the human body.[24]

The **EWG** found that 80% of cosmetics contain one or more of the recognised impurities in mineral oils that are connected to cancer and other health problems. One of them is 1,4-dioxane. They found 34% of all body lotions, 57% of all baby soaps, 36% of facial moisturisers and 33% of eye creams contained it, along with a host of other products.

Besides 1,4-dioxane, there are over 2 dozen other **carcinogenic** impurities in mineral oils. **EWG** surveyed 2,300 people in 2004 to find out which personal care products they used. They found one in 5 adults was potentially exposed to all of the top 7 **carcinogenic** impurities every day, and 94% of all women and 69% of all men were exposed to hydroquinone, the most common one.[25] You'll find mineral oil listed in the ingredients in a number of ways, including:

- mineral oil
- petrolatum
- paraffin oil
- liquid paraffin
- petroleum jelly.

Mineral oils have been connected with non-melanoma skin cancers[26], although this relates to occupational exposure.

Oxybenzone

Oxybenzone is commonly found in sunscreens, which are important for the prevention of skin cancers (although see my warning in Chapter 2 under vitamin D). Laboratory tests by the **EWG** show oxybenzone is absorbed substantially through the skin. It disrupts hormones because it's mildly oestrogenic and strongly anti-androgenic (in other words, it reduces testosterone). This is especially worrying in children.[27] **EWG** has been supported by the **FDA** and they're currently proposing significant changes to how sunscreen safety is evaluated.[27]

Oxybenzone causes a high percentage of contact dermatitis cases when used in sunlight – rather odd for a sunscreen.[28] It has a higher rate of contact dermatitis than para-aminobenzoic acid (PABA)[28], which was virtually outlawed in the 1980s because of contact dermatitis issues.[29]

Oxybenzone isn't as effective as zinc oxide or titanium oxide at blocking UVA rays.[28] Given that chemo and radiation predispose you to all types of cancers, including skin cancers, in my view this could make its use dangerous for cancer patients and survivors. It also damages our marine environment, affects fish reproductive systems and promotes coral bleaching. In 2017, Hawaii passed legislation designed to ban its use, or at least put warnings on packaging about its ability to disrupt marine life.[28]

Parabens

Parabens are used as preservatives because they're antimicrobial, but they're also oestrogenic and oestrogen is known to be central to the development, growth and progression of breast cancers. Tissue samples from mastectomies performed on women with breast cancer showed 99% of them contained parabens. Some of the women had never used underarm cosmetics. The researchers suggested that low concentrations of personal products absorbed through the skin of their breasts over long periods may have contributed to their cancers.[30]

It's believed that everyone is exposed to parabens, in food as well as personal care products. Although we can detoxify parabens from the body through our kidneys, constant exposure to them means they're likely to build up in the body. One study found that minute amounts are enough to stimulate breast cancer growth.[31] Another study suggests that environmental oestrogen sources could explain hormonal therapy failure in some breast cancer patients.[32]

Perfluorooctanoic acid (PFOA)

PFOA is a synthetic organic acid that has a wide range of uses, including:

- non-stick surfaces like Teflon®
- stain and water repellents
- cosmetics, shampoo and toothpaste
- waxes and polishes
- flame repellents
- electronics

- paints, sealants and varnishes
- surfactants, emulsifiers and lubricants
- food containers
- pesticides
- foams used in firefighting
- leather and textiles, such as Gore-Tex®
- cleaning products
- plumbing tape.[33]

PFOA's average half-life in the human body is 2.3 years, and because of its wide range of uses, you're likely to be continually exposed to it. This is a huge problem, as it's been shown to cause kidney and liver damage, developmental problems, effects on the immune system, and cancer.[33]

Pesticides

The dangers of pesticides, which include insecticides and herbicides, have been highlighted regularly but many people are still exposed to them fairly often, either through their work, in the garden or to kill insects at home. A group of doctors, oncologists and **epidemiologists** in Canada conducted a **systematic review** of the research linking pesticides to cancer between 1992 and 2003. In the 83 studies they used, they found positive associations between pesticide exposure and 9 different cancers: breast, lung, pancreas, leukaemia, non-Hodgkin lymphoma, prostate, brain, kidney and stomach. Most of the studies looked at use of multiple pesticides, and the dose determined the level of risk. They concluded that there was sufficient evidence to recommend that everyone reduce exposure to pesticides, especially children and pregnant women.[34] Another review looked at chronic exposure to pesticides. It found sufficient evidence to link many pesticides with non-Hodgkin lymphoma, Hodgkin disease, leukaemia, multiple myeloma, soft tissue sarcoma, and cancers of the prostate, pancreas, lung, ovary, breast, testes, liver, kidney, rectum, brain, stomach and endometrium.[35]

Phthalates

Phthalates are often found in fragrance and perfume (also known as 'parfum'). They disrupt hormones in both women and men, which can cause breast cancer[36] and prostate cancer.[37] They're easy to identify on a product label. If the label lists 'fragrance' or 'perfume', the product almost certainly contains phthalates.

Polycyclic aromatic hydrocarbons (PAH)

PAHs are chemical pollutants commonly found in the environment. There are a number of different types, some of which are used to make certain medicines, plastics, dyes and pesticides. The **IARC** classified one of them as a human **carcinogen**, and several others as probable or possible human **carcinogens**. Testing in animals and population studies shows they're linked with bladder, lung and skin cancers.[38]

Radon

Radon is a radioactive gas that occurs naturally. It comes from the radioactive decay of radium, which is contained in rocks and soil in small amounts. You can't see, smell or taste it. As it decays, it releases radioactive particles, which can damage lung tissue if they're breathed in. That damage can lead to lung cancer, and radon is the second most common cause after smoking, with 3–20% of lung cancer deaths associated with it.[39]

The Australian Radiation Protection and Nuclear Safety Agency (ARPANSA) conducted a nationwide survey of radon in homes. They found the levels of radon in Australia are generally fairly low, about a quarter of the levels worldwide. However, about one in a thousand homes might have high levels of radon. This is more likely in homes built on concrete slabs with brick walls than in timber homes or those built on stumps, and the level of home ventilation also affects radon levels. ARPANSA recommends that homes should contain less than 200 Becquerels per square metre and workplaces less than 1,000 Becquerels per square metre. To check the levels in your home, you can hire a radon meter from ARPANSA[40] at: https://www.arpansa.gov.au/our-services/equipment-hire.

The New Zealand Ministry of Health conducted a survey in 1986–87 and found that radon levels in New Zealand are about the same as elsewhere in the world with no evidence of 'hot spots'.[41]

In the United States, though, about one in 15 homes is estimated to have high radon levels and it's estimated to cause about 21,000 lung cancer deaths per year. The **EPA** recommends that everyone has their home tested, which is easy, quick and relatively inexpensive. People should take remedial action if the levels are higher than 4 picocuries per **litre** (one Becquerel is equivalent to about 27 picocuries). Radon reduction systems are effective and not too expensive. Some can reduce levels by up to 99%.[42]

If you're resident elsewhere, a 2007 **WHO** report can help you identify whether radon is a problem and whether there's an action program available, but the list isn't exhaustive.[43]

Roundup

Roundup is an organophosphorus herbicide containing glyphosate. At very low concentrations, glyphosate has been classified as safe to use. But Roundup also has chemicals designed to increase glyphosate's absorption by about 100-fold, both in plants and humans. At those levels, glyphosate is very dangerous and the **IARC** has classified Roundup as a probable **carcinogen**. The European Food Safety Agency (EFSA) doesn't, probably because it evaluates individual ingredients rather than the whole formula. Roundup disrupts hormones, even though glyphosate alone doesn't. Tests show it contains levels of arsenic, chromium, lead and nickel much higher than those allowed in water. All these heavy metals are toxic.[44]

Various different glyphosate-based herbicides killed human embryonic kidney cells in under 90 minutes, although glyphosate alone didn't. At levels 50–90% less than that, glyphosate-based herbicides disrupted hormone levels. All except 3 of the formulas contained arsenic at levels 5–53 times higher than allowed in water in the European Union or the USA. Almost all contained nickel, 19 of them containing up to 62 times the permitted levels. Six contained up to 11 times the levels of lead allowed. All except one contained higher levels of chromium (up to 62 times) than allowed. These herbicides cause disruption of membranes, affect **apoptosis**, damage **DNA** and affect energy production.[44, 45]

Those exposed to glyphosate-based herbicides as part of their work have a higher incidence of non-Hodgkin lymphoma (NHL), a type of blood cancer.[46] In the US, NHL patients who were exposed to these herbicides won court cases brought against Monsanto, the makers of Roundup.

On 29 July 2021, Bayer, who bought Monsanto in 2018, announced that it was withdrawing the sale of glyphosate-containing products, including Roundup, to US home gardeners. They did this because they were being sued by around 30,000 customers who believed that use of those products had caused them to develop cancer.[85] I hope that this will extend to the rest of the world soon.

Talc

Cancer linked to the use of talc in the genital area was highlighted in some well-publicised legal cases brought by women against Johnson & Johnson, where significant damages were awarded to the women. In a review, exposure to talc in the genital area was associated with a small to moderate increase in risk of most types of ovarian cancer.[47]

Trichoroethylene / Perchloroethylene (TCE, aka PCE)

TCE is a colourless, volatile liquid that's chemically synthesised. Its primary use is in making hydrofluorocarbons and refrigerants, and as a solvent for degreasing metal equipment. It's also used in some household products, such as carpet shampoos, waterproofing agents and adhesives, and as a spot remover by commercial drycleaners. You can be exposed to it by inhaling its vapours or by absorption through the skin. Water contaminated with it is found in areas surrounding industrial plants producing it.

TCE is classified as a known human **carcinogen** by the **NTP** and as a probable **carcinogen** by the **EPA**. There's sufficient evidence to show that it causes kidney cancer, limited evidence to show a link with non-Hodgkin lymphoma, and a possible link to liver cancer.[48] **Epidemiological studies** show a likely link to bladder cancer, multiple myeloma and non-Hodgkin lymphoma too.[49]

Triclosan

Triclosan is a broad-spectrum antibacterial widely used in personal care products. Recent laboratory evidence shows it might play a role in cancer development, perhaps because of its ability to mimic oestrogen or maybe because it inhibits fatty acid synthesis. It's easily absorbed through the skin and mucous membranes, and has been found in blood, urine and breast milk, despite the fact that it's metabolised quite quickly in the body. This could be because it's used so frequently. No human studies have been done to establish a connection with cancer, but the researchers suggested that they should be, to clarify the size of the problem.[50] In laboratory studies and mouse models, though, it's been established that triclosan promotes the growth of breast cancer cells, so it might also promote it in humans.[51]

Volatile organic compounds (VOCs)

VOCs encompass a wide range of chemicals that are emitted as gases from some solids and liquids. They're used in many different household products, including

- glues
- varnishes
- paints and paint strippers
- waxes
- solvents
- aerosols
- cleaners and disinfectants
- air fresheners
- moth repellents
- car parts and stored fuel
- dry-cleaned clothing
- pesticides
- hobby supplies.[52]

We tend to think that volatile chemicals give off gases quite quickly, so all you have to do is use them in an open space or ventilate the area. In reality, some of them give off gases for years. Our homes tend to be full of them. According to the **EPA**, levels of many **VOCs** are up to 10 times higher inside than outside.[52]

The health effects of **VOCs** include:

- Headaches, nausea and loss of coordination.
- Irritation of nose, throat and eyes.
- Damage to the central nervous system, kidneys and liver.

- Some are known to cause cancer in animals and humans. Others are suspected of it.[52]

Personal care products

Antiperspirants and deodorants

The sweat glands in our armpits and groins differ from the rest of the body. They produce sweat that contains more oil, which makes a great meal for bacteria. The smell of body odour comes from toxins produced by these bacteria.

There are 2 ways to prevent this: antiperspirants block sweat from leaving the glands, whereas deodorants stop growth of bacteria. Unfortunately both can have unfortunate effects if you don't choose carefully.

Most antiperspirants contain aluminium salts. Most also contain parabens and fragrance. The action of blocking sweat glands removes one route for toxins to be excreted from the body.[53]

Deodorants prevent bacterial growth, so sweat is still produced. However, most deodorants contain parabens and fragrance.

Natural deodorants are easily available. Most contain sodium bicarbonate (baking soda), which is effective but can cause a rash. You can make these yourself. A typical recipe is:

- 90 **ml** coconut oil
- 60 **ml** organic cornflour or arrowroot
- 60 **ml** sodium bicarbonate
- 10–12 drops of essential oils, if you want a fragrance.

Melt the coconut oil. Mix together the cornflour or arrowroot and sodium bicarbonate. Add the dry mix to the oil and add any essential oils you want.

If you get a rash, try reducing the amount of bicarbonate of soda. You could omit it altogether, as coconut oil has antibacterial properties. Wait for it to be absorbed before dressing, as you can get oily marks on your clothes if you don't.

Alternatively, try magnesium oil. It isn't an oil at all but a suspension of magnesium chloride with an oily texture. It's an effective deodorant and also supplements your magnesium stores, which relaxes your muscles. It may tingle slightly on first use, especially if you're deficient in magnesium, but this should wear off and shouldn't cause irritation.

Some people swear by diluted lemon juice or apple cider vinegar. These inhibit bacterial growth but they can irritate sensitive skin. Lemon juice can also cause skin photosensitivity, so be careful if you sunbathe after using it.

Others use a combination of essential oils with mixed results. Some essential oils have the power to kill bacteria but the effects may not last all day, and they can irritate sensitive skin.

Body washes and liquid soaps

These can be a bit of a chemical soup. Most contain parabens as preservatives, and other preservatives that release formaldehyde, such as:

- quaternium-15
- diaziolidinyl urea (Germall)
- DMDM hydratoin

- sodium hydroxymethyl glycinate
- sodium hydroxymethyl glycinate (suttocide).

On top of these, they may contain sodium lauryl sulphate, which can cause irritation, and fragrances. Antibacterial soaps and body washes are also popular these days. Most contain triclosan. You don't need an antibacterial soap to remove bacteria. Ordinary soap and water is as effective and avoids potential problems.

Many body washes and soaps are marketed as 'natural'. Some are better than others and I recommend you check the ingredients on the **EWG's** Skin Deep database (https://www.ewg.org/skindeep/) before buying them. They vary in price too, and most are significantly dearer than supermarket brands. However some are excellent, and will leave your skin feeling good and smelling lovely. Bear in mind that they may not last as long as those containing parabens, as natural preservatives aren't as effective.

If your budget is tight, invest in a large bottle of Castile soap. This isn't a brand name but was named after Castile in Spain, where it originates. It's made from olive oil, sometimes other vegetable oils (never animal), sodium or potassium hydroxide for the saponification process, and water. There are recipes for it online. It goes a very long way, so it's an incredibly cost-effective alternative. My preference is for a fragrance-free one and I add various essential oils to it. I use a foam dispenser for hand soap, which makes it last longer. As well as washing your body and hands with it, it can be used for washing dishes, clothes and hair, making it a good option when travelling.

Facial skincare and makeup

Facial cleansers, toners, moisturisers and makeup can be a source of many toxins, particularly parabens, phthalates and sulphates. This has been recognised in the industry and it's now easier to find toxin-free alternatives. To be sure, check the ingredients on the Skin Deep database.

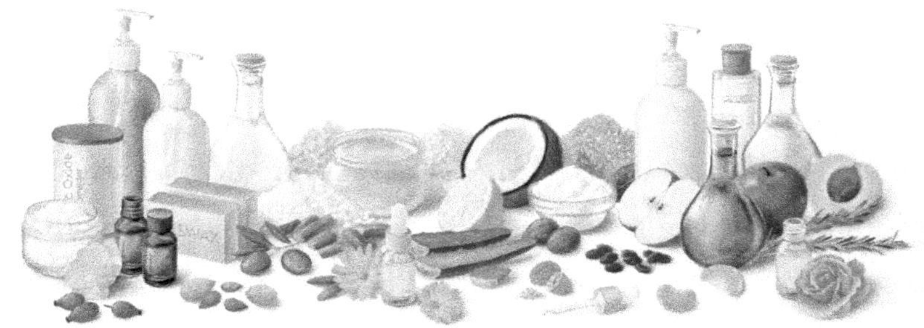

Hair colourants

The links between hair colourants and cancer have been raised numerous times. Before 1980, some chemicals used were definitely linked to cancer, usually bladder cancer. Anyone who used permanent hair colours then may have a higher risk. Manufacturers changed their products' formulations when this was made public and now the links are harder to find.

If you use a dark shade of permanent colour your risk of breast cancer could be increased, although the researcher stresses that the link is an association and doesn't necessarily indicate cause.[54] Some studies also link hair dye use to leukaemia and non-Hodgkin lymphoma but others don't.[54]

More recent analysis of a long-term study shows a slightly increased risk of basal cell carcinoma, especially in natural blondes. More frequent and longer use shows a slightly higher risk of ovarian cancer and breast cancer, particularly oestrogen receptor negative, progesterone receptor negative and hormone receptor negative breast cancers.[55]

There are certainly some toxic chemicals used in them, though, including sulphates, parabens and ethanolamines.[56]

If you've been used to colouring your hair, though, you probably won't want to stop. There are so-called natural products stocked by health food stores but even they aren't completely toxin-free. Henna is another option but it can have unpredictable results on grey hair and it's pretty messy, and very long-lasting, so regrowth can be a problem. It's possible to use plants to colour your hair safely. The effects don't last long and may not cover grey hairs, but they're safe. You could try the following:

- Blueberries, blackberries and cranberries give dark hair some extra colour and shine. Mash with a little water and some apple cider vinegar, apply to damp hair and leave for 15–20 minutes before rinsing.
- Cherries, cranberries and raspberries give brown hair auburn highlights. Use the same method as above.
- Walnut shells or leaves and chamomile can darken brown hair. Infuse in boiling water until it reaches a deep colour. Add apple cider vinegar once it's cooled. Apply to damp hair and leave for 15–20 minutes before rinsing.
- Freshly ground ginger root can enliven red hair. Take care not to get it in your eyes, as it will sting. Use the same method as for the walnut and chamomile colouring.

- Marigold flowers add deep blonde tones to blonde hair. Use the same method as for the walnut and chamomile colouring.

You shouldn't colour your hair for 6 months after chemo because the hair becomes very fragile, particularly if you lost it and it's regrowing. The plant options above are safe, though.

If you've finished treatment, waited 6 months and want to stick with your usual colouring product, I recommend you:

- Stick with lighter hair dyes.
- Leave it as long as you can between colourings to avoid exposure.
- Don't wash your hair for a few days before colouring, as the natural oils help protect your scalp, where the chemicals are absorbed.
- Drink a **litre** of water over the hour after colouring to help flush out any toxins you've absorbed.
- If you colour your hair yourself or you work in a hairdressing salon, use rubber gloves to avoid absorption through your hands.
- Alternatively, foils can help avoid the colourant getting onto the skin, so it can't be absorbed.

Perfume

Most perfumes aren't good if you're battling cancer. They generally contain phthalates. I found this difficult, as I'd been wearing perfume daily for many years. I tend to stick with essential oils now and have some lovely combinations to ring the changes. I find most synthetic perfumes overpowering now and they can give me a headache. There are plenty of websites to guide you with good suggestions for combinations. You'll need to experiment to find the right combination for you. Bear in mind that most essential oils need diluting with a carrier oil, like fractionated coconut oil or sweet almond oil. I suggest using 8 drops of essential oil in a 10 **ml** rollerball or spray bottle, topped up with carrier oil. The oils deteriorate quickly, particularly if you use a rollerball bottle, because your skin oils will contaminate it. So make up small quantities.

You can find helpful advice on the safety of essential oils and the dilutions that are recommended at https://theherbalacademy.com/a-guide-to-essential-oil-safety/ and naturallivingfamily.com

Alternatively, there are companies that make natural perfumes. Search for them online, but check the ingredients to make sure they really are natural.

Shampoo and conditioner

Most shampoos and conditioners contain lauryl or laureth sulphates, parabens, polyethylene glycol (PEG) compounds, triclosan and fragrance, which is likely to contain phthalates unless the label says that it comes from essential oils. It isn't hard to find natural brands of shampoo and conditioner these days. Even supermarkets stock some, but check the ingredients on the Skin Deep database. Alternatively, you can make your own.

Castile soap can be used as a shampoo, although it can be drying. Add an equal amount of coconut milk for moisturising. Essential oils can make it smell good. Rosemary is good for itchy scalps and promoting hair growth. Lavender is often used for soothing the scalp.

If you're brunette, a rinse of equal quantities of apple cider vinegar and water helps remove soap, rebalance pH, and gives a good shine. If you're blonde, the juice of a lemon to a cup of water does the same. You can add raw organic honey, aloe vera gel, essential oils and whole milk for a more luxurious conditioner.

Shaving foam

Products available in supermarkets generally contain **TEA**, lauryl or laureth sulphates, fragrance and polyethylene glycol (PEG) compounds, which are a cocktail of toxins you should avoid. Toxin-free shaving foams, gels and creams are available from health food stores and online. They vary in price but are more expensive than the supermarket brands. In some cases, though, a small amount goes a long way.

There are many recipes for making shaving creams online. A word of warning: many use shea butter. This makes a wonderfully creamy shaving cream, but it's a solid fat and very likely to clog your pipes if used regularly. These recipes can be put into a foam dispenser:

Honey and oil combo

- 60 **ml** cocoa butter (melted)
- 60 **ml** Castile soap
- 125 **ml** sweet almond oil
- 60 **ml** raw honey

- 10 drops essential oils of your choice
- 180 **ml** warm water.

Put cocoa butter into a heat-resistant glass measuring jug and place in a saucepan of boiling water. Add soap, sweet almond oil, honey and essential oils. Pour into a foam dispenser and top up with warm water. Shake well to combine. After use, flush drain with plenty of hot water.

Soap and aloe vera gel

- 60 **ml** aloe vera gel
- 60 **ml** liquid Castile soap
- 30 **ml** sweet almond oil
- 125 **ml** filtered water
- 10 drops essential oils of your choice.

Mix all the ingredients and pour into a foam dispenser.

Bear in mind that these don't contain preservatives. I'd suggest using lavender and sweet orange essential oils, as they have antimicrobial properties, particularly when used together.[57]

Tattoos

Although not strictly a personal care product, tattoos are a common way of decorating the body. Carbon Black ink, often found in tattoos, is classified by the **IARC** as possibly **carcinogenic**, and also contains about 20 different **PAH**s, many of which are also considered probable or possible **carcinogens**. These can be found in tattooed skin and in the nearby **lymph** nodes, from where they could conceivably be transported to other parts of the body.[38] I suggest avoiding tattoos, as they could potentially cause tumours. Use temporary tattoos instead.

Toothpaste

You probably think you can't absorb chemicals from toothpaste. After all, you don't (or at least shouldn't) swallow it. But the mucous membranes in your mouth absorb all sorts of toxins. Toothpaste isn't required to have ingredients listed, but most contain:

- triclosan
- sodium lauryl sulphate, which could contain 1,4-dioxane
- aspartame
- propylene glycol, a skin irritant
- fluoride.

Fluoride was originally considered a pollutant, a by-product of fertiliser manufacturing and smelting of aluminium and other metals. Then in small doses it was shown to give some protection against tooth decay. Too much, though, causes fluorosis, which discolours teeth and causes bone malformations. The evidence for its protective abilities is actually pretty tenuous. It improves enamel strength slightly in children, but doesn't help adults and can produce brittle teeth.[58] In animal tests, male fertility is reduced.[59] More worryingly, there's evidence that it's a neurotoxin, and it's been linked to Alzheimer's disease.[60] Colgate has recognised that its neurotoxicity is dangerous to children and now recommend that only a smear be used for children under 2, whereas they used to recommend a pea-sized amount.[61]

Health food stores stock many toothpastes that don't contain these toxins. Generally, these products **do** list their ingredients. They're usually priced slightly higher than the cost of supermarket brands.

There's some good advice on what should and shouldn't be included in homemade toothpastes, together with some good recipes, on this website: https://askthedentist.com/diy-toothpaste/. They're dentists and offer unbiased advice.

Oil pulling involves swishing oil around your mouth. Any good quality oil works, but I recommend organic unrefined virgin coconut oil because it not only cleans but is antibacterial. Take about 1–2 tablespoons of oil in your mouth and swish it around your teeth. Start with 5 minutes and work your way up to around 20 minutes. You can do this while you're in the shower. Spit it out into a cup rather than down the washbasin because it can clog your pipes. Once it's hardened, it's easy to dispose of. Then brush your teeth. This will remove stains like coffee or tea, and freshens and whitens your teeth. Add a little clove oil for sweet smelling breath.

Household products

Air fresheners, candles and incense

All these products contain fragrance, typically containing a mixture of several dozen to several hundred chemicals, details of which are never revealed. However, perfume contains phthalates. They also contain a range of volatile organic compounds (**VOCs**) which can generate toxins such as formaldehyde, a known **carcinogen**. Besides raising cancer risk, they can also cause asthma attacks, migraine headaches, breathing difficulties and neurological problems.[62] Some candles, usually the cheap household ones, are made from paraffin wax, which is derived from petroleum products. When they burn, they produce toluene and other harmful chemicals.[63] Many also contain lead in the wicks, although some have pure cotton wicks. Incense burning, including mosquito coils, produces numerous toxic substances and some are **carcinogens.**[64]

Opening your windows for a minimum of half an hour a day will freshen the air instead. If it's freezing outside, try boiling a halved lemon for 10–15 minutes. Fresh, scented flowers also freshen the air as well as brightening your home. Alternatively, use a diffuser with your choice of essential oils. Many have therapeutic effects and good quality, pure essential oils don't contain toxins.

Bathroom mould remover

Bathroom mould removers are usually made from chlorine bleach. Aside from being toxic, chlorine bleach isn't effective at killing mould. It can even provide it with a nutrient source. It just bleaches the visible mould, so you won't see it for a few weeks until the mould recovers.[65]

For small spots of mould, tea tree[66] or clove[67] essential oils effectively kill it, but for larger areas the amounts needed can be toxic to children or those sensitive to chemicals.[65] A solution of one cup vinegar to 3 cups water is effective for small areas.

Nicole Bijlsma is a building biologist experienced in mould removal. She recommends what she refers to as 'a HEPA sandwich'. This involves:

- Vacuuming the affected area with a vacuum cleaner with a HEPA filter.
- Wiping with a damp microfibre cloth soaked in ½ **litre** of water with a good squirt of dishwashing liquid. This removes any biofilm, a colony of microbes that forms a protective film around itself.
- Vacuuming the area again.
- Discarding the cloth, the HEPA filter and the vacuum bag if using one. If not using a vacuum bag, ensure that the dust canister is thoroughly washed.[65]

This procedure removes the mould itself but may still leave black marks, particularly on porous surfaces like grouting. You can safely use hydrogen peroxide or a paste of oxygen bleach to remove them.

With a particularly bad mould problem, though, it's safest to employ a professional.

Mould needs food and water to survive. Remove those and you remove the problem. Rinse off any soap deposits, which feed moulds, then thoroughly dry the area after each time you use it. Use an extractor fan to remove humidity and keep the area well ventilated.

Dishwasher detergent

These usually have warning labels on them because they're full of toxic ingredients that will, at the very least, cause respiratory and skin problems. These include:

- Ammonia, a good cleaning agent but highly volatile, so in a hot environment you get ammonia gas in your home. This is extremely irritating to the respiratory system, the eyes and skin.

- Dyes and colourants, usually made from coal tar and often contaminated with heavy metals.
- Chlorine bleach.
- Ethanolamines.
- Formaldehyde.
- Lauryl and laureth sulphates.
- Fragrance.
- Glycol ethers, used to cut through grease. Overexposure to these can cause anaemia, skin and eye irritation, and reproductive damage in men.
- Phosphates, although these levels are much lower than they used to be.

Non-toxic dishwasher detergents are available but some use borax. There are recipes for non-toxic detergents online, such as this one:

- ¼ cup citric acid
- ¼ cup coarse salt
- 1 cup sodium bicarbonate
- 10–15 drops lemon essential oil
- distilled white vinegar.

In a glass container, mix the first 3 ingredients, then add the essential oil and mix again. For an average load, use one teaspoon. For greasy or extra dirty loads, use one tablespoon. Fill the rinse aid compartment with vinegar. It's cheaper than commercial rinse aids and works better.[68]

General household cleaners

Many household cleaners contain fragrance with phthalates, triclosan (especially any marked as antibacterial), lauryl or laureth sulphates, and chlorine bleach.

You can clean bench tops with hot water with a dash of Castile soap. This effectively removes bacteria likely to cause food poisoning. Castile soap also removes soap scum from shower screens and washbasins. Add essential oils for a pleasant smell. Lemon and other citrus oils smell fresh and have antibacterial properties. For tougher jobs, a paste of sodium bicarbonate has a gentle scouring effect as well as removing grease and oils.

Castile soap can be used as dishwashing soap for handwashing dishes. It's a good option for your budget, health reasons and environmentally, and is better than most shop-bought dishwashing liquids, particularly antibacterial ones.

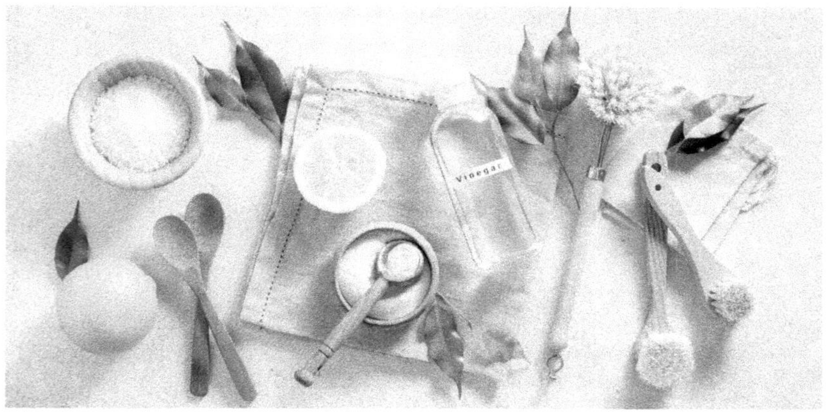

Insect sprays

These are particularly dangerous to children, as the spray invariably falls onto the floor or carpet where children play. Chronic exposure to indoor pesticides in children is linked to a 47% increase in the risk of childhood leukaemia and a 43% increase in childhood lymphoma, and there's a positive association with childhood brain tumours.[69]

You can knock out insects without resorting to chemical sprays. A mixture of white vinegar and Castile soap kills flying and crawling insects almost instantly. The smell of vinegar fades really quickly, but add a few drops of your favourite essential oil for a pleasant smelling spray. Lemon is particularly good. Even on its own, lemon oil deters crawling insects.

Laundry products

The smells in the laundry aisle in the supermarket can be overpowering. Fragrances are one of several toxins in laundry products, which mostly contain phthalates. They're obvious toxins but it's less easy to identify the rest because of poor labelling laws. It's likely, though, that they contain:

- **DEA** (diethanolamine), which is used as a surfactant to remove grease
- quaternium-15, which releases formaldehyde
- petroleum distillates
- chlorine bleach.

Manufacturers are starting to develop more natural alternatives that are just as effective, but you should check the ingredients.

If you'd rather devise your own washing products, other options include soapberries, sometimes known as soap nuts. These are real berries that release saponins, chemicals similar to soap. You can reuse them several times. You can also make detergent from unscented Castile bar soap and sodium bicarbonate.

For brightening, add a cupful of lemon juice to your whites for a natural bleaching effect. Oxygen bleach safely brightens coloured laundry items and lifts stains. A little sodium bicarbonate does the same.

Instead of fabric softener, which coats laundry with noxious fragrances and oils, add half a cup of white vinegar to the rinse cycle. For a pleasant fragrance, add a few drops of essential oils.

If you want to avoid static, instead of dryer sheets try dryer balls, which you can find online. They vary in effectiveness on static cling, but are reputed to speed up drying and soften laundry too.

I prefer to dry my laundry outside. The UV light kills bacteria, fungi and dust mites, and the laundry smells fresh when it's line-dried. It also saves electricity.

Oven cleaner

Instructions for most oven cleaners suggest using rubber gloves and a face mask when using them. No wonder, as they contain such toxic ingredients. These include:

- Sodium hydroxide, which is a wonderful degreaser but extremely corrosive.
- Ethers, which are solvents and highly volatile.
- Ethylene glycol, commonly used in antifreeze.
- Methylene chloride, an excellent degreaser and a solvent often used in paint strippers, but irritating, smelly and volatile. It's considered by the US Occupational Safety and Health

Administration to be a workplace **carcinogen.**[70]

- Petroleum distillates.

There are a couple of safe, natural oven cleaners. If it isn't too dirty and you clean it regularly, try this:

- Halve 2 lemons and squeeze their juice into an oven dish. Put the squeezed halves into the dish and fill it about one third full with water.
- Bake in the oven at 120°C for 30–45 minutes to soften the grime.
- Let the oven cool and remove the dish, keeping the contents.
- Remove the grime with a non-scratch scouring pad.
- Use a sponge and the lemon water to rinse the oven clean
- Dry the oven with a towel.

If there's significant build-up this method works best:

- Soak the oven racks in the bathtub with some dishwashing liquid or Castile soap.
- Mix a cup of sodium bicarbonate, ½ cup coarse sea salt and ¼ cup dishwashing liquid to make a paste. Add a little water if it's too thick.
- Spread the paste over the oven and leave for several hours or overnight, if possible.
- With a sponge dipped in warm water, wipe down the oven. Use a scouring pad if necessary to remove baked-on grime.
- Spray the oven interior with distilled white vinegar and wipe dry with a clean sponge. Dry with a towel.
- Use a scouring pad to clean the soaked oven racks. Dry before replacing in the oven.

Toilet cleaner

Most toilet cleaners have warnings on the label about getting burned if it contacts the skin, or not mixing with other chemicals. It's obvious that they're poisonous. Many contain hydrochloric acid to remove limescale and some contain chlorine bleach or other antibacterial agents, such as triclosan. Others use ammonia. Because of poor labelling laws, it's difficult to know what they contain, but it's safe to say that they're toxic.

Plain white distilled vinegar is all that you need to clean the toilet. It removes limescale, deodorises and kills bacteria. If you feel the need to scrub, sprinkle sodium bicarbonate and brush the bowl before you add vinegar. It fizzes up but it's only producing carbon dioxide, so it's quite safe. If you want a pleasant fragrance, cinnamon, clove and orange essential oils will not only freshen the air but have been shown to kill *Staphylococcus aureus* and *E. coli*, the 2 main bacteria in toilets.[71]

If you like using a gel that clings to the bowl, try the following:

- 1 tsp glycerine
- ½ tsp xanthan gum
- ½ cup distilled white vinegar
- 1 cup water.

Blend all the ingredients. Add essential oils if you want.

Window cleaners

Most commercial window cleaners contain toxins, such as:

- 2-butoxyethanol, a glycol ether, which is a powerful solvent that causes anaemia, skin and eye irritation, and causes

reproductive damage in men
- ammonia
- phthalates.

Newspaper and vinegar do an excellent job on windows and mirrors, and are much cheaper. They can leave streaks, though. For a better option, try this:

- ¼ cup isopropyl alcohol (rubbing alcohol)
- ¼ cup distilled white vinegar
- 15 **ml** cornflour (prevents streaking by filling the pits in the glass)
- 2 cups water
- 10 drops essential oil (the best are orange, lemon or lavender).

Mix the ingredients, ensuring the cornflour is fully dissolved, and fill a spray bottle.

Home furnishings

Beds and bedding

We spend about a third of our lives in bed and we breathe very close to it, so it's important that it's safe. Many of us, though, sleep on a cocktail of chemicals.

Bed frames are usually made from particleboard, which contains **VOCs**, including formaldehyde. If your bed frame is more than 5 years old, many of the **VOCs** will have finished off-gassing, so the danger period is more or less over. If it's newer, you could consider replacing it with a solid wood frame. I recommend a bed with wooden slats, as that also allows the mattress to breathe. If that isn't an option, consider buying a second-hand bed frame, the older the better, as it will have finished off-gassing. You can also buy sealants that don't contain **VOCs**, which seal the wood, preventing off-gassing. That assumes you can access the frame. With a divan bed, that's tricky.

I recommend you avoid polyurethane foam mattresses, which are highly flammable and must be treated with flame retardants. Memory foam is very popular but can also contain **VOCs**. I suggest sniffing any mattress you intend to buy: the smell tells you whether it's high in **VOCs**. If your mattress is more than 5 years old, it's probably relatively safe. If it's newer than that and you don't want to replace it, take it outside and expose it to full sun for as long as possible to speed up the off-gassing. The best mattresses with no **VOCs** or flame retardants are made from pure, natural latex. Not all latex mattresses are natural latex. Synthetic latex, known as talalay, contains petrochemical additives. They're easy to differentiate: you can smell the additives in the synthetic version, and the natural one will be more expensive. If you need more support, a sprung mattress with a natural latex mattress topper would be the best option.

Pillows can be toxic too. Many people use memory foam, which off-gas high levels of **VOCs**. Again, airing them in full sun will speed up the off-gassing if you want to keep them. If you don't suffer from allergies, natural fibres such as feather and wool are safe. If you do suffer, natural latex pillows can be found that are relatively inexpensive.

For bedding, natural fibres are best, such as cotton, hemp,

linen, silk and bamboo. Bamboo is particularly good because it's naturally antibacterial and antifungal, so no pesticides are used in its cultivation. Cotton is heavily sprayed with them unless it's organic.[65] Bamboo sheets are very soft and lightweight and have thermo-regulating properties, but they tend to wrinkle easily and are usually more expensive than cotton.

Blankets made in Asia, particularly China, may contain high levels of formaldehyde. In 2007, this was investigated in Australia and New Zealand.[72] They're also likely to contain fumigants[65], so they're best avoided.

Furniture

Like bed frames, other wooden furniture is commonly made of particleboard. The same advice applies.

Cushioning on chairs and sofas is usually made from polyurethane foam, which must be treated with fire retardants because it's highly flammable. It breaks down over time, causing dust that contains fire retardant chemicals. If you live in the US, you can take part in a free study conducted by Duke University to test for fire retardants.[73] In Australia, you can get testing done by the Australian Wool Testing Authority (AWTA), although it can be expensive.[74] Testing may be available in other countries too.

PFCs are often used in stain-resistant finishes. Similar to Teflon®, these have been linked by some researchers to birth defects and cancer.[75] The risk in furniture is likely to be lower than in cookware, though, which is heated and so off-gases more.

The adhesives, polishes and sealants used in furniture

manufacture contain **TCE**. You're likely to find benzene too.

The risks come not just from the items themselves, but also the volatile chemicals they release and the dust that they generate. To reduce your risk, do the following:

- Opt for less flammable fabrics, such as cotton, wool and leather.
- Leave furniture in the sun during warm, dry weather for as long as possible (several weeks is ideal) to enable off-gassing.
- Avoid furniture made in Asia, which is likely to contain formaldehyde.
- Wash your hands regularly to reduce exposure to flame retardants.
- Dust surfaces and floors with a damp microfibre cloth.
- Vacuum carpets and furniture using a cleaner with a HEPA filter.
- Clean heating vents and inlets, air conditioning and ducts regularly.
- Open your windows for at least 30 minutes a day to air the house.

Garden chemicals

Pesticides and herbicides

The main pesticide widely used is Roundup, which is covered extensively at the beginning of this chapter. I can't stress strongly enough how dangerous this is. I encourage you to dispose of any you've stored, immediately, by contacting your local waste management company and following their advice for toxic waste.

Weed problems are solved pretty easily with white vinegar in areas where you want plantings, sprayed directly on the weeds. On paths, a salt water solution is really effective and helps prevent weeds regrowing.

Ant colonies can be eliminated by pouring boiling water into their nests. It is safer (and cheaper) than ant powder, which usually contains borax. Don't use petrol! Apart from being toxic to you as well as the ants, it poisons the ground. Recently, someone used petrol on an ant-hill and lit it. He now has a ready-made hole in his garden for a pool, after it exploded.

Another useful substance is diatomaceous earth, which is the fossilised remains of algae. It's completely safe to humans and pets, and it doesn't poison insects – its abrasive surface and ability to absorb waxes from insects' exoskeletons kills them by dehydration. It repels, but doesn't kill, slugs and snails, so it's worth sprinkling around plants that are being attacked by them. The only drawback is that rain or watering washes it away, so it needs redoing each time it gets wet.

To get rid of slugs and snails, spread espresso coffee grounds around your vulnerable plants. The caffeine from the coffee disrupts their mucus glands and they die. It smells good too.

Neem oil is effective at disrupting insects at each stage: egg, larvae and adult. It acts as a hormone disruptor on insects, but not on humans, pets, fish and other wildlife. It discourages insects from eating the leaves of sprayed plants. It's a natural insecticide against leaf-sucking and chewing insects, and nematode worms (but not earthworms). It's biodegradable, and can also combat powdery mildew, black spot and other plant fungal infections.

To discourage flies and other insects around a barbecue area or outdoor seating, consider planting pyrethrum daisies. Insects hate pyrethrum. Planting them near your front and back doors also deters them from coming into your home.

To prevent aphids, mites and fungal infections in your garden, the following recipe, courtesy of one of my friends, is very effective:

- First make a supply of organic white oil by mixing 4 parts of sunflower oil and one part of Castile soap.
- Cut a head of garlic across the middle and boil it in about a **litre** of water for 10 minutes.
- When the water has cooled, add a teaspoon of organic white oil, a teaspoon of neem oil, a teaspoon of sodium bicarbonate and a teaspoon of Castile soap or dishwashing liquid.
- Pour into a spray bottle, shake well and spray your plants all over, including the underside of leaves.
- Use every fortnight for continued protection or more often if it's wet.

Pool chemicals

Most people disinfect their pools with chlorine, which is absorbed by the skin and can affect the gut microbiome. That's why I recommend using a shower filter. Even salt water pools can have this effect because chlorine is released by electrolysis from the sodium chloride (salt), albeit at lower levels. However, chlorine is the least of your worries if you're a regular swimmer because many pool chemicals react with organic material in the water like urine, sweat, dirt and skin moisturisers. The reaction produces hundreds of disinfection by-products (DBPs), some of which can cause cancer.[76] One such group is trihalomethanes. Long-term exposure to these is associated with doubling the risk of bladder cancer.[77]

I'm not suggesting for a moment that you forgo your swims. The exercise is beneficial and it's enjoyable. If possible, swimming in the sea is preferable to a pool. If that's not possible, ensure you shower just before each swim and train yourself and your family not to pee in the pool, as this produces the most DBPs.[76] Avoid swimming regularly in public pools, as neither of these precautions protects against other people's habits.

General advice on keeping your home safe from toxins

According to the **EPA**, the air inside our homes has levels of some organic compounds 2–5 times greater than those outside.[52] This is general advice for minimising the impact:

- Open doors and windows as much as possible, at least 30 minutes each day. My grandmother was English and she opened the doors and windows every morning, even with snow on the ground. Her home always smelled fresh and clean.
- Whenever you use toxic chemicals, such as paint, ventilate the area.
- Buy an air filter that removes **VOCs**, dust, pet hair, dander, pollen, bacteria and fungi. Shop around, as prices vary and the best ones aren't necessarily the most expensive.

- Remove your shoes at the door. Shoes carry fungi, bacteria, viruses and chemicals into your home.
- Mop and dust regularly with a damp cloth to remove household dust, which contains pesticides, flame retardants and lead. Use a vacuum cleaner with a HEPA filter on carpets.
- Grow indoor plants. RMIT and the University of Melbourne found that one houseplant reduced **VOCs** by 25% in a 20 square metre room. Five houseplants reduced them by 75% and 10 gave maximum health and wellness.[78] Not all plants are equal at **VOC** removal. The top 10 for removing carbon monoxide, benzene and formaldehyde are:
- Areca Palm (*Chrysalidocarpus lutescens*) – semi-sun
- Lady Palm (*Rhapis excelsa*) – semi-sun
- Bamboo Palm (*Chamaedorea seifrizii*) – semi-sun
- Rubber Plant (*Ficus robusta*) – semi-sun to semi-shade
- Dracaena 'Janet Craig' (*Dracaena deremensis 'Janet Craig'*) – semi-shade
- Philodendron (*Philodendron sp.*) – semi-shade
- Dwarf Date Palm (*Phoenix roebelenii*) – semi-sun
- Ficus Alii (*Ficus macleilandii 'Alii'*) – full sun and semi-sun
- Boston Fern (*Nephrolepis exaltata 'Bostoniensis'*) – semi-sun
- Peace Lily (*Spathiphyllum 'Mauna Loa'*) – semi-shade.

Technology

We're surrounded by electromagnetic radiation. It's generated by electrical wiring, electrical appliances, transformers, meter boxes and power lines. Electromagnetic fields at higher frequencies, also known as radiofrequency (RF) radiation, are emitted by wireless devices – mobile phones, modems, cordless phones, baby monitors, PCs and laptops, tablets, microwave ovens, smart devices like smart meters, and smart TVs.

A review of numerous studies shows that RF radiation, which is non-ionising, generates free radicals that damage **DNA**, contributing to **carcino**gene**sis**.[79] In 2011, the **IARC** categorised RF radiation as a 'possible human **carcinogen**'. In 2018, a review of **epidemiological studies** concluded the **IARC** should re-categorise it as '**carcinogenic** to humans'. They found mobile phone use increased the risk of brain cancer, particularly gliomas. Glioma numbers have been increasing in UK and other countries. Four studies showed increased risk of vestibular nerve tumours. These benign tumours in the nerves control balance and hearing in the inner ear. There were also associations with thyroid, testicular, and breast cancers in both men and women, and with leukaemia.[80]

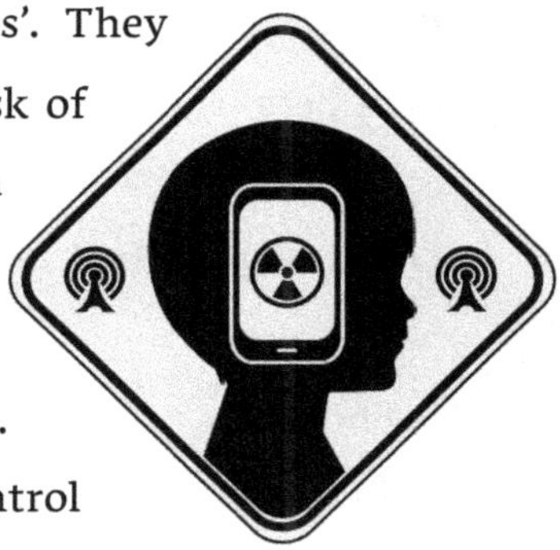

This research has been buried by the telecommunications industry and international governments, like the dangers of tobacco were in the 1950s. It's inconvenient to them to acknowledge the dangers of these products, as big money is involved, in profits to the manufacturers and taxes by governments. In 1996, the US Federal Communications Commission (FCC) established the 'specific absorption rate' (SAR) as a measure of safety of mobile phones.[81] SAR is used internationally. It measures the thermal effects, which are quite different from the mechanism outlined above. Also, mobile phone manufacturers self-report SAR levels, which aren't independently confirmed, and the levels aren't required to be shown on packaging. It's been a very effective cover-up, as numbers of mobile phones have rocketed since they first appeared.

The problem isn't confined to mobile phones. Your Wi-Fi modem at home is probably constantly on, emitting RF radiation. Cordless phones continually emit RF radiation. Smart TVs do too. Baby monitors are placed alongside our most vulnerable family members. Developing brains are particularly susceptible.

It isn't only cancer that's been associated with RF radiation. **IARC** have linked fertility problems, and damage to sight and hearing to it.[80]

I hope you get the picture, but I'm no Luddite. I'm not advocating living without the internet or your mobile phone. It wouldn't really help anyway, as radiation from our neighbours' devices can penetrate our homes. Even shopping centres are introducing Wi-Fi. We must try to reduce our exposure as much as possible.

Turn off Wi-Fi when you aren't actively using it. Wired connections are significantly safer, although not as convenient (but they are faster). An Ethernet home network connects multiple users.

Site your router/modem where people don't spend much time, if possible, and unplug it at night. This prevents melatonin reduction, which will help with sleep.

Avoid carrying your mobile phone on your person. Some women

have slipped theirs inside their bra and subsequently developed primary breast cancers in exactly the same spot.[80] Similarly, men often carry theirs in their breast pockets. Men can also get breast cancers. Phones carried in pants pockets affect sperm quality, damaging men's fertility.[82]

Use speakerphone if possible. Bluetooth headsets don't necessarily minimise exposure. Among 9 headsets, RF radiation emissions varied widely, and were significantly increased in poor reception areas.[83] If you're somewhere public, plug in an Air Tube headphone set instead. These conduct sound through hollow tubes instead of a wire, eliminating the antenna effect. They're easily available and are inexpensive. If you already have a pair of wired headphones, clip on a ferrite bead. This reduces RF radiation by about 95%. They're also easily available and cost less than Air Tubes.

Avoid making calls in poor reception areas. RF radiation is significantly stronger to maintain the signal.

Turn your phone to flight mode when travelling by car, train or tram, as in these conditions it emits more radiation to maintain the signal.

Keep children under 15 away from phones except in emergencies. Texting is safer than making calls. For playing games, switch to flight mode to avoid a wireless connection. If they need the internet, encourage them to use a wired PC.

Turn off Bluetooth on devices unless you need it.

Switch to a wired home phone. If you want a cordless phone, remove any handsets in the bedroom, where you spend many hours a day. You can buy analogue cordless phones that have an ECO mode which powers them down when not being used.

Don't keep your mobile phone by your bed. If you've been using yours as an alarm clock, switch to a battery operated or wind up one. Charge your mobile as far away as possible from the bedroom.

Stand a metre or more away from the microwave when it's cooking.

Use a corded baby monitor rather than a wireless one, placed at least a metre away from baby's bed. If you need a wireless one, use analogue in preference to digital – they have fewer channels and use a lower frequency. Use voice activation mode to avoid transmitting continuously.

Position your smart meter at least 2 metres away from where you sleep, study or work. Ensure the meter box is enclosed in a metal box to reduce RF emissions.

Keep your computer CPU (box) at least 30 centimetres from your body.

Use your laptop on a table top or a laptop stand, ensuring it's at least 10 centimetres from your body.

Avoid wireless keyboards and mice.

If you're moving house, check the location of nearby phone towers. Try to ensure that you're at least 400 metres away from them. This becomes more problematic with the introduction of 5G, as the towers are more densely located, small and less easy to identify. Many are attached to lamp posts. To find out the location of 5G towers in Australia, check: http://web.acma.gov.au/pls/radcom/site_proximity.main_page

If you're close to a tower and can't move, install thick metal blinds to reduce the radiation.

References

1. Coussens L, Werb Z. Inflammation and cancer. *Nature*. 2002;420(6917):860-867. doi:10.1038/nature01322

2. Darbre P. Underarm antiperspirants/deodorants and breast cancer. *Breast Cancer Research*. 2009;11(S3). doi:10.1186/bcr2424

3. American Cancer Society. Arsenic and Cancer Risk. American Cancer Society. https://www.cancer.org/cancer/cancer-causes/arsenic.html. Published 2020. Accessed August 23, 2021.

4. International Agency for Research on Cancer. Arsenic and Arsenic Compounds. International Agency for Research on Cancer. https://monographs.iarc.fr/wp-content/uploads/2018/06/mono100C-6.pdf. Published 2018. Accessed August 23, 2021.

5. Stayner L, Welch L, Lemen R. The Worldwide Pandemic of Asbestos-Related Diseases. *Annu Rev Public Health*. 2013;34(1):205-216. doi:10.1146/annurev-publhealth-031811-124704

6. Environmental Protection Agency. Benzene. Environmental Protection Agency. https://www.epa.gov/sites/production/files/2016-09/documents/benzene.pdf. Published 2012. Accessed August 23, 2021.

7. EWG's Skin Deep®. Top Tips For Safer Products || Skin Deep® Cosmetics Database | EWG. EWG's Skin Deep®. https://www.ewg.org/skindeep/top-tips-for-safer-products/. Accessed August 23, 2021.

8. Godt J, Scheidig F, Grosse-Siestrup C et al. The toxicity of cadmium and resulting hazards for human health. *Journal of Occupational Medicine and Toxicology*. 2006;1(1):22. doi:10.1186/1745-6673-1-22

9. Brennan J. Toxicity of Household Bleach. Sciencing. https://sciencing.com/toxicity-household-bleach-21461.html. Published 2017. Accessed August 23, 2021.

10. Odabasi M, Elbir T, Dumanoglu Y, Sofuoglu S. Halogenated volatile organic compounds in chlorine-bleach-containing household products and implications for their use. *Atmos Environ*. 2014;92:376-383. doi:10.1016/j.atmosenv.2014.04.049

11. Environmental Protection Agency. Chloroform. Environmental Protection Agency. https://www.epa.gov/sites/production/files/2016-09/documents/chloroform.pdf. Published 2000. Accessed August 23, 2021.

12. Agency for Toxic Substances and Disease Registry. Carbon Tetrachloride | Public Health Statement | ATSDR. Agency for Toxic Substances and Disease Registry. https://wwwn.cdc.gov/TSP/PHS/PHS.aspx?phsid=194&toxid=35. Published 2011. Accessed August 23, 2021.

13. Garone M, Howard J, Fabrikant J. A review of common tanning methods. *J Clin Aesthet Dermatol*. 2015;8(2):43-47. https://pubmed.ncbi.nlm.nih.gov/25741402/. Accessed August 23, 2021.

14. Campaign for Safe Cosmetics. Ethanolamine Compounds (MEA, DEA, TEA And Others) - Safe Cosmetics. Campaign for Safe Cosmetics. http://www.safecosmetics.org/get-the-facts/chemicals-of-concern/ethanolamine-compounds. Accessed August 23, 2021.

15. EWG's Skin Deep®. EWG Skin Deep® | What is TRIETHANOLAMINE. EWG's Skin Deep®. http://www.ewg.org/skindeep/ingredient/706639/Triethanolamine/. Accessed August 23, 2021.

16. Silent Spring Institute. A previously unrecognized flame retardant found in Americans for the first time. Science Daily. https://www.sciencedaily.com/releases/2014/11/141112084506.htm. Published 2014. Accessed August 23, 2021.

17. Hoffman K, Lorenzo A, Butt C et al. Exposure to flame retardant chemicals and occurrence and severity of papillary thyroid cancer: A case-control study. *Environ Int.* 2017;107:235-242. doi:10.1016/j.envint.2017.06.021

18. Deziel N, Yi H, Stapleton H, Huang H, Zhao N, Zhang Y. A case-control study of exposure to organophosphate flame retardants and risk of thyroid cancer in women. *BMC Cancer.* 2018;18(1):637. doi:10.1186/s12885-018-4553-9

19. Gorini F, Iervasi G, Coi A, Pitto L, Bianchi F. The Role of Polybrominated Diphenyl Ethers in Thyroid Carcinogenesis: Is It a Weak Hypothesis or a Hidden Reality? From Facts to New Perspectives. *Int J Environ Res Public Health.* 2018;15(9):1834. doi:10.3390/ijerph15091834

20. American Cancer Society. Formaldehyde. American Cancer Society. https://www.cancer.org/cancer/cancer-causes/formaldehyde.html. Published 2014. Accessed August 23, 2021.

21. Pope S. Organic Furniture: Going Nontoxic on a Budget. The Healthy Home Economist. https://www.thehealthyhomeeconomist.com/organic-furniture-sustainable-nontoxic/. Published 2016. Accessed August 23, 2021.

22. Environmental Protection Agency. Basis of OSHA Carcinogen Listing for Individual Chemicals. Environmental Protection Agency. https://www.epa.gov/sites/production/files/2018-08/documents/osha_carcinogen_basis_august_2018.pdf. Published 2018. Accessed August 23, 2021.

23. Vrabie C, Candido A, van Duursen M, Jonker M. Specific in vitro toxicity of crude and refined petroleum products: II. Estrogen (α and β) and androgen receptor-mediated responses in yeast assays. *Environ Toxicol Chem.* 2010;29(7):1529-1536. doi:10.1002/etc.187

24. Concin N, Hofstetter G, Plattner B et al. Evidence for Cosmetics as a Source of Mineral Oil Contamination in Women. *J Womens Health.* 2011;20(11):1713-1719. doi:10.1089/jwh.2011.2829

25. Environmental Working Group. EWG Research Shows 22 Percent of All Cosmetics May Be Contaminated With Cancer-Causing Impurity. Environmental Working Group. https://www.ewg.org/news/news-releases/2007/02/08/ewg-research-shows-22-percent-all-cosmetics-may-be-contaminated-cancer?_ga=2.219734992.852698033.1565248591-1708371622.1565248591. Published 2007. Accessed August 23, 2021.

26. National Cancer Institute. Mineral Oils: Untreated and Mildly Treated - Cancer-Causing Substances. National Cancer Institute. https://www.cancer.gov/about-cancer/causes-prevention/risk/substances/mineral-oils. Published 2019. Accessed August 23, 2021.

27. Environmental Working Group. EWG's Guide to Safer Sunscreens. Environmental Working Group. https://www.ewg.org/sunscreen/report/the-trouble-with-sunscreen-chemicals/. Published 2021. Accessed August 23, 2021.

28. DiNardo J, Downs C. Dermatological and environmental toxicological impact of the sunscreen ingredient oxybenzone/benzophenone-3. *J Cosmet Dermatol*. 2017;17(1):15-19. doi:10.1111/jocd.12449

29. Ngan V. Allergy to PABA | DermNet NZ. DermNet NZ. https://www.dermnetnz.org/topics/allergy-to-paba/. Published 2012. Accessed August 23, 2021.

30. Barr L, Metaxas G, Harbach C, Savoy L, Darbre P. Measurement of paraben concentrations in human breast tissue at serial locations across the breast from axilla to sternum. *Journal of Applied Toxicology*. 2012;32(3):219-232. doi:10.1002/jat.1786

31. Goodman B. FAQ: Parabens and Breast Cancer. WebMD. https://www.webmd.com/breast-cancer/news/20151027/parabens-breast-cancer. Published 2015. Accessed August 23, 2021.

32. Gonzalez T, Rae J, Colacino J. Implication of environmental estrogens on breast cancer treatment and progression. *Toxicology*. 2019;421:41-48. doi:10.1016/j.tox.2019.03.014

33. Environmental Protection Agency. Drinking Water Health Advisory for Perfluorooctanoic Acid (PFOA). Environmental Protection Agency. https://www.epa.gov/sites/production/files/2016-05/documents/pfoa_health_advisory_final-plain.pdf. Published 2016. Accessed August 23, 2021.

34. Bassil K, Vakil C, Sanborn M, Cole D, Kaur J, Kerr K. Cancer health effects of pesticides: Systematic review. *Canadian Family Physician*. 2007;53(10):1704-1711. https://europepmc.org/article/PMC/2231435. Accessed August 23, 2021.

35. Alavanja M, Hoppin J, Kamel F. Health Effects of Chronic Pesticide Exposure: Cancer and Neurotoxicity. *Annu Rev Public Health*. 2004;25(1):155-197. doi:10.1146/annurev.publhealth.25.101802.123020

36. Breast Cancer Prevention Partners (BCPP). Phthalates - Breast Cancer Prevention Partners (BCPP). Breast Cancer Prevention Partners (BCPP). https://www.bcpp.org/resource/phthalates/. Published 2021. Accessed August 23, 2021.

37. Zhu M, Huang C, Ma X et al. Phthalates promote prostate cancer cell proliferation through activation of ERK5 and p38. *Environ Toxicol Pharmacol*. 2018;63:29-33. doi:10.1016/j.etap.2018.08.007

38. Lehner K, Santarelli F, Vasold R et al. Black Tattoos Entail Substantial Uptake of Genotoxicpolycyclic Aromatic Hydrocarbons (PAH) in Human Skin and Regional Lymph Nodes. *PLoS One*. 2014;9(3):e92787. doi:10.1371/journal.pone.0092787

39. Kim S, Hwang W, Cho J, Kang D. Attributable risk of lung cancer deaths due to indoor radon exposure. *Ann Occup Environ Med*. 2016;28(8). doi:10.1186/s40557-016-0093-4

40. Australian Radiation Protection and Nuclear Safety Agency. Radon exposure and health. Australian Radiation Protection and Nuclear Safety Agency. https://www.arpansa.gov.au/understanding-radiation/radiation-sources/more-radiation-sources/radonhttps://www.arpansa.gov.au/understanding-radiation/radiation-sources/more-radiation-sources/radon. Published 2021. Accessed August 23, 2021.

41. Ministry of Health NZ. Radon (radioactive gas). Ministry of Health NZ. https://www.health.govt.nz/your-health/healthy-living/environmental-health/

radiation-environment/radon-radioactive-gas. Published 2013. Accessed August 23, 2021.

42. Stöppler M. Radon (A Citizen's Guide to Radon). MedicineNet. https://www.medicinenet.com/radon_symptoms_poisoning_tests_cancer_causes/article.htm. Published 2021. Accessed August 23, 2021.

43. Zeeb H. International Radon Project: Survey on Guidelines, Programmes and Activities. WHO. https://www.who.int/ionizing_radiation/env/radon/IRP_Survey_on_Radon.pdf. Published 2007. Accessed August 23, 2021.

44. Defarge N, Spiroux de Vendômois J, Séralini G. Toxicity of formulants and heavy metals in glyphosate-based herbicides and other pesticides. *Toxicol Rep*. 2018;5:156-163. doi:10.1016/j.toxrep.2017.12.025

45. Mesnage R, Defarge N, Spiroux de Vendômois J, Séralini G. Potential toxic effects of glyphosate and its commercial formulations below regulatory limits. *Food and Chemical Toxicology*. 2015;84:133-153. doi:10.1016/j.fct.2015.08.012

46. Schinasi L, Leon M. Non-Hodgkin Lymphoma and Occupational Exposure to Agricultural Pesticide Chemical Groups and Active Ingredients: A Systematic Review and Meta-Analysis. *Int J Environ Res Public Health*. 2014;11(4):4449-4527. doi:10.3390/ijerph110404449

47. Terry K, Karageorgi S, Shvetsov Y et al. Genital Powder Use and Risk of Ovarian Cancer: A Pooled Analysis of 8,525 Cases and 9,859 Controls. *Cancer Prevention Research*. 2013;6(8):811-821. doi:10.1158/1940-6207.capr-13-0037

48. National Toxicology Program. Report on Carcinogens, Fourteenth Edition Trichloroethylene. National Toxicology Program. https://ntp.niehs.nih.gov/ntp/roc/content/profiles/trichloroethylene.pdf. Published 2016. Accessed August 23, 2021.

49. Guyton K, Hogan K, Scott C et al. Human Health Effects of Tetrachloroethylene: Key Findings and Scientific Issues. *Environ Health Perspect*. 2014;122(4):325-334. doi:10.1289/ehp.1307359

50. Dinwiddie M, Terry P, Chen J. Recent Evidence Regarding Triclosan and Cancer Risk. *Int J Environ Res Public Health*. 2014;11(2):2209-2217. doi:10.3390/ijerph110202209

51. Lee H, Hwang K, Nam K, Kim H, Choi K. Progression of Breast Cancer Cells Was Enhanced by Endocrine-Disrupting Chemicals, Triclosan and Octylphenol, via an Estrogen Receptor-Dependent Signaling Pathway in Cellular and Mouse Xenograft Models. *Chem Res Toxicol*. 2014;27(5):834-842. doi:10.1021/tx5000156

52. Environmental Protection Agency. Volatile Organic Compounds' Impact on Indoor Air Quality | US EPA. Environmental Protection Agency. https://www.epa.gov/indoor-air-quality-iaq/volatile-organic-compounds-impact-indoor-air-quality. Published 2021. Accessed August 23, 2021.

53. Genuis S, Birkholz D, Rodushkin I, Beesoon S. Blood, Urine, and Sweat (BUS) Study: Monitoring and Elimination of Bioaccumulated Toxic Elements. *Arch Environ Contam Toxicol*. 2010;61(2):344-357. doi:10.1007/s00244-010-9611-5

54. Fillon M. Examining the Link Between Hair Chemicals and Cancer. *JNCI: Journal of the National Cancer Institute*. 2017;109(9). doi:10.1093/jnci/djx202

55. Zhang Y, Birmann B, Han J et al. Personal use of permanent hair dyes and cancer risk and mortality in US women: prospective cohort study. *BMJ*. 2020;370:m2942.

doi:10.1136/bmj.m2942

56. Bray K, Smith G. Should I use box dye to colour my hair at home? | CHOICE. CHOICE. https://www.choice.com.au/health-and-body/beauty-and-personal-care/hair-care-and-removal/articles/chemicals-in-hair-dye. Published 2020. Accessed August 23, 2021.

57. de Rapper S, Kamatou G, Viljoen A, van Vuuren S. The In Vitro Antimicrobial Activity of Lavandula angustifolia Essential Oil in Combination with Other Aroma-Therapeutic Oils. *Evidence-Based Complementary and Alternative Medicine*. 2013;2013:852049. doi:10.1155/2013/852049

58. Peckham S, Awofeso N. Water Fluoridation: A Critical Review of the Physiological Effects of Ingested Fluoride as a Public Health Intervention. *The Scientific World Journal*. 2014;2014:293019. doi:10.1155/2014/293019

59. Jeremy D. The 9 Dangers of Fluoride in Toothpaste. Holistic Dental Institute. https://holisticdentalinstitute.com/dangers-of-fluoride-in-toothpaste/. Published 2018. Accessed August 24, 2021.

60. Goschorska M, Baranowska-Bosiacka I, Gutowska I, Metryka E, Skórka-Majewicz M, Chlubek D. Potential Role of Fluoride in the Etiopathogenesis of Alzheimer's Disease. *Int J Mol Sci*. 2018;19(12):E3965. doi:10.3390/ijms19123965

61. Colgate. Pediatric Guidelines For Using Toothpaste In Young Children. Colgate. https://www.colgate.com/en-us/oral-health/life-stages/infant-kids/pediatric-guidelines-for-using-toothpaste-in-young-children-0614. Published 2021. Accessed August 24, 2021.

62. Steinemann A. Fragranced consumer products: exposures and effects from emissions. *Air Quality, Atmosphere & Health*. 2016;9(8):861-866. doi:10.1007/s11869-016-0442-z

63. South Carolina State University. Frequent use of certain candles produces unwanted chemicals. South Carolina State University. http://www.scsu.edu/news_article.aspx?news_id=832. Published 2009. Accessed August 24, 2021.

64. Jilla A, Kura B. Particulate Matter and Carbon Monoxide Emission Factors from Incense Burning. *Environment Pollution and Climate Change*. 2017;1(4). doi:10.4172/2573-458x.1000140

65. Bijlsma N. *Healthy Home Healthy Family*. 3rd ed. Warrandyte, VIC: Red Planet Print Management; 2018.

66. Carson C, Hammer K, Riley T. Melaleuca alternifolia (Tea Tree) Oil: a Review of Antimicrobial and Other Medicinal Properties. *Clin Microbiol Rev*. 2006;19(1):50-62. doi:10.1128/cmr.19.1.50-62.2006

67. Nazzaro F, Fratianni F, Coppola R, De Feo V. Essential Oils and Antifungal Activity. *Pharmaceuticals*. 2017;10(4):86. doi:10.3390/ph10040086

68. DailyHealthPost. Toxic Dishwasher Capsules are Loaded With Chemicals That Cause Severe Respiratory Issues and Cancer. DailyHealthPost. https://dailyhealthpost.com/toxic-dishwasher-capsules/. Published 2016. Accessed August 24, 2021.

69. Chen M, Chang C, Tao L, Lu C. Residential Exposure to Pesticide During Childhood and Childhood Cancers: A Meta-Analysis. *Pediatrics*. 2015;136(4):719-729. doi:10.1542/peds.2015-0006

70. US Occupational Safety and Health Administration. Methylene Chloride. US Occupational Safety and Health Administration. https://www.osha.gov/methylene-chloride. Accessed August 24, 2021.

71. Prabuseenivasan S, Jayakumar M, Ignacimuthu S. In vitro antibacterial activity of some plant essential oils. *BMC Complement Altern Med*. 2006;6(1). doi:10.1186/1472-6882-6-39

72. The Sydney Morning Herald. Poison blanket recall. The Sydney Morning Herald. https://www.smh.com.au/national/poison-blanket-recall-20070823-gdqxcx.html. Published 2007. Accessed August 24, 2021.

73. Duke University Pratt School of Engineering. How does the Duke University Foam Project work? | Superfund Analytical Chemistry Core. Duke University Pratt School of Engineering. http://foam.pratt.duke.edu/. Accessed August 24, 2021.

74. Australian Wool Product Testing Authority. Product Testing Fees Price List Structure. Australian Wool Product Testing Authority. https://awtaproducttesting.com.au/index.php/component/edocman/fees-list-2020-21. Published 2020. Accessed August 24, 2021.

75. Medical Daily. 9 Toxic Chemicals Found In Furniture: Is Your Home A Hazard Zone?. Medical Daily. https://www.medicaldaily.com/9-toxic-chemicals-found-furniture-your-home-hazard-zone-256572. Published 2013. Accessed August 24, 2021.

76. Arnaud C. The chemical reactions taking place in your swimming pool. Chemical and Engineering News. https://cen.acs.org/articles/94/i31/chemical-reactions-taking-place-swimming.html. Published 2016. Accessed August 24, 2021.

77. Villanueva C, Cantor K, Grimalt J et al. Bladder Cancer and Exposure to Water Disinfection By-Products through Ingestion, Bathing, Showering, and Swimming in Pools. *Am J Epidemiol*. 2006;165(2):148-156. doi:10.1093/aje/kwj364

78. Plant Life Balance. The Simple Science. Plant Life Balance. https://plantlifebalance.com.au/the-science/. Published 2020. Accessed August 24, 2021.

79. Havas M. When theory and observation collide: Can non-ionizing radiation cause cancer?. *Environmental Pollution*. 2017;221:501-505. doi:10.1016/j.envpol.2016.10.018

80. Miller A, Morgan L, Udasin I, Davis D. Cancer epidemiology update, following the 2011 IARC evaluation of radiofrequency electromagnetic fields (Monograph 102). *Environ Res*. 2018;167:673-683. doi:10.1016/j.envres.2018.06.043

81. Hertsgaard M, Dowie M. How Big Wireless Made Us Think That Cell Phones Are Safe: A Special Investigation. The Nation. https://www.thenation.com/article/how-big-wireless-made-us-think-that-cell-phones-are-safe-a-special-investigation/. Published 2018. Accessed August 24, 2021.

82. Al-Bayyari N. The effect of cell phone usage on semen quality and fertility among Jordanian males. *Middle East Fertil Soc J*. 2017;22(3):178-182. doi:10.1016/j.mefs.2017.03.006

83. Wall S, Wang Z, Kendig T, Dobraca D, Lipsett M. Real-world cell phone radiofrequency electromagnetic field exposures. *Environ Res*. 2019;171:581-592. doi:10.1016/j.envres.2018.09.015

84. Environmental Working Group. EWG Skin Deep® | What is BHA. Environmental Working Group. https://www.ewg.org/skindeep/ingredients/700740-bha/. Published 2021. Accessed August 24, 2021.

85. Bayer Global. Bayer Provides Update on Path to Closure of Roundup™ Litigation. Bayer Global. https://www.media.bayer.com/baynews/baynews.nsf/id/Bayer-Provides-Update-on-Path-to-Closure-of-Roundup-Litigation. Published 2021. Accessed August 24, 2021.

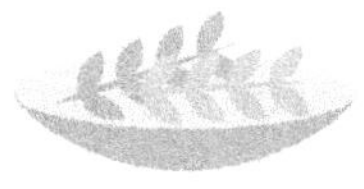

Chapter 7

Helpful nutritional supplements

'If we could give every individual the right amount of nourishment and exercise, not too little and not too much, we would have the safest way to health.'

– **Hippocrates**

Why should you consider taking supplements?

That's a good question. As a naturopath, I'd prefer that people use food for their nutrients wherever possible. Foods contain many different nutrients that work best together. But there are good reasons why a supplement can be useful:

- You might not like the foods containing the nutrients you need.
- The side-effects of cancer treatments, such as nausea, vomiting, changes in taste and smell, **mucositis**, constipation and diarrhoea, make eating unappealing and your body might absorb fewer nutrients if your gut has been badly affected.
- The quality of food isn't particularly good. Modern farming methods produce foods with fewer nutrients.[1] They may be

picked too early, before some nutrients peak. Some plants have been bred to produce increased yields, sacrificing nutrient quality.

- Soil quality has declined, so nowadays plants absorb fewer nutrients than they used to.[2]
- You might need higher amounts of a particular nutrient than it's feasible to get from food.

Not all supplements are created equal, though. Sadly, many of those available contain poor quality ingredients. For example, did you know that most vitamin C is created in factories, rather than being sourced from plants, and 85–95% is manufactured in China?[3] In some cases, they don't contain absorbable forms or therapeutic doses. Also, many vitamin supplements contain either synthetic forms of the vitamin, which can be detrimental to your health, or the wrong form of the vitamin, which your body can't absorb well.

The research, on vitamin supplements particularly, is difficult to interpret. Generally, the form of the supplement used isn't specified and sometimes dietary and supplement use is grouped together. We know that vitamins in food are beneficial but it isn't easy to differentiate between benefits you get from food and benefits from supplements. For example, if someone taking part in a study of vitamin C is also consuming a lot of foods containing high levels of vitamin C, it is difficult for the researchers to distinguish between the effects of the vitamin supplement and the foods. Wherever possible, I've used studies that treat them separately, but usually people eat normally alongside the supplements being researched and this can affect the outcomes.

To add to the confusion, some nutrients (vitamins, minerals and other dietary supplements) can interact with your prescribed medications, some beneficially but some not. Although the interactions are included here, it's impossible to ensure that every medication is listed. New drugs come to market all the time, and new research may find new interactions with existing drugs.

I strongly recommend you consult a naturopath, a nutritionist, a pharmacist or an integrative doctor before taking any supplements. They can check the interactions with your medications and ensure that the correct dosage is prescribed for your needs. They can also access high quality products that are restricted to natural medicine practitioners.

The antioxidant controversy

A number of the supplements that I cover in this chapter have antioxidant properties:

- vitamin A
- vitamin C
- vitamin D
- vitamin E
- co-enzyme Q10 (CoQ10)
- glutamine
- N-acetyl cysteine (NAC)
- melatonin
- fish oils (Omega 3 fatty acids)
- selenium
- zinc.

There is much debate amongst oncologists about whether antioxidants interfere with chemo and radiation therapy. Some researchers say that radiation and chemo drugs act by producing free radicals that kill cancer cells. From that, they theorise that taking antioxidants, and so neutralising the free radicals, would interfere with chemo and radiation. Others argue that chemo and radiation attack cancer cells by causing **mutations** in their **DNA** that cause **apoptosis**. Those **mutations** usually occur when cells divide. Since chemo and radiation generally create a lot of free radicals, those free radicals slow down the rate of division. That makes it more difficult for the treatments to work. By mopping up the free radicals, antioxidants may actually increase the effectiveness of chemo and radiation because they help to remove the barriers to cell division.

A **systematic review** conducted in 2011 explains the arguments on both sides and looked at some useful studies on glutathione, Vitamin E and NAC, but didn't reach a definitive conclusion.[4]

One clear outcome is that smokers who take beta (β)-carotene (a type of vitamin A) or alpha (α)-tocopherol (a type of vitamin E) whilst going through chemo and/or radiation therapy for head and neck cancers have significantly worse outcomes than non-smokers.[5]

The controversy hasn't been resolved yet. In a 2015 **systematic review**, some antioxidants were very positive, helping both survival and side-effects, whilst others, although they helped with side-effects, didn't affect survival rates.[5]

For safety, skip antioxidant supplements for a week before treatment and for a week afterwards. This should ensure that they're not in your system when the treatment is doing its work but will help mop up the free radicals afterwards and help with any side-effects.

Vitamin A

Vitamin A, like some other vitamins, comes in different forms.

The type found in animal proteins is ready for the body to use – often referred to as 'pre-formed'. Most of it is retinol. Pre-formed vitamin A is fat-soluble, so your body can store it.[6] This means it can potentially build up in the body and become toxic.

Vitamin A in colourful vegetables and fruit are in the form of carotenoids, and these must be converted before the body can use them. They're often known as 'pro-vitamin A'. There are various classes of carotenoids and they work together in the body to provide health benefits. Too much pro-vitamin A can turn your skin yellow but can't cause toxicity. The best known form in supplements is β-carotene.

Vitamin A is important for a number of functions in the body, including:

- Cancer prevention – it helps induce **apoptosis**, boosts immunity by activating **B** and **T** cells (white blood cells) and reduces infection risk.
- Skin – it maintains integrity of skin and mucous membranes, so it helps with healing after surgery.
- Blood – it's needed for development of red blood cells. If you have anaemia after treatment, this is crucial: iron and Vitamin A work more effectively together to treat anaemia.

- Antioxidant – it's a powerful antioxidant. Cancer treatments generate high levels of free radicals, which antioxidants neutralise.

There's been concern over vitamin A supplementation since the CARET trial in 2004[7], which showed that synthetic β-carotene significantly increased the lung cancer incidence in female smokers and those who'd been exposed to asbestos at work. Those who'd stopped smoking before the trial had no increased risk. β-carotene from fruit and vegetables lowers cancer risk, but this may be connected with other nutrients in them, which are protective.[8]

However, in another trial, patients with head and neck cancer (60%) or with lung cancer (40%), most of whom were previous or current smokers, were given supplements of a megadose of vitamin A and/or a regular dose of NAC. There was no significant difference in overall survival between the groups that received the supplements and those that didn't.[9]

In 2017, Cancer Therapy Advisor, a website designed for oncologists, concluded that supplementation with vitamin A doesn't reduce the effectiveness of chemotherapy and was unlikely to harm most patients.[10]

There's evidence that supplemental vitamin A increases chemo effectiveness for chronic myelogenous leukaemia.[11]

After removal of polyps, a precursor to bowel cancer, vitamin A plus vitamins C and E, selenium and zinc reduced the risk of recurrence by 39%.[12]

Bladder cancer patients were treated with immunotherapy plus either a multivitamin, or a multivitamin plus megadoses of vitamins A, B6, C, E and zinc. The recurrence rate after 5 years was 91% in the first group but 41% in the megadose group.[13]

After surgery for stage I non-small cell lung cancer (**NSLC**), patients were given either megadoses of retinol palmitate (a form of vitamin A) or nothing for 12 months. After almost 4 years, the group given vitamin A had a lower rate of recurrence or new primary tumours than the **control group**.[14]

This isn't a complete list of all the research on vitamin A and cancer. However in all the research I've seen, except in the case of smokers taking β-carotene supplements, cancer survival has either been improved or not affected, and treatment side-effects have been reduced. So if you aren't eating enough fruit and vegetables, supplementing may be helpful.

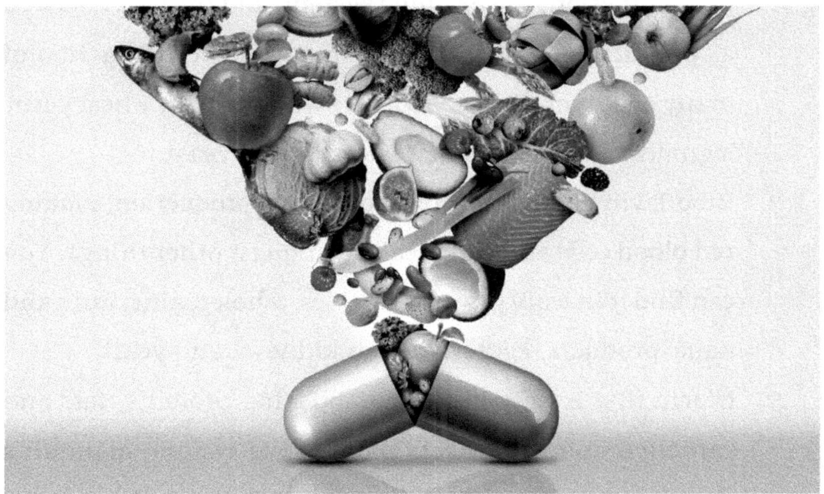

Dosage

Stick to α- and β-carotene, which aren't stored in the body. Up to 7 **mg** per day is considered safe.[15]

Interactions, contraindications and side-effects

Vitamin A reduces the effectiveness of 5-fluorouracil, a chemotherapy drug, so it shouldn't be used during chemo.

Ideally, during chemo it should be taken under the supervision of a healthcare practitioner.[16]

B vitamins

B vitamins are water-soluble, so you need a constant supply because most of them can't be stored. Each is dependent on others in the group to carry out their functions, most of which are related to energy production. So it's best to take a B complex if you need more. There are 7 vitamins in the B group:

1. Thiamine (B1) is involved in many body functions, including nerve function, the immune system, and the heart, as well as producing energy. It's also important for the action of many enzymes. Best sources are wholegrains, wheat germ, legumes, red meats, nuts, and brewer's yeast.
2. Riboflavin (B2) is important for energy production, making red blood cells and skin health, amongst other things. You can find it in leafy green vegetables, wholegrains, milk and dairy products, eggs, liver and kidneys, and yeast.
3. Niacin (B3) is needed for metabolising proteins, fats and carbohydrates. It protects the nervous system, maintains the digestive system and skin, helps **DNA** repair and may play a part in reducing skin cancers other than melanoma. Good sources include chicken, meat, eggs, fish, legumes, nuts and wholegrains.

4. Pantothenic acid (B5) is required for metabolising fats, proteins and carbohydrates. It's involved in antibody production, improves resistance to stress, and is needed for steroid hormone and vitamin D production. It's widely found but good sources are green vegetables, liver, heart and kidney, legumes, and eggs.
5. Pyridoxine (B6) is essential for metabolising proteins, fats and carbohydrates. It supports the nervous system, is involved in red blood cell production, inhibits **angiogenesis**, and sensitises cancer cells to chemo. It can be found in fish, beans, poultry, eggs, legumes, nuts and seeds.
6. Folate (B9) is used for **DNA** repair, cell growth, formation of red blood cells, and to make some neurotransmitters. It's probably best known for preventing neural tube defects in the foetus during pregnancy. Best sources are green leafy vegetables, legumes, liver, eggs and yeast.
7. Methylcobalamin (B12) is important for maintaining normal bone marrow, skin and the lining of the gut, and for healthy cell production. It's also used for metabolising fat, protein and carbohydrate. Good sources include any animal products, so vegans are at particular risk of deficiency.

Most vitamin B supplements use synthetic forms of the individual B vitamins. This can be a problem because some **genetic mutations** reduce the ability of the body to break down those synthetic forms. One group of **mutations** is on the **MTHFR gene**, which controls production of an enzyme that breaks down folic acid, the synthetic form of folate, causing high levels of serum folate. About 55% of the population have some form of **mutation** on this **gene.**[17] This is particularly relevant for cancer patients because some cancers have been linked to these **mutations.**[18] All bread-making flour except organic flour in Australia has been fortified with folic acid since 2009.

Activated B complex contains forms of B vitamins in the form the body can use without any, or much, conversion. They're better for everyone, even those without **MTHFR mutations**, because they're easier for the body to absorb.[17] They're available from naturopaths, good chemists or health food shops.

Taking B vitamin supplements isn't risk-free and should only be done under professional supervision. There's conflicting evidence for cancer risk with many B vitamins.

Thiamine (B1) supplementation is linked to tumour growth in some cancers.[19, 20]

Riboflavin (B2) is associated with a reduced risk of bowel cancer[21] and high blood levels of riboflavin reduced breast cancer risk in pre-menopausal, but not post-menopausal, women.[22] These studies didn't differentiate between dietary and supplemental intake, though, and many of the foods containing riboflavin have anti-cancer properties. Riboflavin deficiency has been linked to a raised oesophageal cancer risk, increases in cervical dysplasia, the precursor to cervical cancer, but the presence of riboflavin increases **DNA** damage when exposed to liver **carcinogens.**[23]

Niacinamide, a form of niacin (B3), can be useful in cream form for breast cancer patients. Some chemo can cause dry, itchy skin and niacinamide cream is protective for this.[24] Nicotinamide, another form of niacin, taken orally is effective for reducing rates of non-melanoma skin cancers in high-risk patients.[25]

Pyridoxine (B6) was studied in a very large **systematic review** and **meta-analysis** in which over 96,000 participants had some form of cancer. There was a significant relationship between higher levels of active pyridoxine (pyridoxal-5'-phosphate) in the blood and reduced cancer risk, particularly in cancers of the digestive tract. Dietary levels showed the risk reduction. However, when they examined dietary **and** supplement levels there was no reduction in risk.[26] Maybe the supplements included other B vitamins which increased the risk, or perhaps a synthetic form of pyridoxine was used and it wasn't well absorbed.

Folate (B9) has a narrow dosage range that's protective. For example, a **meta-analysis** found that a dose of 200–320 **microgram**s a day resulted in a lower risk of breast cancer, but doses over 400 **microgram**s a day increased the risk significantly.[27] High levels of circulating folate can increase the risk of breast cancer in women with the BRCA **mutations.**[28] This is very likely to be because of the **MTHFR gene mutations** mentioned above. Dietary folate reduces bowel cancer by 40–60%, with lesser protection for cancers of the throat, oesophagus, stomach, pancreas, cervix, ovary, lung, leukaemia and neuroblastoma.[29] Large doses of supplemental folic acid increase the growth of existing tumours.[29] Since folic acid is routinely added to bread-making flour and cereals in many industrialised countries, this raises significant concerns for eating bread and cereals. No tests on supplements of the activated form of folate have been conducted to date.

Methylcobalamin (B12), folate (B9) and pyridoxine (B6) work closely together and most studies relating to methylcobalamin's effects on cancer include folate and pyridoxine. Ten years use of B complex supplements containing higher doses of pyridoxine and methylcobalamin increased lung cancer risk in men, particularly in smokers. There was no such link in women, though.[30]

Given the potential risks of vitamin B supplements, I'd recommend you get a good supply of the dietary sources listed above, unless you're being supervised by a qualified person. Stress increases the need for B vitamins, though, so you would probably benefit. If you choose to take a supplement, make sure that it contains the activated forms of the B vitamins.

Vitamin C

Vitamin C is probably the best-known of the vitamins. It's important for many different functions, including:

- supporting the immune system
- improving wound healing
- increasing iron absorption
- protecting against free radicals: at normal doses it's a powerful antioxidant
- helping maintain bones, teeth and cartilage
- formation of collagen
- helping to make some hormones.

We need about 100–200 **mg** per day to avoid scurvy, but low levels of vitamin C are common, even in industrialised countries.

In the United States, vitamin C deficiency is the fourth leading nutrient deficiency.[31]

Cancer patients have low levels of vitamin C in their bodies compared with healthy people.[32] This isn't surprising: anyone under stress, physical or mental, produces more free radicals, so vitamin C is depleted more quickly.

Vitamin C is helpful after surgery, as it speeds up wound healing time.[31]

Methotrexate is often used in chemo but side-effects include kidney and liver damage. In a laboratory study, vitamin C helped methotrexate work more effectively, so that lower doses killed liver cancer cells. Lower doses of methotrexate could help reduce side-effects.[33]

High doses of oral vitamin C aren't absorbed well but intravenous infusions work effectively. At the high doses used, the effects are pro-oxidant, not antioxidant. A number of human trials show that infusions increase some chemo's effectiveness and help reduce its side-effects.[34, 35] A number of case reports show cancers going into remission after intravenous vitamin C.[36, 35]

Intravenous vitamin C has also been shown to improve quality of life in terminal cancer patients[37], to prolong their lives[38, 39], and to reduce fatigue, pain, nausea, insomnia, depression and dizziness in chemo patients.[40] No major side-effects were reported.

Intravenous vitamin C shouldn't be used by anyone who has glucose-6-phosphate deficiency, a **genetic** enzyme deficiency that's common in people of African, Asian and Mediterranean descent, because it can cause blood clots.[41]

You can't get intravenous vitamin C treatment from mainstream doctors in Australia, as it isn't covered by Medicare, but it's available at Integrative Medicine centres and a partial refund may be available from private health insurers.

Laboratory testing shows that Vitamin C can increase the rate of growth of some blood cancers.[42-44]

A study was conducted on smokers to learn the effects of vitamin C on one of the risk factors for tobacco-related cancers. They used doses of 1, 2 or 4 **g** per day but there was no response.[45] Smokers need large amounts of vitamin C to counter the free radicals produced by tobacco, so it's possible that all of it was used by the body for that purpose.

If you're currently having chemo or radiotherapy, it would be unwise to take vitamin C without professional supervision. Individual chemo drugs may react with it, and it needs to be carefully timed with radiotherapy. If you've just had surgery and no other treatment is currently planned, vitamin C will help with healing. If you're post-treatment, it's a helpful addition to a healthy diet.

Dosage

500 **mg** to 3 **g** per day, divided into 3 doses. Higher doses cause laxative effects in some people, although others can tolerate them, particularly if they're low in vitamin C. If you take more than your body needs, it's simply excreted. If you find you're getting diarrhoea, reduce the dose.

Interactions, contraindications side-effects

Taken at the same time as beta-blockers, vitamin C could interfere with their action. Separate the doses of each by 2 hours to avoid this.[16]

Vitamin D

Vitamin D is important for many reasons, including:

- supporting the immune system
- preventing and treating chronic diseases
- assisting the nervous system
- strengthening the respiratory system
- protecting the heart
- building healthy bones and teeth
- healthy brain function, by influencing levels of hormones that affect social behaviour[46]
- supporting the digestive system and food absorption.

There are 2 dietary forms of vitamin D:

1. D3, also known as cholecalciferol, which comes from dairy, fish, eggs and meat
2. D2, also known as ergocalciferol, which is found in yeast and fungi that have been exposed to UV light.

Our main source of vitamin D is made by our own bodies, in response to sunlight. The amount of sunlight you need depends on your skin colour (darker skins make less vitamin D), where you live and the strength of the sun. It's best to avoid the middle of the day in summer, as the sun can be too strong and you could burn. Aim to get into the sun at about 10 am or 2 pm (11 am or 3 pm in Daylight Savings areas). In winter, midday is the best time for boosting vitamin D. If you're living in Australia, expose your arms, or an equivalent amount of skin, for the following periods.[47]

Location	Summer (10 am or 2 pm)	Winter (midday)
Cairns	6–7 minutes	7 minutes
Townsville	5–7 minutes	7 minutes
Brisbane	6–7 minutes	10 minutes
Perth	5–6 minutes	15 minutes
Sydney	6–8 minutes	15 minutes
Adelaide	5–7 minutes	20 minutes
Melbourne	6–8 minutes	25 minutes
Hobart	7–10 minutes	30 minutes

I'm not recommending you stay in the sun long enough to burn. Sun damage should be avoided, as it increases skin cancer risk. If your skin is very fair, stay outside only as long as your skin can tolerate before it burns.

Vitamin D deficiency is now very common in developed countries, probably because we've been told to cover up and use sunscreen before we even venture outside. According to the Australian Bureau of Statistics, about 23% of Australians are deficient. They define deficiency as having levels of less than 50 nmol/**litre** in the blood.[48] Most experts believe a level of 100–120 nmol/**litre** is needed to give significant protection against cancers of the breast, colon, pancreas, prostate, ovary and lungs.[49] To achieve that, you'd need a dietary intake of between 1,000 and 4,000 IU per day. That's a lot of salmon, which is the richest food source.

A number of **epidemiological studies** have found a reduced risk of cancers, especially prostate and bowel cancers, when sun exposure is higher.[50]

A large study showed that 1,500 **mg** of calcium together with 1,100 IU of vitamin D3 substantially reduced the risk of all cancers. One group in the study took just calcium but didn't have the same risk reduction.[51]

Vitamin D is a fat-soluble vitamin, so it can be stored in the body and overdosing can be toxic, although this only occurs with very high doses for a period of months and is very rare. When your body makes it, though, it only makes enough for its needs.[52] Before taking a supplement, have your vitamin D levels tested and only take a supplement if you're deficient. Many doctors will not order vitamin D tests unless they see a need. If yours refuses, a naturopath can order the test for you.

The most effective (and cheapest) way of getting sufficient vitamin D is from sunlight. However, a supplement is helpful if you can't get outside, or if you choose not to, and you're shown to be deficient.

Dosage

Use cholecalciferol, vitamin D3. To work out the dosage you need, use the following calculation.[49]

(75 – (your blood vitamin D level in nmol/**litre**)) divided by 0.7, then multiplied by 40 to get the IU level that your body needs

Get retested after 3 months and continue until your levels reach 100–120 nmol/**litre**.

Interactions, contraindications and side-effects

Cholecalciferol (vitamin D3) reduces the effectiveness of thioridazine, an anti-psychotic drug.[16]

Calcium channel blockers, such as Verapamil, are blocked by supplemental vitamin D.[16]

Vitamin E

Vitamin E comes in a number of forms. It's made up of 2 groups, each of which has 4 different types. These are:

1. Tocopherols: alpha tocopherol (α-tocopherol), beta tocopherol (β-tocopherol), gamma tocopherol (γ-tocopherol) and delta tocopherol (δ-tocopherol)
2. Tocotrienols: α-tocotrienol, β-tocotrienol, γ-tocotrienol and δ-tocotrienol.

Each works slightly differently. All forms are fat-soluble and antioxidant. The most common is α-tocopherol, which is the form most easily absorbed by the body.

Its functions in the body include:

- reducing inflammation
- lowering risk of blood clots, which are common in cancer patients
- helping the liver to detoxify
- involvement in immune function.

α-tocopherol is found naturally in high amounts in nuts, seeds, and sunflower and safflower seed oils, but green leafy vegetables also contain significant amounts. American diets are high in γ-tocopherol, which is mainly found in oils such as canola, soybean and corn, and also in nuts. Tocotrienols are mainly found in palm oil, but there are trace amounts in rice bran oil and wheat germ.

Dietary vitamin E reduces the risk of oesophageal cancer.[53] Some studies showed a reduction in risk of breast, prostate, lung and colon cancers, but others didn't find a link between dietary vitamin E and cancer, although most studied α-tocopherol. Results were much more promising where γ-tocopherol was used.[54]

α-tocopherol succinate

Most supplements contain synthetic forms of α-tocopherol, which are more stable and don't have any antioxidant properties.[55] One of them is α-tocopherol succinate, which has been extensively studied for anti-cancer effects, although human trials haven't been conducted yet. In large oral doses (800 IU per day) α-tocopherol succinate is absorbed into the bloodstream, although some is converted to α-tocopherol, which is antioxidant.[56] So where cancer cells have been used in testing, they should translate to human trials.

α-tocopheryl succinate improved breast cancer cells' sensitivity to doxorubicin, a common chemo drug, and reduced their ability to survive.[57] It stops breast cancer cells from growing, and it affects the **gene** governing production of a growth factor involved in **angiogenesis**.[58]

It also stopped the growth of melanoma cells in mice[59,] and, in a separate study, growth of malignant mesothelioma cells.[60]

For lung cancer cells, there was some reduction in growth but α-tocopheryl succinate didn't completely stop growth.[61]

The growth of colon cancer cells was inhibited by nearly 80%, with **apoptosis** occurring. It was non-toxic to normal cells.[62]

α-tocopheryl succinate caused prostate cancers in mice to shrink significantly, by about 70%.[63, 64] This may explain why people receiving long-term vitamin E supplements have a low incidence of prostate cancer.[65] In laboratory tests, **metastasis** of prostate cancer was reduced.[65]

α-tocopheryl succinate also has a protective effect in radiotherapy. In a mouse study, it protected them against lethal radiation doses. It also stimulated the bone marrow cells, reducing loss of platelets and **neutrophils** that radiation often causes.[66]

These results were only found with α-tocopherol succinate. α-tocopherol acetate, another commonly found synthetic form of vitamin E, didn't show the same effects.[67]

Tocotrienols

Because α-tocopherol is the most easily absorbed type of vitamin E, tocotrienols were mostly ignored by researchers until the 1980s. But they've been found to have powerful effects in the body, from anti-cancer to anti-inflammatory, while lowering cholesterol and protecting nerve tissue. They're able to enter cells easily and are much better absorbed into fatty tissues like the brain and the liver.[68]

Tocotrienols can stop **angiogenesis**, a process that is crucial for cancer growth.[69]

Human trials on tocotrienols have begun. One study of women with early oestrogen receptor positive breast cancers used tamoxifen, either with or without tocotrienols. After 5 years, the number of deaths was 60% lower in the group using tocotrienols. The incidence of recurrence was similarly reduced.[70]

Another trial involving pancreatic cancer patients used δ-tocotrienol before surgery to find out the effects of different doses on safety, blood levels of the compound, and whether it caused **apoptosis** of the cancer cells. There were no adverse effects. Blood levels were high enough to match the effectiveness in pre-clinical trials, and after surgery a significant level of **apoptosis** was found.[71] This was a Phase I trial, so it was quite small, but the results were very positive.

Numerous trials in animals and on human cancer cells show that tocotrienols are effective in reducing both cancer incidence and in treating existing cancers.[68, 72]

Dosage

If taking α-tocopheryl succinate: 400 mg per day[73]

If taking tocotrienols: ideally use delta and gamma tocotrienols, about 160 mg per day.[73]

Interactions, contraindications and side-effects

Tocopheryl succinate has a protective effect on bone marrow, so it shouldn't be used during blood cancer treatment.[66]

Vitamin E is an antioxidant vitamin, so some oncologists may veto its use during chemo. However, there's no conclusive evidence that it interferes with chemo drugs.[16]

High doses of vitamin E can increase the effects of anticoagulants, such as warfarin. If you're taking anticoagulants, ensure that this is carefully monitored.[16]

Stop taking vitamin E one week prior to surgery.

Vitamin K

Vitamin K comes in 3 forms:

1. Vitamin K1, also known as phylloquinone, is found in green leafy vegetables, mostly in the green outer leaves, with lower amounts in vegetable oils like soybean and olive oils.
2. Vitamin K2, also known as menaquinone, is commonly found in fermented foods like cheese, curds and natto (a Japanese fermented soybean product). Bacteria in the colon produce some but, because K2 is absorbed in the small intestine, any produced in the colon may not be absorbed.
3. Vitamin K3, or menadione, is a synthetic form of vitamin K that's often added to animal feeds. It is found in meats and the body converts it into K2 so it can be absorbed.

As it's a fat-soluble vitamin, eat it with oil to improve absorption. It isn't stored in large amounts in the body and needs regular top-ups from the diet. The body is able to recycle a small amount. It's easier to absorb vitamin K from supplements rather than food.

It's important for blood clotting. Without it, you bleed longer. It's also needed for bone health, because it helps your body absorb calcium. Sufficient vitamin K reduces risk of heart disease by 22% and reduces all-cause mortality by 15%.[74]

Vitamin K2 increases **apoptosis** in cancer cells, making it valuable in fighting cancer. It's effective at killing both human liver and colon cancer cells implanted in animals, and, together with sorafenib, a chemo drug, was more effective in treating liver cancer than the drug alone.[75]

In laboratory studies, vitamin K2 had an anticancer effect on cancer cells of the liver, bile duct, bowel, ovaries and pancreas, and leukaemia.[75]

In a human study, patients with acute myeloid leukaemia following myelodysplasia, where immature blood cells in the bone marrow don't mature properly, were treated with vitamin K2. Fewer immature cells were produced, along with higher **neutrophils.**[75]

In several other studies patients at high risk of contracting liver cancer had a reduced risk after being treated with vitamin K2.[75]

Since vitamins K1 and K2 do not appear to be toxic, even at high doses, a vitamin K2 supplement in particular would be helpful to support cancer treatment.

Dosage

Recommended dosage is 20 mg per day for anti-cancer effects.[73]

Interactions, contraindications and side-effects

Do not take with anticoagulant medications such as warfarin and heparin.[73]

Calcium

It's well known that calcium is important for bones but it has other uses including:

- muscle contraction
- nerve function
- blood clotting
- communication between cells
- activating some enzymes
- maintaining a regular heartbeat.
- helping to reduce the risks of some cancers.

If you're on hormonal treatments, you're at higher risk of osteoporosis, so I would encourage you to get a DEXA scan to measure your bone density every 1–2 years. If your bone density is reduced, calcium supplements (with vitamin D) are essential.

People with bowel polyps are at higher risk of developing bowel cancer. In a study of people who'd recently had polyps removed, 1200 **mg** of elemental calcium (3 **g** of calcium carbonate) daily reduced the risk of further polyps by about 20%.[76] Those with a lower body mass index (**BMI**) have a better response to calcium supplementation.[77] A recent study, though, showed that those taking calcium with a history of serrated sessile polyps, particularly in women and current smokers, significantly increased the risk of developing further polyps of this type. The researchers suggested that this group should avoid using calcium supplements.[78]

Another trial looked at the effects of 1,400–1,500 **mg** of calcium daily (either calcium citrate or calcium carbonate) on cancer incidence generally, over a period of 4 years. It reduced the frequency of non-skin cancers by almost half.[51] However, a **meta-analysis** found that using 400 **mg** or more of calcium daily had no effects on the incidence of cancers.[79] This suggests you need a higher dose to reduce cancer risk.

Men given 1200 **mg** of calcium for 4 years had almost half the rate of prostate cancer after 6 years, 2 years after they stopped taking it, than men taking a **placebo**. The effects were reduced after 10 years.[80]

There is growing evidence that calcium supplements, taken alone, can raise heart disease risk and, to a lesser extent, stroke. They can also raise blood pressure. This doesn't apply to dietary calcium. A high intake of calcium-rich foods causes a reduction in calcium absorption in the intestines and an increase in the amount excreted via the kidneys. It's thought that supplements are absorbed differently from food.[81]

Taking calcium with magnesium supplements in a calcium/magnesium ratio of 1.7 or above is associated with reduced risks of both total mortality and cardiovascular mortality.[82] This is because calcium and magnesium have opposing effects in many things, including **apoptosis**, **angiogenesis**, **DNA** repair and other factors involved in cancer development and growth.[82]

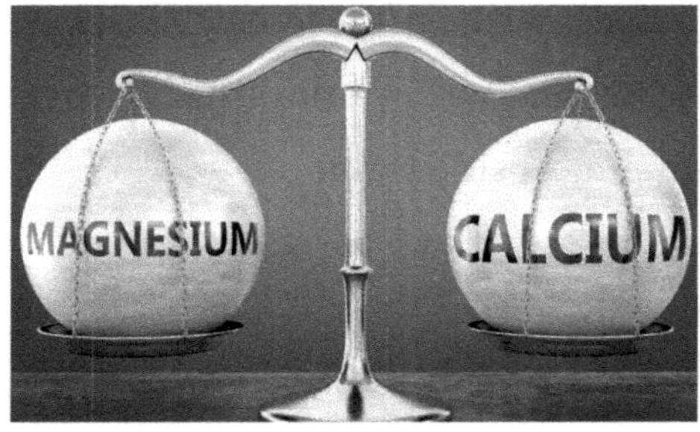

Dosage

Different calcium supplements are available using differing types of calcium salts. Calcium carbonate is the commonest, and cheapest, form. However, if you have low stomach acid it's hard to absorb because it needs acid to break it down.[83] As we age, we tend to produce less stomach acid. Many people take antacid medications, some of which are designed to reduce the production of stomach acid. I recommend you avoid calcium carbonate supplements. If you choose to use them, take them with food because the body produces more stomach acid when you eat.

Better forms are calcium citrate or calcium malate. Although they both contain lower amounts of elemental calcium, both are absorbed more easily.[83]

Avoid calcium supplements made from dolomite or bone, as they may contain heavy metals such as lead.

If you take calcium supplements, ensure you take a magnesium supplement too, in the ratio of 1.7 **mg** of calcium to each milligram of magnesium.

My personal preference is for calcium supplements made from powdered algae. These contain other trace minerals, including magnesium, iodine, selenium, strontium and boron, all in the proportions the body needs. Because they're effectively a foodstuff, they're easier to absorb. You can find them in health food stores, both in powder and capsule form.

I recommend a dose of at least 1,200 **mg** per day, preferably divided into 2 doses.

Interactions, contraindications and side-effects

Calcium supplements can cause mild gastro-intestinal problems, such as abdominal pain, wind and constipation.

If blood tests show you have too much or too little phosphate, calcium supplements should be used under medical supervision, so that it can be monitored. Calcium and phosphate must be kept in balance.

If you're taking thyroid hormone replacement medication, separate it from calcium supplements by 4 hours.

Avoid taking calcium supplements if your blood calcium levels are high, such as in sarcoidosis or parathyroid disorders.

Poor kidney function can result in too much calcium in the blood if taking calcium supplements, so you'll need regular blood tests.

Thiazide diuretics can increase blood calcium levels, so this should be monitored if you take supplements.

Calcium can interact with some antibiotics, especially quinolones and tetracyclines. Avoid taking them together. Separate calcium from quinolones by an hour, either before or after, and take calcium either 2 hours before or 4 hours after tetracyclines.

Separate beta-blockers by 2 hours from calcium.

Take bisphosphonate medications for bone loss 30 minutes before calcium or later in the day.

If you're taking lithium, calcium may already be raised, so get calcium levels checked before taking supplements.

Co-enzyme Q10 (CoQ10)

CoQ10 is made by the body and stored in the mitochondria, where energy is produced. It's needed to make **ATP**, the storage form of energy in the body, so it's found in almost every cell in the human body and is essential for our health. It's particularly important in parts of the body needing high energy levels, especially the heart, liver, kidneys and lungs. We produce less as we age and it's been suggested that this may be one of the causes of ageing.

It's found in these foods:

- liver, kidney and heart
- pork, chicken and beef, especially in the leg meat
- oily fish, such as salmon, sardines, trout, mackerel and herring
- broccoli, cauliflower and spinach
- strawberries and oranges
- legumes, such as soybeans, lentils and peanuts
- pistachios and sesame seeds.

CoQ10 benefits us in a number of ways by helping to:

- treat heart failure
- reduce migraine incidence
- increase power and reduce fatigue during exercise
- improve blood sugar levels and increase insulin sensitivity
- protect the brain from oxidative damage
- reduce inflammation and oxidative damage in the lungs, helping prevent lung disease.[84]

CoQ10 is an antioxidant, so it reduces oxidative damage, which can cause cancers. Cancer patients' levels are low, especially in cancers of the pancreas, lung and breast, and in melanoma patients. In melanoma, low levels are also associated with **metastasis.**[85] High CoQ10 levels are associated with higher breast cancer risk in post-menopausal women[86], which suggests that there's a middle range that's protective.

As well as affecting melanoma risk, melanoma patients treated with recombinant interferon-alpha plus CoQ10 for 3 years had a significantly reduced recurrence rate, compared with those treated with recombinant interferon-alpha alone.[87]

Liver cancer patients given 300 **mg** per day of CoQ10 for 12 weeks after surgery had significantly reduced inflammatory markers (which are usually high after surgery). Higher CoQ10 levels resulted in lower levels of free radicals and higher levels of antioxidant enzymes.[88] Higher levels of inflammation and free radicals are associated with liver cancer progression, so this suggests CoQ10 treatment can help prevent progression.

The chemo drug doxorubicin (Adriamycin®) can reduce CoQ10 in the body and in high doses can damage the heart. Supplementing with 100–200 **mg** per day of CoQ10 can prevent that damage[89] and doesn't alter the effectiveness of doxorubicin.[90] Doxorubicin can also damage the kidneys, but CoQ10 protects them too.[91] Doxorubicin belongs to a family of chemo drugs called anthracyclines. Other anthracyclines will also affect the heart and kidneys, and CoQ10 can help to prevent this. Higher dosages of the drugs can be used when taking CoQ10 without these side-effects.

In an animal study of breast cancer, tamoxifen together with vitamins B2 and B3 and CoQ10 made the tamoxifen more effective.[92] In a human study of breast cancer patients taking tamoxifen with CoQ10, it reduced **angiogenesis**, which could contribute to reducing **metastasis**. There were also fewer inflammatory markers and other markers involved in cancer growth.[93]

Patients with various types of end-stage cancers received CoQ10 and a mixture of other antioxidants, including selenium, beta-carotene, folic acid and vitamin C, and were followed up until they died. Each had the median survival time for their particular type of cancer calculated at the start. For 76%, survival was longer than predicted. Five had particularly interesting case histories:

1. A 57 year old woman had a second breast cancer after having one breast removed. She had metastases in her ovaries, rectum and in the abdominal cavity. She wasn't offered any conventional treatment but was given the antioxidant therapy. She felt well and was active for 3 years until she died of a **metastasis** in her brain.
2. A 37 year old woman with breast cancer developed metastases in her pelvis, skull, bone marrow, and the **lymph** glands in her neck 4 years later. After chemo and radiation to her ovaries, she went into partial remission. About 29 months later she joined this study, and continued to live an active life, including continuing to work, until a few months before she died, almost 7 years later. Only about 10% of patients with stage 4 breast cancer like hers survive that long.
3. A 57 year old man had a kidney removed due to cancer but developed a **metastasis** in his liver. He joined the study a year later with a predicted survival time of 9 months but survived for 25 months.
4. A 47 year old man had an inoperable lung cancer with a lot of fluid collecting around his lungs. He wasn't given

therapy except regular drainage of the fluid. He was included in the study a month after diagnosis. For just over a year he continued to work and was fairly well. The fluid gradually disappeared without treatment. He then developed a **metastasis** in his brain and was given radiation treatment. He died about 6 months later, after surviving for 22 months. His predicted survival time when he entered the study was 9 months.

5. A 60 year old woman had pancreatic cancer with fast growing **metastasis** in her liver. She was included in the study a month after diagnosis but received no conventional treatment. Her predicted survival was 5 months but a year later she was still fully mobile and her liver wasn't enlarging. She survived 25 months.[93]

Since CoQ10 is involved in energy production, you'd expect it would alleviate fatigue in cancer patients. But a study showed it didn't help treatment-related fatigue in newly diagnosed breast cancer patients.[94]

Dosage

There's no recommended dose for CoQ10. In human studies, dosages have ranged from 90—390 mg per day.[95] I suggest starting with 100 mg and slowly increasing it to 300 mg per day. Don't exceed 600 mg per day.[73] If you experience dizziness, upper abdominal discomfort, diarrhoea or nausea, reduce the dose and/or take smaller doses 3 times a day

CoQ10 is fat-soluble, making it better absorbed with fat. So supplements should be taken with food. Take it with breakfast, as it can increase energy levels and may cause insomnia if taken at night.

Interactions, contraindications and side-effects

There's a theoretical possibility that CoQ10 could interfere with warfarin, although in a trial there was no significant effect. This effect may only exist in certain genetic types, so if you're taking warfarin, ensure you're carefully monitored.[16]

Glutamine

Glutamine is an amino acid, which are the building blocks of proteins. It's the most abundant amino acid in the human body. It's found in meat, poultry, fish, eggs, dairy products, beans and legumes, and vegetables like cabbage, Brussels sprouts, beetroot, carrots and green vegetables. Nuts and seeds are also a good source.

Generally speaking, the body makes all the glutamine it needs from proteins you eat, but glutamine can help with faster recovery after surgery or infections.

Glutamine is the main food source for cells lining the gut. Some immune cells use it as their main fuel source too. It also helps the liver with detoxification.

Glutamine helps prevent **mucositis**, a miserable condition resulting from destruction of cells in the gut by chemo and radiation. It results in ulceration, which can occur throughout the gut, from mouth to anus. It's very painful, with raw open sores in the mouth and throat, a sensation like sunburn throughout the gut, nausea and vomiting, and bowel irritation with either constipation or diarrhoea. Sometimes it results in bleeding, particularly in those with low platelets. The open sores can become infected, which can be serious when patients' immunity is reduced. Eating becomes very difficult, which causes muscle and weight loss.

Glutamine helps repair **mucositis** damage. This has been demonstrated in animal studies and in a small study on humans. Patients who suffered oral and throat **mucositis** on their first rounds of chemo were recruited before their next round. They received a suspension of 4 **g** of glutamine twice daily, which they used as a mouthwash then swallowed, from day one of chemo for 28 days or until any **mucositis** had healed. The severity and duration of **mucositis** in most of the participants was reduced. There were no signs of toxicity and it didn't cause any further drop in **neutrophils**. The study cited a number of other trials using intravenous glutamine instead of oral. These had no effect on **mucositis** but did help to prevent infections and reduced hospitalisation time. This suggests it's the physical presence of glutamine in the gut that reduces **mucositis**. They also quoted another study using a lower dose of oral glutamine, which had no effect on **mucositis**, suggesting it's dose-dependent.[96]

Another trial on head and neck cancer patients receiving chemo and radiation therapy found glutamine delayed **mucositis** onset and significantly reduced its severity.[97]

A **systematic review** studied the effect of glutamine on treatment complications for colorectal and colon cancers:

- One trial assessed oral glutamine's effects on patients with metastatic colorectal cancers. It found the intestinal lining was significantly improved, whereas in the **control group** it was damaged, and there was less **mucositis** in the stomach and small intestine.

- Another investigated oral glutamine's effects on peripheral neuropathy (nerve damage) caused by chemo in colorectal cancers, finding it significantly reduced the incidence and severity of neuropathy.
- Another evaluated oral glutamine as protection against chemo toxicity. It found oral glutamine prevented **mucositis** in the intestines and reduced diarrhoea. It also discovered a protective effect on the intestine's ability to absorb nutrients and against damage to the gut lining.
- Prevention of **mucositis** and neutropenia was found in another trial using large doses of glutamine.
- In a study of those receiving radiotherapy and chemo before surgery, large doses of glutamine didn't result in reduction of diarrhoea incidence or severity, and inflammatory markers were unchanged.
- Two studies using intravenous glutamine on patients undergoing surgery for colorectal cancers found the incidence of infections was significantly reduced and hospital stays were shorter.
- Those going through colorectal surgery often have reduced immune systems, making them susceptible to infections. So one trial evaluated the effects of intravenous glutamine on T-cell production. T-cells are white blood cells that directly kill bacteria, viruses and cancer cells. They found T-cell production increased and immunity was improved.

- Another small study of patients undergoing surgery reported that intravenous glutamine didn't reduce any of the usual complications. However, incidence of complications after surgery was 33.3% in the study group compared with 50% in the **control group**.[98]

A **systematic review** found 2 studies confirming the significant effects of glutamine on reducing chemo-induced neuropathy.[99]

A **meta-analysis** found that glutamine significantly reduced duration of chemo-induced diarrhoea but didn't affect its severity.[100]

Radiation treatment can be painful, often causing the treatment to be delayed, and scarring from it is often a problem. A study conducted on women with Stage I and II breast cancers undergoing radiation treatment following surgery and chemo found oral glutamine resulted in less pain, swelling and scarring, resulting in no delays to radiation therapy. Cosmetically, the glutamine group had excellent results, compared with fair to good for the **placebo** group. The researchers noted that glutathione levels were reduced in the tumour but increased in the rest of the body.[101] Glutamine is used by the body to make glutathione. High levels of glutathione in tumours reduce chemo and radiation effectiveness, so glutamine may decrease chemo and radiation resistance.

Patients with Stage IV stomach cancer fed a normal diet with a mixture of arginine (an amino acid), glutamine and omega 3s added had a significant improvement in short-term survival. In the first 3 months there were no deaths in the study group but 9 in the standard diet group, and there was a significant reduction in the first 6 months. Sadly, long-term survival in both groups was the same.[102]

There is debate over using glutamine during active cancers. Many tumours contain high levels of glutamine, which they can use to grow when glucose isn't available. Some can make glutamine themselves, whilst others use what's available from dietary and supplemental sources. It's difficult to make broad statements about which cancer types can use supplemental glutamine because it depends on the location of the cancer, the environment surrounding it, its particular subtype, and the patient's physiology and diet collectively.[103] So despite all of its potential for reducing side-effects, improving chemo and radiation resistance, and improving survival, it could theoretically encourage cancer growth. If you want to use it, I strongly encourage you to discuss with your oncologist whether you could benefit from it or not.

Once you've completed your treatment, glutamine may help repair the damage to your gut.

Dosage

20–30 **g** per day, with supplementation continuing for at least 5 days.[104, 73] Take half the dose twice a day. Swish the solution around your mouth before swallowing it.

Glutamine is most beneficial during treatment if taken in conjunction with a low carbohydrate diet, and glutamine and glucose levels should be carefully monitored.[105]

Interactions, contraindications and side-effects

In some people, doses above 300 mg can cause mania, a psychiatric disorder typically with excessive physical activity, rapidly changing ideas and impulsive behaviour.[73] If you're affected, stop taking it.

If you have kidney disease don't take glutamine.[73]

Those with liver problems shouldn't take glutamine.[106]

If you're sensitive to MSG, you may also be sensitive to glutamine, as it's converted to glutamate in the body.[106]

If you're prone to seizures, glutamine may increase their occurrence, and it may affect medications designed to prevent seizures.[106]

Glutamine makes lactulose less effective.[106]

Glutamine reduces elimination of methotrexate from the body, so the effects and side-effects of it could be increased.[73]

Iodine

Iodine is important for:

- Healthy thyroid function. The thyroid produces hormones that control our metabolism.
- Development of healthy brains and nervous systems in babies and children.
- Helping regulate blood pressure and maintaining normal heartbeat.
- Detoxification of heavy metals, especially mercury.
- Development and maintenance of healthy breast tissue.
- Breaking down oestrogen. High levels of iodine are found in the ovaries.
- Healthy prostate glands.

We get iodine from food and we need a regular supply to maintain optimum levels. The best sources are:

- Seafood, including canned fish and shellfish such as oysters. Eating it twice a week is sufficient for most adults, but vary the type, as they contain varying amounts of iodine and many, especially oysters and large fish like tuna, contain high levels of toxins, pollutants and heavy metals.
- Seaweed, including kelp.
- Bread in Australia (and some other countries) has been fortified with iodine since 2009, except for organic and gluten free breads.
- Some fruit and vegetables, but it depends on the iodine content of the soil they're grown in.
- Eggs.
- Dairy foods used to be a good source, as equipment was sanitised with iodine products. Since modern sanitisers were introduced, they're less helpful.
- Iodised salt. Salt in processed foods is rarely iodised.

Some foods block the absorption of iodine. They're known as goitrogens. Most are in the Brassica family, which includes:

- cabbage
- brussels sprouts
- spinach
- kale
- cauliflower
- Chinese greens
- radishes
- swede
- turnip.

Cooking reduces this effect, though, so don't avoid them. Unless you're eating a lot of raw brassicas, perhaps in smoothies, the goitrogenic effect isn't likely to affect you, and, as outlined in Chapter 2, they're important for cancer prevention.

Along with the thyroid, iodine accumulates in other tissues, including:

- breast tissue
- prostate
- ovaries
- uterus
- pancreas
- thymus
- salivary glands
- tear glands
- lining of the stomach
- parts of the brain
- parts of the eye
- skin
- placenta.[107]

Iodine protects against development of fibrocystic breast tissue and breast cancer. Consumption of iodine is very high in Japan, because they eat a lot of fish and seaweed, and the rate of benign and cancerous breast disease in Japanese women is substantially lower than in the West.[108] When Japanese women migrate to the West and adopt a Western diet, the incidence of breast cancer rises. Iodine deficiency has also been associated with more aggressive forms of breast cancer in younger women, who tend to have lower levels of iodine than older women. It's thought that deficiencies make breast tissue more sensitive to oestrogen.[109]

Studies into iodine's effects on prostate cancer aren't as advanced as breast cancer studies. Laboratory tests on 3 different human prostate cancer types show that iodine induces **apoptosis** and prevents their growth.[110] Japanese men have lower rates of prostate cancer than men in the West, and this is likely to be from their high intake of iodine from fish and seaweed, just as in women and breast cancer.[111] Men with the highest iodine intake have approximately 25% fewer prostate cancers.[111]

Iodine levels are low in stomach cancer tissue, suggesting that iodine may have a protective effect against stomach cancer.[112]

Increasing iodine levels has been shown to cause **apoptosis** in some non-small cell lung cancers.[112]

Molecular iodine, as opposed to sodium iodide, was effective in reducing the growth and killing cancer cells in laboratory studies. The cells were from breast, lung, pancreatic and melanoma cancers.[113] Whilst human trials haven't been conducted, these areas of the body are all those where iodine accumulates.

Ideally, you should get iodine from food. But, if you don't eat foods that contain iodine, supplementing is a good idea.

Dosage

You can use iodine **topically**, because it's easily absorbed by the skin. This is particularly helpful if you have skin cancers, but it's more difficult to get the right dosage. That's important because overdosing can cause hyperthyroidism. If you decide to use it

topically, get your iodine levels checked regularly. It's a simple urine test. If your doctor won't order it, a naturopath can.

It's easy to find iodine supplements in tablet form. Molecular iodine is more effective than potassium iodide. To maintain iodine levels you need 150 **micrograms** a day. To help with cancer treatment or prevention, though, it's safe to use up to one milligram (1,000 **micrograms**) a day.[114]

Interactions, contraindications and side-effects

Do not use iodine if you have hyperthyroidism (an over-active thyroid).

Avoid using iodine if you have Hashimoto's disease (autoimmune hypothyroidism).

If you have kidney disease or damage, talk to your doctor before using iodine.

Taking iodine with lithium can cause your thyroid to become underactive (hypothyroid).

Iodine can interact with anti-arrhythmic drugs.

ACE inhibitors and angiotensin-receptor inhibitors, both used for high blood pressure, taken with potassium iodide can cause your potassium levels to rise too high.

Some diuretics taken with potassium iodide can cause potassium levels to increase dangerously.[115]

Melatonin

In Chapter 5, we discussed melatonin's effects on sleep, but melatonin is now also considered to be a cell protector that's antioxidant, balances the immune system and is involved in blood production. On top of that it's been shown to stop the spread of cancer.[116] It's also prescribed for its sedative effects, for anxiety, for pain relief, to reduce blood pressure, as an anti-inflammatory, to improve brain functioning and for depression.[117] These effects are helpful during cancer treatment.

Melatonin has a role in cancer prevention. There is a higher incidence of breast, bowel and endometrial cancer in night shift workers, who are exposed to light at night and therefore have lower melatonin levels. The rise in melatonin at night is therefore considered to act as a 'natural restraint' on tumours starting and growing.[117] It may, of course, be due to the lack of sleep that night shift workers suffer. The importance of sleep was covered in Chapter 5. Either way, in 2007 the **IARC** classified shift work that involves night work as 'probably **carcinogenic** to humans'.[118] If you're a night shift worker and have trouble sleeping during the day, it would be worth trying melatonin to help with sleep and avoid the increased risk.[119] Melatonin supplements only help insomnia sufferers, though. If you normally sleep well, it won't help you get to sleep faster or sleep longer.[120]

Melatonin also prevents overproduction of oestradiol, the oestrogen type that stimulates breast cell division.[121] This makes it particularly helpful for prevention of women's hormonal cancers, such as breast, ovarian and endometrial cancers.

A study of metastatic breast cancer patients receiving tamoxifen who hadn't responded to treatment showed that taking melatonin for a week before starting tamoxifen improved response rates.[122]

Cancer's effects on sleep and depression come not just from treatment but also insomnia caused by drug treatments, anxiety, pain, trouble breathing in some cases, nausea and itchiness. All these have a significant effect on patients' quality of life and many can be helped by melatonin's ability to help with sleep.[117]

Prostate and bowel cancer survival can be improved with melatonin. Patients with these cancers have extremely low levels of night-time melatonin, and they drop even further as their tumours grow. Taking melatonin at night reduces growth of the tumours, whereas taking it in the morning increases growth.[121]

A review of melatonin's effects on cancer showed it reduced the toxicity of various chemo drugs, including:

- cisplatin
- anthracyclines, such as doxorubicin
- Etoposide
- 5-fluorouracil.[117]

This allows larger doses of the drugs to be used safely, giving better results.

The studies also showed a reduction in side-effects, such as:

- nerve damage
- heart damage
- kidney damage
- bone marrow suppression
- loss of energy and strength.[117]

An interesting **meta-analysis** looked at the effects of melatonin on 643 patients who hadn't responded to conventional therapy. They included people with breast, skin, kidney, brain and lung cancers. They were given large doses of 1040 **mg** per day of melatonin as their sole treatment and followed for a year. Survival rates over the year were 66%.[123]

A review of patients with a wide range of solid tumours looked at the effects of melatonin in conjunction with chemo, radiation, supportive care or palliative care. They were given oral doses of melatonin in the evening ranging from 10–40 **mg**. They showed a significant positive effect on survival rates, treatment response rates, disease progression and side-effects. It reduced hair loss, fatigue, anaemia and loss of platelets.[124]

Melatonin is safe for most people. Women treated with 75 **mg** per night of melatonin for 4 years showed no sign of ill effects.[125] Another study looked at the effects of very high doses (1–6.6 **g** per day) for 30–45 days and followed it with a range of biochemical tests for toxicity. Their conclusion was that, apart from drowsiness, all the findings were normal.[125] There's some evidence it may affect men's fertility and it could accelerate autoimmune conditions.[125] In some (but not all) people with depression, including bipolar disorder, it may make it worse, particularly if taken during the day.[125] In animals, fairly large doses (equivalent to about 30 **mg** per day in humans) increased eye damage caused by light.[125] Another animal study found that those with high cholesterol levels who were given high doses of melatonin had increased rates of atherosclerosis, which can cause heart attacks.[126]

Dosage

Importantly, if you have an existing tumour, you should only take melatonin in the evening. If you take it in the morning, it can make the tumour grow faster, and if you take it in the afternoon, it will have no effect on your tumour but may make you drowsy.[121]

If not receiving treatment, start with around 0.2 **mg** per night, taken about an hour before sleep. If it's ineffective, slowly increase the dose until you feel the benefits. Typical doses range up to 5 **mg** per night.

If you're receiving treatment for an active tumour, doses of 10–40 **mg** per night are appropriate.[124] Again, start with a low dose and increase it if you can tolerate it.

In Australia, New Zealand, the UK and maybe some other countries, melatonin is only available over the counter in homeopathic form. This may be helpful for insomnia but maybe not for its anti-cancer effects. If you want normal doses it's available by prescription from a medical doctor. It's freely available in the US.

Interactions, contraindications and side-effects

Side effects are usually minimal but can include:

- drowsiness
- changes to sleep patterns
- disorientation
- rapid heartbeat
- flushing
- itching
- stomach cramps
- headaches
- nightmares

- insomnia
- abnormally low body temperature.[127]

Don't use melatonin during treatment for blood cancer because of its protective effects on bone marrow.

Melatonin may reduce the effectiveness of immune-suppressing drugs.[128]

If you're taking any kind of sedative medication, melatonin may cause too much sleepiness, which could be dangerous.

Contraceptive pills increase the amount of melatonin made by the body, so taking more might result in undesirable higher melatonin levels.[128]

Fluvoxamine, an antidepressant, can increase absorption of melatonin, which could increase its effects.[128]

Melatonin may increase blood sugar. If you're taking medication for diabetes, melatonin could reduce its effectiveness, so monitor blood sugar carefully.[128]

Blood clotting could be slowed down by melatonin, so taking anticoagulant or antiplatelet drugs, such as warfarin, Coumadin, heparin, aspirin, diclofenac (Voltaren), or ibuprofen, with it could result in bleeding and bruising.[128]

Nifedipine GITS, which is used to reduce blood pressure, may be less effective if taken with melatonin.[128]

Verapamil, a calcium channel blocker, reduces melatonin's effectiveness.[128]

Flumazenil, which is used to reverse the effects of benzodiazepines like Valium, may reduce the effects of melatonin.[128]

Methamphetamine's effects and side-effects might be increased if you take melatonin.[129]

Fluoxetine, an antidepressant, and melatonin can interact to make both less effective.[16]

N-acetyl cysteine (NAC)

NAC is a nutritional supplement that's converted by the body into the amino acid L-cysteine and glutathione, the body's major antioxidant. It isn't something the body produces naturally and it isn't available from food sources, but it's easily found in health food stores.

Its benefits are:

- Antioxidant, reducing oxidative stress in the body. Many chronic diseases are associated with oxidative stress: cancer, heart disease, lung diseases, diabetes, cataracts and Parkinson's disease.
- Anti-inflammatory.
- Protects the liver, so it's helpful for detoxification of drugs and heavy metals. It's often used in hospitals for people who've overdosed on paracetamol (acetaminophen).
- Breaks down thick mucus, so it's used in conditions like chronic obstructive pulmonary disorder, asthma and bronchitis.
- Helps with drug addictions (including giving up smoking) and compulsive behaviour, because of its effects on the brain.
- Improves effects of pharmaceutical treatment for polycystic ovary syndrome (PCOS).
- Increases sensitivity of cancers to chemo and reduces chemo

side-effects.

- Prevents cancers from forming.

Colon cancer is often treated with fluorouracil and leucovorin, but adding oxaliplatin makes these drugs more effective. Although it improves disease-free survival, it often causes severe neuropathy. In colon cancer patients with metastases, **NAC** was shown to reduce neuropathy side-effects significantly.[130]

Oral **mucositis** is a side-effect of high dose chemo. It's often severe and very painful. In a study, leukaemia patients about to start chemo prior to a stem cell transplant were either given **NAC** at a dose of 100 **mg** per **kg** per day or a **placebo**, from the first day of chemo until 15 days after the transplant. The incidence of severe oral **mucositis** was significantly lower in the **NAC** group (23.7%) compared with the **placebo** group (45.3%), and on average it lasted for 2 days less.[131] This is significant, as I can attest. I suffered oral **mucositis** after my stem cell transplant. On a scale of one to 10, with 10 being highest, I rated the pain at 10 whenever I swallowed, and no amount of the various opioids that I received reduced the pain, which lasted for about 8 days.

Children with acute lymphoblastic leukaemia (ALL) were treated with a combination of 400 IU of vitamin E and 600 **mg** of **NAC** each day, alongside their usual chemo and radiotherapy, or chemo or radiotherapy alone. The supplements reduced the level of toxic hepatitis and elevation of liver enzymes, which indicate liver damage. They also reduced the number of fevers caused by infection and the number of platelet and blood transfusions that the children needed. The effect increased as treatment progressed.

The researchers concluded that the supplements had significantly reduced the free radicals normally produced by the treatment.[132]

Chemo is known for causing cognitive impairment, commonly referred to as 'chemo brain'. An animal trial showed that **NAC** prevented free radical production and partially reversed the cognitive problems caused by cisplatin in the animals.[133]

Pancreatic cancer is usually treated with gemcitabine but tumours quickly become resistant to it. In an animal study, 100 **mg** of **NAC** per **kg** of body weight, taken daily in addition to gemcitabine significantly reduced tumour growth. The researchers concluded that gemcitabine had a paradoxical effect on tumours, actively promoting a signalling chemical that increased their growth, and that **NAC** inhibited that chemical.[134]

Liver cancer is generally treated with Interferon Alpha 2A (IFN), a drug that activates the body's immune response against cancer and affects cancer cell growth. A combination of IFN and **NAC** reduced cancer cells' survival by about 50% in 96 hours, which was more effective than IFN alone.[135]

NAC is also effective for cancer prevention. A trial was conducted on healthy smokers (if there is such a thing) with no history of cancer. Half were given 600 **mg** of **NAC** twice a day and the other half a **placebo**. They were then monitored for various markers connected with cancer. The **NAC** group had a significant reduction in many of those markers.[136] So if you're a smoker, **NAC** could help prevent cancer.

This preventive effect in smokers contrasts with the EUROSCAN trial, conducted on patients with lung cancer or head and neck cancers, most of whom were previous or current smokers. They were given either high doses of Vitamin A (retinyl palmitate), 600 **mg** of **NAC**, a combination of both, or a **placebo** for 2 years. There was no difference in findings between any of the study groups.[9] In response to this, it was suggested that **NAC** detoxified the **carcinogens** causing cancer, and once cancers start growing this doesn't help.[137] An animal study showed that **NAC** (and vitamin E) increased the growth of lung cancers[138] but this research may not translate to humans.

Dosage

600 **mg** once or twice a day, which is sufficient for an antioxidant effect. The safe range is up to 2,500 **mg** per day.[73]

Interactions, contraindications and side-effects

NAC is considered very safe, but possible side-effects include:

- digestive problems, including nausea, vomiting, diarrhoea or constipation
- low blood pressure, headache, fever, rashes, drowsiness or liver problems, all of which are rare
- bronchospasm in asthma patients.

NAC can increase the effects of nitroglycerin and therefore its side-effects, such as headache, light-headedness and dizziness.[139]

With medications for high blood pressure, NAC could cause your blood pressure to drop too low.[139]

NAC can slow blood clotting, so it may increase the effects of any blood thinning medication, such as warfarin, heparin, aspirin, ibuprofen and diclofenac. Stop taking it 2 weeks prior to surgery.[139]

Omega 3 fatty acids

The most common source of omega 3 fatty acids is in fish oils, which are supplements used for many conditions. Many plant foods, like flaxseed oil and chia seeds, contain high levels of alpha-linolenic acid (ALA). The body can convert ALA to docosahexaenoic acid (**DHA**) and eicosapentaenoic acid (**EPA**), the omega 3 fatty acids in fish oils, but the conversion isn't very efficient at only 15%. The best food sources are Atlantic salmon, sardines and herrings, but most seafood contains some fish oils. In order to get therapeutic levels, though, you need a supplement.

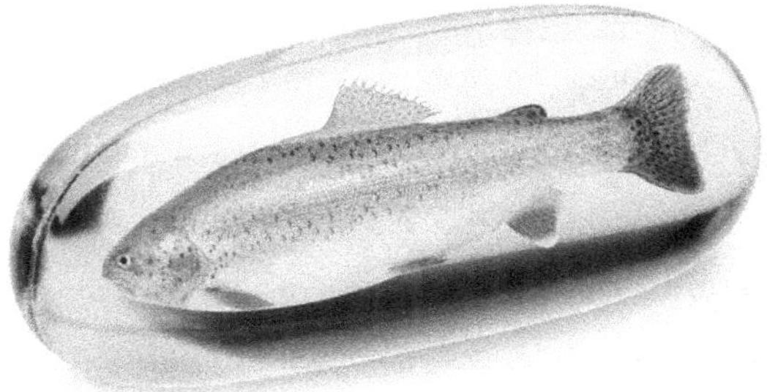

They are powerful anti-inflammatories and are used, amongst other things, to help with:

- reducing cholesterol levels and improving heart health
- reducing pain in rheumatoid arthritis
- reducing risk of cognitive decline in older populations
- lowering risk of macular degeneration
- dry eye disease

- depression
- ADHD
- reducing risk of childhood allergies in offspring when the pregnant mother takes fish oils, although results are inconclusive
- possibly improving lung function in cystic fibrosis sufferers.[140]

The effects of omega 3 fatty acids on cancer risk are unclear. Whereas in animal studies and in the laboratory they reduce the risk, in human studies it's less clear. Some people are able to absorb them better than others, depending on their **genetics**. Those who absorb them well seem to have a reduced risk of cancer.[141]

One study found that higher blood levels of omega 3s equated to a higher risk of prostate cancer.[142] A **meta-analysis** of studies using both blood levels and diet reporting noted that blood levels only show intake over the previous one or 2 days. It's what people do over 10 years plus that really shows a reduction in cancer risk. They concluded that there's no evidence of a statistical link between omega 3s and prostate cancer. They also quoted another study showing that prostate cancer itself increased blood levels of omega 3s.[143]

A large trial studied the effects of omega 3s on cancers and found no reduction in cancer risk. However, they used a dose of just 460 **mg** of **EPA** and 380 **mg** of **DHA** daily.[144] This isn't considered a therapeutic dose. Generally 3—3.5 **g** of combined **EPA** and **DHA** is used daily in chronic inflammatory conditions, including cancer.[145]

In animal studies, omega 3s reduced PGE2, an inflammatory marker which is related to colon cancer risk. A human study found the same, but the reduction was only fully effective in people of normal weight. It wasn't as effective in overweight and obese participants, even when they received a higher dose than those of normal weight.[146] This could explain why being overweight is linked to higher colon cancer risk.

The mechanisms of how omega 3s reduce cancer risk are clearly understood:

- They reduce cancer growth by changing the way that cell membranes work.
- They're antioxidant.
- They're anti-inflammatory.
- They change the amount of calcium entering cells. Calcium is essential for the growth of cancer cells.[147]

A study of women with metastatic breast cancer showed that 1.8 **g** of **DHA** can improve their sensitivity to anthracycline drugs, such as doxorubicin, epirubicin and mitoxanthrone, without any adverse effects.[148]

In a study on rats with breast cancer, **DHA** improved sensitivity to radiation. Tumours were reduced by 60% in rats fed **DHA** compared with 31% in the **control group.**[149]

Patients who had chemo following surgery to remove gastrointestinal cancers were given 2 **g** of fish oils a day for 8 weeks. This stopped reduction of **neutrophils,** whereas in the controls they dropped 30%. This means they're less likely to suffer infections. The fish oils also helped them gain 1.7 **kg** weight on average, whereas those in the **control group** lost an average of 2.5 **kg.**[150] A similar study of the effects of taking fish oils before surgery found it was equally effective in reducing post-operative infections and reducing hospital stays.[151]

When the body metabolises **EPA**, it produces a prostaglandin that kills leukaemia stem cells in mice.[152]

A study of patients newly diagnosed with blood cancers (acute and chronic leukaemia, Hodgkin lymphoma and non-Hodgkin lymphoma) evaluated the effects of fish oils during the beginning of their chemo. They found inflammatory markers were lower, they tolerated more chemo, and survival rates at 14 months were significantly better (no deaths in the fish oil group but 8 in the **control group**).[153]

In laboratory tests, multiple myeloma cells treated with **EPA** and **DHA** undergo **apoptosis** and are more sensitive to bortezomib, a multiple myeloma treatment.[154]

A review on use of omega 3s during chemo showed omega 3s are effective across a number of cancers and a range of drugs, both increasing chemo's efficiency and reducing toxic side-effects.[155] If side-effects are reduced, higher doses and/or longer treatment times can be used to make the drugs more effective and increase life expectancy. It also means patients' quality of life is improved.

A big problem in cancer patients is unintentional loss of weight, with loss of both fat and muscle, known as **cachexia**. This makes patients tired and weak, and reduces their ability to move around. It's also a sign of cancer progression and is often linked to a poor prognosis. **EPA** supplements of 2.2 **g** per day are effective in reversing this weight loss.[156]

Dosage

A dosage of 3–4 **g** per day of **EPA/DHA** combined has been used in a number of clinical trials, but 1–2 **g** may be sufficient. Generally, this would be in capsule form. Some people experience fishy burps after taking them, but capsules containing fish oils and citrus oils usually prevent this.

Interactions, contraindications and side-effects

At high doses, some people experience gastrointestinal problems, usually nausea, diarrhoea, indigestion, reflux or bloating. These are generally not serious and reducing the dose usually resolves the problem. Taking the capsules with food, starting with low doses and increasing them gradually helps avoid this.

They help prevent clotting, which is helpful for cardiovascular problems. Logically, you'd think that this could be problematic if you're undergoing surgery. However, a **systematic review** of patients undergoing surgery found no increase in bleeding or need for transfusions, either during or after surgery.[157]

There's no evidence of any reduction in warfarin levels in patients taking fish oil supplements compared with controls. Nor was there any statistically significant difference in the number of minor bleeds between the 2 groups. Neither group had any major bleeds.[158] These results confirmed a previous trial of warfarin patients taking 4 **g** of fish oils a day. No additional bleeding events were found in the group taking the fish oils compared with the controls.[159]

Probiotics

Probiotics are live micro-organisms that improve gut health. This is a short list of some of their actions:

- They help balance the bacteria in your gut. An imbalance happens when there are too many bad bacteria and not enough good ones. It can happen when you've been taking antibiotics, if you've been ill, or when you haven't eaten healthily, amongst other things. When an imbalance occurs, you can develop digestive problems, allergies, put on weight, suffer mental health problems, and much more.
- They can help to prevent and treat diarrhoea. Good bacteria usually control the bad ones by crowding them out. When you've taken antibiotics, though, they kill the good bacteria as well as the bad, and this can result in too many bad bacteria, causing diarrhoea.
- They can improve some mental health conditions. The health of our guts and brains are closely interlinked. In fact, more serotonin, a feel good neurotransmitter, is secreted in the gut than in the brain. Research shows that conditions like anxiety, depression, memory loss and stress can all be improved with probiotics.
- Some probiotics can help keep your heart healthy by reducing **LDL** ('bad') **cholesterol** and blood pressure.
- Certain probiotics can also help reduce allergies and eczema.
- Some probiotics can reduce symptoms of some digestive problems, such as ulcerative colitis and irritable bowel syndrome (IBS).

- Probiotics can boost your immune system. They increase natural antibodies, white blood cells and **NK cells**. *Lactobacillus GG* reduces the incidence and gravity of respiratory infections by 17%.[160]
- Some probiotics help with weight loss. They prevent the absorption of fat in the intestines, burning more energy, making you feel less hungry and storing less fat. *Lactobacillus rhamnosus* and *L. gasseri* have been shown to help, but *L. acidophilus* can have the opposite effect.
- There's evidence that probiotics can help prevent cancers, reduce treatment-related diarrhoea and reduce infections in cancer surgery, as outlined below.

In animal testing, *Lactobacillus casei BL23* significantly protected against bowel cancer by reducing inflammatory messengers.[161]

Another animal study showed that probiotics reduced liver cancer growth by 40% compared with the control.[162]

A **systematic review** and **meta-analysis** looked at use of probiotics to prevent diarrhoea from chemo or radiation in abdominal and pelvic cancer patients. Probiotics helped about half the patients.[163] Another **systematic review** and **meta-analysis** studying various cancer types found probiotics prevented treatment-related diarrhoea in around half the patients.[164]

When patients undergo surgery for bowel cancer, they're prone to infections at the incision site. The risk is higher when the levels of certain intestinal bacteria are unbalanced.[165] A study of the use of probiotics taken before and after the surgery found that 6.7% of patients in the probiotic group developed an infection, compared with 19.8% in the **placebo** group.[166]

If you've been hospitalised during treatment, there's a good chance you'll have picked up a *Clostridium difficile* infection. This is a serious gastrointestinal infection that can result in a perforated bowel in extreme cases. Even mild infections cause ongoing diarrhoea, which can upset electrolyte balance. This could be life-threatening. The usual treatment is antibiotics but the bacterium is resistant to most of them. One successful treatment is a probiotic called *Saccharomyces boulardii*. A **meta-analysis** showed about 40% of patients treated with *S. boulardii* responded.[167] It's even more effective when combined with high doses of vancomycin, an antibiotic commonly used for severe recurrent infections. It was 67% more effective in preventing further bouts than vancomycin alone.[168] If you choose to use this, use a supplement that doesn't need refrigerating (lyophilised), because they're more effective.

Dosage

Each species of probiotic has a different effect on the body and even within the same species there are different strains that act in particular ways. I recommend consulting someone who's familiar with all the different species and strains to ensure you get the right one for your needs. If you're not able or willing to do that, then alternate different broad spectrum probiotics with high colony numbers. That increases your chances of getting the particular strain that you need. Be warned, though, it may take a lot longer and you could spend a lot of money on 'frogs' before you find your 'prince'.

For treating gastrointestinal symptoms, I recommend up to 10 billion colony forming units (CFU) in each capsule, taken daily for about 4 weeks or until symptoms resolve. For maintenance of general health, a capsule containing 2 million should be sufficient.

Interactions, contraindications and side-effects

A **systematic review** looked at the safety of probiotics. This can be an issue with immunocompromised people, as very occasionally the probiotics get into the bloodstream and cause sepsis. To put this into perspective, the review included 2,242 patients and there were only 5 reports of infection from the probiotics, or 0.22% of the patients.[164] *S.boulardii* carries a particular risk: patients taking it who then touched their chemo port with unwashed hands have contracted sepsis. So I strongly suggest that you wash your hands after taking probiotics.

Selenium

Selenium is a mineral the body needs in small amounts from our diet. It's important because:

- It's a powerful antioxidant that works by increasing glutathione levels.
- It can help reduce heart disease risk by reducing inflammation. Inflammation and oxidative stress are linked to the build-up of plaque in the arteries, known as atherosclerosis. Atherosclerosis can result in strokes, heart attacks and coronary artery disease.

- It helps prevent Alzheimer's disease, multiple sclerosis and Parkinson's disease.
- It boosts the immune system.
- It's involved in production of thyroid hormones and helps keep the thyroid healthy.
- It helps reduce asthma symptoms.
- It may help reduce the risks of some cancers.
- It helps with the side-effects of radiation therapy.

Selenium levels around the world vary according to soil levels. In Australia and New Zealand, the main sources are seafood, eggs and poultry. Other muscle meats contribute smaller amounts. Dietary selenium levels in New Zealand tend to be lower because soil levels are low.[169] However, 2 Brazil nuts per day provide the recommended amount of selenium.[170] If you like Brazil nuts and are prone to eating handfuls, stick to eating them occasionally, as more than 6 daily takes you over the safe level of selenium.

The Nutritional Prevention of Cancer Study researched whether selenium supplements reduced recurrence of non-melanoma skin cancer. It didn't, but it was effective in reducing the risk of prostate, lung and colon cancers.[171] On further analysis, the effects were only found in men who had low selenium levels (below 123.2 nanograms per millilitre, at the outset).[172] In men with normal selenium levels at the outset, there wasn't any reduction, either in prostate cancer, bowel, lung or overall cancer rates. In fact, those with higher selenium levels at the outset had a higher risk of non-melanoma skin cancer.[173, 174] If you want to use selenium supplements for preventive treatment, I recommend you get your levels checked beforehand. Hair or nail analysis is the best way to check long-term selenium status, because blood and urine tests only show consumption over the previous few days. Naturopaths can organise hair and nail analysis.

Cancer patients receiving radiation therapy could benefit from selenium supplementation if their levels are low, which they generally are in cancer patients. Two trials demonstrated this:

- Gynaecological cancer patients, all of whom had low selenium at the outset of treatment, were given selenium supplements during radiotherapy after surgery. Generally, patients given radiation therapy in the pelvic area suffer from diarrhoea. In the selenium group, levels of diarrhoea were less frequent and severe, and their 10 year survival rate increased significantly.[175]
- A second trial involved patients with head and neck cancers. Radiation therapy in this part of the body often causes problems swallowing and loss of taste. In the selenium group, both side-effects were reduced.[175]

A review looked at studies of selenium supplements and radiotherapy from 1998—2010 and found it was helpful for:

- Brain tumour, by reducing intracranial pressure.
- Head and neck cancer. In one study, it helped immune responsiveness, and in the other it reduced problems with swallowing (this trial was mentioned in the previous paragraph).
- Secondary lymphoedema. It improved quality of life.
- Oral cancer. It improved the body's defence systems.
- Cervical and uterine cancer. It reduced the incidence and severity of radiotherapy-induced diarrhoea.

There was no reduction in radiotherapy effectiveness, nor were there any toxic signs or complications with the supplements.[176]

Dosage

There are different kinds of selenium:

- Organic, found in meat and to a lesser extent plants. These include selenomethionine and selenocysteine
- Inorganic, found in soil. These include sodium selenite and sodium selenate.

You can buy supplements of both types. For cancer prevention and treatment, selenomethionine is the most effective: it prevents cancer growth and reduces **metastasis**. Those who used selenised yeast as a supplement, mostly as selenomethionine, in doses of 200 **microgram**s a day, reduced their overall cancer risk by almost half.[73]

All the radiotherapy studies used sodium selenite and dosages ranged from 200–500 **microgram**s per day.[176] However, it's considered to be less bioavailable[16] and only delays tumour growth in the short term.[73]

Interactions, contraindications and side-effects

Selenium can slow blood clotting, so taking it with blood thinning and anticoagulant medications, such as warfarin, may increase the chance of bruising and bleeding.

A combination of selenium, vitamins C and E, and beta-carotene can make cholesterol lowering medications less effective. Niacin, sometimes used for raising **HDL cholesterol**, may also be less effective with this combination.[177] It isn't known whether selenium alone has this effect.

Selenium may slow down breakdown of barbiturates, increasing their effects and possible side-effects.[177]

Zinc

Zinc is a mineral that's essential to good health and it's found in every cell in the body. We can only get it from food or supplements. It's necessary for:

- The actions of over 300 enzymes in the body that help with digestion, metabolism, nerve function and many more processes
- The function and development of immune cells
- **DNA** synthesis
- Skin health, including wound healing
- Protein production
- Growth and development
- Our senses of smell and taste
- Battling oxidative stress and inflammation[178].

The best sources of zinc in order of their content are:

- Oysters, which contain about 5 times a man's daily needs per dozen. Bear in mind, though, that because they're bottom feeders they do contain a lot of toxins, pollutants and heavy metals. Indulging occasionally is good, but not too often.
- Red meat.
- Seafood.
- Fortified breakfast cereals.

- Pork.
- Chicken, with dark meat containing more than breast.
- Pumpkin seeds.
- Dairy foods.
- Legumes, such as baked beans, chickpeas, kidney beans and peas.
- Nuts.[178]

Severe zinc deficiency is quite rare, but even mild deficiency can cause symptoms. These include:

- Lowering of immunity, with more coughs and colds
- Poor wound healing
- Hair loss
- Diarrhoea
- Brittle nails
- Poor mood, including depression and a loss of cognitive function
- Skin problems, such as acne and dermatitis
- Loss of taste and smell
- Loss of appetite.

If these symptoms sound familiar to you, you won't be surprised to hear that chemo and radiation reduce your ability to absorb zinc, mainly by their effects on the gut. What's surprising, though, is that population studies suggest that at least one in 5 people in the general population suffers from a zinc deficiency.[179] People most at risk are those who don't eat much red meat or seafood, and those who have a lot of phytates in their diet.

Phytates are chemicals that bind to zinc and prevent its

absorption (and also iron and manganese). They're found in plant foods, such as grains, legumes, nuts and seeds. That isn't to say that these foods are bad. They have cancer-fighting properties because they increase NK cells and slow down tumour growth. They also help prevent formation of blood clots and hardening of the arteries. They bind to cadmium and lead, heavy metals that are toxic. And they're antioxidant.[180]

For most people, phytates are unlikely to cause zinc deficiency. But if you're a vegetarian or vegan, you'll need to consume twice as much zinc to counteract the phytates you probably eat.[181] You can lower the levels of phytates to a manageable level by:

- soaking (particularly legumes, nuts and seeds)
- sprouting (especially grains, legumes and seeds)
- fermentation (think sourdough bread)
- adding foods rich in vitamin C to high phytate foods
- using vinegar to dress salads or in cooking
- supplementing with phytase supplements, which break down phytates.

Alternatively, take a zinc supplement.

Prostate cells accumulate more zinc than the other cells in the body, and zinc inhibits the growth of those cells, including increasing **apoptosis.**[182] The levels of zinc in prostate cancer cells are significantly lower than in surrounding prostate cells. It appears that the cancerous cells actively pump zinc out of the cells to prevent **apoptosis**. The theory is that increasing zinc intake could reduce prostate cancer risk and some researchers are suggesting that it could be used to treat prostate cancer patients.[183,]

[184] This has been demonstrated on prostate cancer cells in the laboratory.[185]

However, all the latest research into prostate cancer cases and dietary zinc intake suggests that higher doses on average actually promote prostate cancer, although at normal levels they only increase less invasive and more localised cancers.[186, 187, 188] One of the papers also looked at **genetic** susceptibility factors for prostate cancer. It showed that men who were **genetically** susceptible and had higher dietary zinc levels ran a higher risk of contracting prostate cancer.[186]

Diets high in zinc generally include a lot of red meat, which we know is a risk factor for cancer. But it could be the quality of that meat that affects cancer risk. For example, a diet high in burgers, sausages and bacon would be high in zinc but is likely to raise cancer risk. However, a diet that includes organic grass-fed red meat, which doesn't contain pesticides and herbicides and is likely to have higher ratios of omega 3s to omega 6s, is much less likely to increase risk.

In fact, a large study looked at people who had the beginnings of age-related macular degeneration. One group used 80 **mg** of zinc supplements and another used zinc supplements plus antioxidants. These 2 groups were asked to restrict their dietary intake of zinc, to avoid any possible ill effects of large doses. Another group used antioxidants alone and there was a **placebo** group. As well as the effects on age-related macular degeneration, they looked at overall mortality. They found that over more than 6 years the 2 groups which used zinc supplements had lower mortality rates than the other groups.[189] This suggests that it might not be the zinc itself but poor quality zinc-rich foods that caused prostate cancer to develop in the prostate cancer studies above.

Another paper looked at whether taking zinc supplements increased prostate cancer rates. It concluded that doses of up to 80 **mg** per day were unlikely to increase the likelihood of prostate cancer and, in fact, could be protective against it. However, at those doses they recommended limiting the amount of dietary zinc with it because of the possibility of overdosing. They also suggested it might not be helpful for men currently suffering from prostate cancer to take zinc.[190]

In a **meta-analysis** of studies using up to 90 **mg** of zinc supplements daily, those who consumed more zinc reduced their risk of pancreatic cancer significantly.[181]

A trial was conducted on patients in Linzhou, an area of China which has some of the highest rates of oesophageal cancer in the world. At the beginning of the 6 year trial, they performed endoscopies and biopsies on 440 individuals. They then followed them for the period of the trial and at the end 88 of them had developed oesophageal cancer, of which 60 had enough tissue from the biopsy to test for zinc in the tissue. They found the risk of developing oesophageal cancer was significantly lower when there were higher levels of zinc in the tissue.[191]

Taking zinc during cancer treatment doesn't appear to have any negative effects on chemo or radiation treatment and can help with some side-effects. One study showed that zinc sulphate helped prevent infections and **mucositis** in patients undergoing radiotherapy for head and neck cancers.[5] This was confirmed in a **systematic review** that looked at 3 studies[192], but a more recent **meta-analysis** of 5 studies found the opposite.[193]

Similarly, there's conflicting evidence for using zinc sulphate to prevent and correct loss of taste from radiotherapy, with 2 small trials showing it's effective[194, 195], and another larger one showing it wasn't.[196]

Two studies looked at the effects of zinc supplements on patients with head and neck cancers.

1. The first one was conducted after radiotherapy. The group that received zinc had a better survival rate than the **placebo** group after 3 years. Those in the group who had Stage III and IV cancers had much better 3 year survival rates when they received chemo and radiation as well as zinc.[197]
2. The other study looked at patients with Stage III and IV nose and throat cancers. They received 75 **mg** per day of zinc for 2 months as well as receiving chemo and radiation. After 5 years, the zinc group had a much better local-free and disease-free survival rate than the **placebo** group. However, there was no significant difference in **metastasis**-free survival rates between the 2 groups. That was believed to be connected with the advanced stage of their disease.[198]

A trial on children and adolescents with acute leukaemia (some lymphocytic and others myeloid leukaemia) studied the effect of zinc supplements on weight gain and infections. They were given 2 **mg** per **kg** of body weight per day for 60 days whilst undergoing chemo. The group given zinc gained an average of 2 **kg**, which is an excellent outcome because most children with leukaemia are undernourished when diagnosed. The zinc group also grew taller and had fewer infections than the **placebo** group.[199]

In 2011–12, the Australian Bureau of Statistics estimated that about 10% of women and about 37% of men in Australia were deficient in zinc.[200] You can get your zinc levels tested. Blood levels tend to reflect recent intake. A more reliable test is hair mineral analysis, which measures long-term zinc intakes, or a naturopath can use a taste test to assess whether or not you're deficient.

Dosage

The **RDA** for zinc is 15 **mg** per day for an adult, but for cancer support you can safely use up to 80 **mg** per day provided that you limit your intake of dietary zinc.

Interactions, contraindications and side-effects

High doses of zinc taken for extended periods can prevent absorption of copper, and too much copper can also prevent absorption of zinc. So if you're taking large doses of zinc, I recommend you do it under the supervision of a qualified health practitioner.

Zinc supplements can affect absorption of quinolone antibiotics, which include ciprofloxacin, gemifloxacin, levofloxacin, moxifloxacin, norfloxacin and ofloxacin. Take zinc supplements several hours away from these antibiotics.[16]

Tetracycline antibiotics can also be affected by zinc, so take them separated by several hours.[16] Doxycycline isn't affected by zinc.[201]

Amiloride, a diuretic or 'water pill', can increase your blood zinc levels, so you shouldn't take zinc with it.[201]

Zinc can reduce the effects of penicillamine, which is used for kidney stones, rheumatoid arthritis and Wilson's disease.[202]

Zinc, or any medication containing zinc, should be separated by about 4 hours from thrombopoietin receptor agonists, such as eltrombopag.[202]

References

1. Davis D, Epp M, Riordan H. Changes in USDA Food Composition Data for 43 Garden Crops, 1950 to 1999. *J Am Coll Nutr.* 2004;23(6):669-682. doi:10.1080/07315724.2004.10719409
2. Johns C. The state of Australia's soils. Apo.org.au. http://apo.org.au/node/54472. Published 2015. Accessed August 24, 2021.
3. Harrison-Dunn A. Made in China: DSM talks vitamin C price pressures. NUTRAingredients.com. https://www.nutraingredients.com/Article/2016/02/17/Made-in-China-DSM-talks-vitamin-C-price-pressures. Published 2016. Accessed August 24, 2021.
4. Nakayama A, Alladin K, Igbokwe O, White J. Systematic Review: Generating Evidence-Based Guidelines on the Concurrent Use of Dietary Antioxidants and Chemotherapy or Radiotherapy. *Cancer Invest.* 2011;29(10):655-667. doi:10.3109/07357907.2011.626479
5. Yasueda A, Urushima H, Ito T. Efficacy and Interaction of Antioxidant Supplements as Adjuvant Therapy in Cancer Treatment. *Integr Cancer Ther.* 2015;15(1):17-39. doi:10.1177/1534735415610427
6. Office of Dietary Supplements. Vitamin A. Office of Dietary Supplements. https://ods.od.nih.gov/factsheets/VitaminA-HealthProfessional/. Published 2021. Accessed August 24, 2021.
7. Goodman G, Thornquist M, Balmes J et al. The Beta-Carotene and Retinol Efficacy Trial: Incidence of Lung Cancer and Cardiovascular Disease Mortality During 6-Year Follow-up After Stopping Beta-Carotene and Retinol Supplements. *JNCI Journal of the National Cancer Institute.* 2004;96(23):1743-1750. doi:10.1093/jnci/djh320
8. Cancer Council Australia. Position statement - Beta-carotene and cancer risk. Cancer Council Australia. https://wiki.cancer.org.au/policy/Position_statement_-_Beta-carotene_and_cancer_risk. Published 2013. Accessed August 24, 2021.
9. van Zandwijk N, Dalesio O, Pastorino U, de Vries N, van Tinteren H. EUROSCAN, a Randomized Trial of Vitamin A and N-Acetylcysteine in Patients With Head and Neck Cancer or Lung Cancer. *J Natl Cancer Inst.* 2000;92(12):977-986. doi:10.1093/jnci/92.12.977

10. Blevins Primeau A. Vitamin A and Cancer. Cancer Therapy Advisor. https://www.cancertherapyadvisor.com/fact-sheets/fact-sheet-vitamin-a-cancer-oncology/article/681266/. Published 2017. Accessed August 24, 2021.
11. Meyskens F, Kopecky K, Appelbaum F, Balcerzak S, Samlowski W, Hynes H. Effects of vitamin A on survival in patients with chronic myelogenous leukemia: A SWOG randomized trial. *Leuk Res.* 1995;19(9):605-612. doi:10.1016/0145-2126(95)00032-j
12. Bonelli L, Puntoni M, Gatteschi B et al. Antioxidant supplement and long-term reduction of recurrent adenomas of the large bowel. A double-blind randomized trial. *J Gastroenterol.* 2012;48(6):698-705. doi:10.1007/s00535-012-0691-z
13. Lamm D, Riggs D, Shriver J, vanGilder P, Rach J, DeHaven J. Megadose Vitamins in Bladder Cancer: A Double-Blind Clinical Trial. *Journal of Urology.* 1994;151(1):21-26. doi:10.1016/s0022-5347(17)34863-2
14. Pastorino U, Infante M, Maioli M et al. Adjuvant treatment of stage I lung cancer with high-dose vitamin A. *Journal of Clinical Oncology.* 1993;11(7):1216-1222. doi:10.1200/jco.1993.11.7.1216
15. Wyss A. Beta-Carotene Safety. Nutri-facts. https://www.nutri-facts.org/en_US/nutrients/items/carotenoids/beta-carotene/safety.html. Published 2017. Accessed August 24, 2021.
16. Stargrove M, Treasure J, McKee D. *Herb, Nutrient And Drug Interactions.* St Louis, Mo: Mosby Elsevier; 2008.
17. Scaglione F, Panzavolta G. Folate, folic acid and 5-methyltetrahydrofolate are not the same thing. *Xenobiotica.* 2014;44(5):480-488. doi:10.3109/00498254.2013.845705
18. MTHFRSupport Australia. Cancer. MTHFRSupport Australia. https://www.mthfrsupport.com.au/cancer/. Published 2014. Accessed August 24, 2021.
19. Lu-ong K, Nguyen L. Open Access The Role of Thiamine in Cancer: Possible Genetic and Cellular Signaling Mechanisms. *Cancer Genomics and Proteonomics.* 2013;10(4):160-185. https://cgp.iiarjournals.org/content/10/4/169.long. Accessed August 24, 2021.
20. Zastre J, Sweet R, Hanberry B, Ye S. Linking vitamin B1 with cancer cell metabolism. *Cancer Metab.* 2013;1(1):16. doi:10.1186/2049-3002-1-16
21. Zschäbitz S, Cheng T, Neuhouser M et al. B vitamin intakes and incidence of colorectal cancer: results from the Women's Health Initiative Observational Study cohort. *Am J Clin Nutr.* 2012;97(2):332-343. doi:10.3945/ajcn.112.034736
22. Lopes C, Dourado A, Oliveira R. Phytotherapy and Nutritional Supplements on Breast Cancer. *Biomed Res Int.* 2017;2017:1-42. doi:10.1155/2017/7207983
23. Mamede A, Tavares S, Abrantes A, Trindade J, Maia J, Botelho M. The Role of Vitamins in Cancer: A Review. *Nutr Cancer.* 2011;63(4):479-494. doi:10.1080/01635581.2011.539315
24. Wohlrab J, Bangemann N, Kleine-Tebbe A et al. Barrier protective use of skin care to prevent chemotherapy-induced cutaneous symptoms and to maintain quality of life in patients with breast cancer. *Breast Cancer: Dove Medical Press.* 2014;6:115-122. doi:10.2147/bctt.s61699
25. Chen A, Martin A, Choy B et al. A Phase 3 Randomized Trial of Nicotinamide for Skin-Cancer Chemoprevention. *New England Journal of Medicine.* 2015;373(17):1618-1626. doi:10.1056/nejmoa1506197

26. Mocellin S, Briarava M, Pilati P. Vitamin B6 and Cancer Risk: A Field Synopsis and Meta-Analysis. *J Natl Cancer Inst*. 2016;109(3):djw230. doi:10.1093/jnci/djw230

27. Zhang Y, Shi W, Gao H, Zhou L, Hou A, Zhou Y. Folate Intake and the Risk of Breast Cancer: A Dose-Response Meta-Analysis of Prospective Studies. *PLoS One*. 2014;9(6):e100044. doi:10.1371/journal.pone.0100044

28. Kim S, Zuchniak A, Sohn K et al. Plasma folate, vitamin B-6, and vitamin B-12 and breast cancer risk in BRCA1- and BRCA2-mutation carriers: a prospective study. *Am J Clin Nutr*. 2016;104(3):671-677. doi:10.3945/ajcn.116.133470

29. Mason J. Folate, cancer risk, and the Greek god, Proteus: a tale of 2 chameleons. *Nutr Rev*. 2009;67(4):206-212. doi:10.1111/j.1753-4887.2009.00190.x

30. Brasky T, White E, Chen C. Long-Term, Supplemental, One-Carbon Metabolism–Related Vitamin B Use in Relation to Lung Cancer Risk in the Vitamins and Lifestyle (VITAL) Cohort. *Journal of Clinical Oncology*. 2017;35(30):3440-3448. doi:10.1200/jco.2017.72.7735

31. Carr A, Maggini S. Vitamin C and Immune Function. *Nutrients*. 2017;9(11):1211. doi:10.3390/nu9111211

32. Nabzdyk C, Bittner E. Vitamin C in the critically ill - indications and controversies. *World J Crit Care Med*. 2018;7(5):52-61. doi:10.5492/wjccm.v7.i5.52

33. Yiang G, Chou P, Hung Y et al. Vitamin C enhances anticancer activity in methotrexate-treated Hep3B hepatocellular carcinoma cells. *Oncol Rep*. 2014;32(3):1057-1063. doi:10.3892/or.2014.3289

34. Ma Y, Chapman J, Levine M, Polireddy K, Drisko J, Chen Q. High-Dose Parenteral Ascorbate Enhanced Chemosensitivity of Ovarian Cancer and Reduced Toxicity of Chemotherapy. *Sci Transl Med*. 2014;6(222):222ra18. doi:10.1126/scitranslmed.3007154

35. Fritz H, Flower G, Weeks L et al. Intravenous Vitamin C and Cancer. *Integr Cancer Ther*. 2014;13(4):280-300. doi:10.1177/1534735414534463

36. El Halabi I, Bejjany R, Nasr R et al. Ascorbic Acid in Colon Cancer: From the Basic to the Clinical Applications. *Int J Mol Sci*. 2018;19(9):2752. doi:10.3390/ijms19092752

37. Yeom C, Jung G, Song K. Changes of Terminal Cancer Patients' Health-related Quality of Life after High Dose Vitamin C Administration. *J Korean Med Sci*. 2007;22(1):7. doi:10.3346/jkms.2007.22.1.7

38. Cameron E, Pauling L. Supplemental ascorbate in the supportive treatment of cancer: Reevaluation of prolongation of survival times in terminal human cancer. *Proceedings of the National Academy of Sciences*. 1978;75(9):4538-4542. doi:10.1073/pnas.75.9.4538

39. Murata A, Morishige F, Yamaguchi H. Prolongation of survival times of terminal cancer patients by administration of large doses of ascorbate. *International Journal for Vitamin And Nutrition Research*. 1982;23:103-113. https://europepmc.org/article/MED/6811475. Accessed August 24, 2021.

40. Carr A, Vissers M, Cook J. The Effect of Intravenous Vitamin C on Cancer- and Chemotherapy-Related Fatigue and Quality of Life. *Front Oncol*. 2014;4(283). doi:10.3389/fonc.2014.00283

41. O'Brien K, Sali A. *A Clinician's Guide To Integrative Oncology*. Cham, Switzerland: Springer International Publishing AG; 2017.

42. Guaiquil V, Vera J, Golde D. Mechanism of Vitamin C Inhibition of Cell Death Induced by Oxidative Stress in Glutathione-depleted HL-60 Cells. *Journal of Biological Chemistry*. 2001;276(44):40955-40961. doi:10.1074/jbc.m106878200

43. Park C, Kimler B, Bodensteiner D, Lynch S, Hassanein R. In vitro growth modulation by L-ascorbic acid of colony-forming cells from bone marrow of patients with myelodysplastic syndromes. *Cancer Res*. 1992;52(16):4458-4566. https://pubmed.ncbi.nlm.nih.gov/1643638/. Accessed August 24, 2021.

44. Park C, Bergsagel D, McCulloch E. Ascorbic Acid: A Culture Requirement for Colony Formation by Mouse Plasmacytoma Cells. *Science (1979)*. 1971;174(4010):720-722. doi:10.1126/science.174.4010.720

45. King T, Trizna Z, Wu X et al. A clinical trial to evaluate the effect of vitamin C supplementation on in vitro mutagen sensitivity. The University of Texas M. D. Anderson Clinical Community Oncology Program Ne2rk. *Cancer Epidemiology, Biomarkers & Prevention*. 1997;6(7):537-542. https://pubmed.ncbi.nlm.nih.gov/9232342/. Accessed August 24, 2021.

46. Patrick R, Ames B. Vitamin D hormone regulates serotonin synthesis. Part 1: relevance for autism. *The FASEB Journal*. 2014;28(6):2398-2413. doi:10.1096/fj.13-246546

47. Healthy Bones Australia. Vitamin D and Bone Health. Healthy Bones Australia. https://healthybonesaustralia.org.au/wp-content/uploads/2020/11/HBA-Fact-Sheet-Vitamin-D.pdf. Published 2020. Accessed August 24, 2021.

48. Australian Bureau of Statistics. Australian Health Survey: Biomedical Results for Nutrients, 2011-12. Australian Bureau of Statistics. http://www.abs.gov.au/ausstats/abs@.nsf/Lookup/4364.0.55.006Chapter2002011–12. Published 2013. Accessed August 24, 2021.

49. Ingraham B, Bragdon B, Nohe A. Molecular basis of the potential of vitamin D to prevent cancer. *Curr Med Res Opin*. 2008;24(1):139-149. https://pubmed.ncbi.nlm.nih.gov/18034918/. Accessed August 24, 2021.

50. Ali M, Vaidya V. Vitamin D and cancer. *J Cancer Res Ther*. 2007;3(4):225-230. doi:10.4103/0973-1482.38998

51. Lappe J, Travers-Gustafson D, Davies K, Recker R, Heaney R. Vitamin D and calcium supplementation reduces cancer risk: results of a randomized trial. *Am J Clin Nutr*. 2007;85(6):1586-1591. doi:10.1093/ajcn/85.6.1586

52. Zeratsky K. Vitamin D toxicity: What if you get too much?. Mayo Clinic. https://www.mayoclinic.org/healthy-lifestyle/nutrition-and-healthy-eating/expert-answers/vitamin-d-toxicity/faq-20058108. Published 2020. Accessed August 24, 2021.

53. Cui L, Li L, Tian Y, Xu F, Qiao T. Association between Dietary Vitamin E Intake and Esophageal Cancer Risk: An Updated Meta-Analysis. *Nutrients*. 2018;10(7):801. doi:10.3390/nu10070801

54. Ju J, Picinich S, Yang Z et al. Cancer-preventive activities of tocopherols and tocotrienols. *Carcinogenesis*. 2009;31(4):533-542. doi:10.1093/carcin/bgp205

55. Kaczor T. Alpha Tocopheryl Succinate in Cancer Care. *Natural Medicine Journal*. 2011;3(6). https://www.naturalmedicinejournal.com/journal/2011-06/alpha-tocopheryl-succinate-cancer-care. Accessed August 24, 2021.

56. Prasad K. *Neurogenerative Disease And Micronutrients*. Boca Raton, Florida: CRC Press; 2015:185.

57. Tam K, Ho C, Lee W et al. Alteration of α-tocopherol-associated protein (TAP) expression in human breast epithelial cells during breast cancer development. *Food Chem*. 2013;138(2-3):1015-1021. doi:10.1016/j.foodchem.2012.09.147

58. Malafa M, Neitzel L. Vitamin E Succinate Promotes Breast Cancer Tumor Dormancy. *Journal of Surgical Research*. 2000;93(1):163-170. doi:10.1006/jsre.2000.5948

59. Malafa M, Fokum F, Mowlavi A, Abusief M, King M. Vitamin E inhibits melanoma growth in mice. *Surgery*. 2002;131(1):85-91. doi:10.1067/msy.2002.119191

60. Stapelberg M, Gellert N, Swettenham E et al. α-Tocopheryl Succinate Inhibits Malignant Mesothelioma by Disrupting the Fibroblast Growth Factor Autocrine Loop. *Journal of Biological Chemistry*. 2005;280(27):25369-25376. doi:10.1074/jbc.m414498200

61. Quin J, Engles D, Litwiller A et al. Vitamin E succinate decreases lung cancer tumor growth in mice. *Journal of Surgical Research*. 2005;121(2):139-143. doi:10.1016/j.jss.2004.07.0

62. Weber T, Lu M, Andera L et al. Vitamin E Succinate Is a Potent Novel Antineoplastic Agent with High Selectivity and Cooperativity with Tumor Necrosis Factor-related Apoptosis-inducing Ligand (Apo2 Ligand) in Vivo. *Clinical Cancer Research*. 2002;8(3):863-869. https://clincancerres.aacrjournals.org/content/8/3/863. Accessed August 24, 2021.

63. Angulo-Molina A, Reyes-Leyva J, López-Malo A, Hernández J. The Role of Alpha Tocopheryl Succinate (α-TOS) as a Potential Anticancer Agent. *Nutr Cancer*. 2013;66(2):167-176. doi:10.1080/01635581.2014.863367

64. Zhang Y, Ni J, Messing E, Chang E, Yang C, Yeh S. Vitamin E succinate inhibits the function of androgen receptor and the expression of prostate-specific antigen in prostate cancer cells. *Proceedings of the National Academy of Sciences*. 2002;99(11):7408-7413. doi:10.1073/pnas.102014399

65. Zhang M, Altuwaijri S, Yeh S. RRR-α-tocopheryl succinate inhibits human prostate cancer cell invasiveness. *Oncogene*. 2004;23(17):3080-3088. doi:10.1038/sj.onc.1207435

66. Singh V, Brown D, Kao T. Tocopherol succinate: A promising radiation countermeasure. *Int Immunopharmacol*. 2009;9(12):1423-1430. doi:10.1016/j.intimp.2009.08.020

67. Dunn B, Richmond E, Minasian L, Ryan A, Ford L. A Nutrient Approach to Prostate Cancer Prevention: The Selenium and Vitamin E Cancer Prevention Trial (SELECT). *Nutr Cancer*. 2010;62(7):896-918. doi:10.1080/01635581.2010.509833

68. Sen C, Khanna S, Roy S. Tocotrienols: Vitamin E beyond tocopherols. *Life Sci*. 2006;78(18):2088-2098. doi:10.1016/j.lfs.2005.12.001

69. Miyazawa T, Shibata A, Nakagawa K, Tsuzuki T. Anti-angiogenic function of tocotrienol. *Asia Pac J Clin Nutr*. 2008;17(51):253-256. https://apjcn.nhri.org.tw/server/APJCN/17%20Suppl%201/253.pdf. Accessed August 24, 2021.

70. Nesaretnam K, Selvaduray K, Razak G, Veerasenan S, Gomez P. Effectiveness of tocotrienol-rich fraction combined with tamoxifen in the management of women with early breast cancer: a pilot clinical trial. *Breast Cancer Research*. 2010;12(5). doi:10.1186/bcr2726

71. Springett G, Husain K, Neuger A et al. A Phase I Safety, Pharmacokinetic, and Pharmacodynamic Presurgical Trial of Vitamin E δ-tocotrienol in Patients with

Pancreatic Ductal Neoplasia. *EBioMedicine.* 2015;2(12):1987-1995. doi:10.1016/j.ebiom.2015.11.025

72. Smolarek A, So J, Burgess B et al. Dietary Administration of δ- and γ-Tocopherol Inhibits Tumorigenesis in the Animal Model of Estrogen Receptor–Positive, but not HER-2 Breast Cancer. *Cancer Prevention Research.* 2012;5(11):1310-1320. doi:10.1158/1940-6207.capr-12-0263

73. Osiecki H. *The Nutrient Bible.* 9th ed. Eagle Farm, QLD: Bio Concepts Publishing

74. Cheung C, Sahni S, Cheung B, Sing C, Wong I. Vitamin K intake and mortality in people with chronic kidney disease from NHANES III. *Clinical Nutrition.* 2015;34(2):235-240. doi:10.1016/j.clnu.2014.03.011

75. Xv F, Chen J, Duan L, Li S. Research progress on the anticancer effects of vitamin K2 (Review). *Oncol Lett.* 2018;6:8926-8934. doi:10.3892/ol.2018.8502

76. Baron J, Beach M, Mandel J et al. Calcium Supplements for the Prevention of Colorectal Adenomas. *New England Journal of Medicine.* 1999;340(2):101-107. doi:10.1056/NEJM199901143400204

77. Baron J, Barry E, Mott L et al. A Trial of Calcium and Vitamin D for the Prevention of Colorectal Adenomas. *N Engl J Med.* 2015;373(16):1519-1530. doi:10.1056/NEJMoa1500409

78. Medscape. Calcium Supplements Up Risk for Precancerous Serrated Polyps. Medscape. https://www.medscape.com/viewarticle/893319. Published 2018. Accessed August 24, 2021.

79. Bristow S, Bolland M, MacLennan G et al. Calcium supplements and cancer risk: a meta-analysis of randomised controlled trials. *British Journal of Nutrition.* 2013;110(8):1384-1393. doi:10.1017/S0007114513001050

80. Baron J, Beach M, Wallace K et al. Risk of Prostate Cancer in a Randomized Clinical Trial of Calcium Supplementation. *Cancer Epidemiology Biomarkers & Prevention.* 2005;14(3):586-589. doi:10.1158/1055-9965.EPI-04-0319

81. Reid I, Birstow S, Bolland M. Calcium and Cardiovascular Disease. *Endocrinology and Metabolism.* 2017;32(3):339-349. doi:10.3803/enm.2017.32.3.339

82. Dai Q, Shu X, Deng X et al. Modifying effect of calcium/magnesium intake ratio and mortality: a population-based cohort study. *BMJ Open.* 2013;3(2):e002111. doi:10.1136/bmjopen-2012-002111

83. Reddy M. Importance of Bioavailable Calcium and Other Minerals to Reduce the Calcium Deficiency Symptoms, Aging, and Other Pertinent Diseases. *Clin Pharmacol Biopharm.* 2017;06(2). doi:10.4172/2167-065x.1000172

84. Semeco A. 9 Benefits of Coenzyme Q10 (CoQ10). Healthline. https://www.healthline.com/nutrition/coenzyme-q10. Published 2017. Accessed August 24, 2021.

85. Rusciani L, Proietti I, Rusciani A et al. Low plasma coenzyme Q10 levels as an independent prognostic factor for melanoma progression. *J Am Acad Dermatol.* 2006;54(2):234-241. doi:10.1016/j.jaad.2005.08.031

86. Chai W, Cooney R, Franke A et al. Plasma Coenzyme Q10 Levels and Prostate Cancer Risk: The Multiethnic Cohort Study. *Cancer Epidemiology Biomarkers & Prevention.* 2011;20(4):708-710. doi:10.1158/1055-9965.epi-10-1309

87. Rusciani L, Proietti I, Paradisi A et al. Recombinant interferon α-2b and coenzyme Q10 as a postsurgical adjuvant therapy for melanoma: a 3-year trial with recombinant interferon-α and 5-year follow-up. *Melanoma Res*. 2007;17(3):177-183. doi:10.1097/cmr.0b013e32818867a0

88. Liu H, Huang Y, Cheng S, Huang Y, Lin P. Effects of coenzyme Q10 supplementation on antioxidant capacity and inflammation in hepatocellular carcinoma patients after surgery: a randomized, placebo-controlled trial. *Nutr J*. 2015;15(85). doi:10.1186/s12937-016-0205-6

89. Chen P, Hou C, Shibu M et al. Protective effect of Co-enzyme Q10 On doxorubicin-induced cardiomyopathy of rat hearts. *Environ Toxicol*. 2016;32(2):679-689. doi:10.1002/tox.22270

90. Greenlee H, Shaw J, Lau Y, Naini A, Maurer M. Lack of Effect of Coenzyme Q10 on Doxorubicin Cytotoxicity in Breast Cancer Cell Cultures. *Integr Cancer Ther*. 2012;11(3):243-250. doi:10.1177/1534735412439749

91. El-Sheikh A, Morsy M, Mahmoud M, Rifaai R, Abdelrahman A. Effect of Coenzyme-Q10 on Doxorubicin-Induced Nephrotoxicity in Rats. *Adv Pharmacol Sci*. 2012;2012:1-8. doi:10.1155/2012/981461

92. Perumal S, Shanthi P, Sachdanandam P. Augmented efficacy of tamoxifen in rat breast tumorigenesis when gavaged along with riboflavin, niacin, and CoQ10: Effects on lipid peroxidation and antioxidants in mitochondria. *Chem Biol Interact*. 2005;152(1):49-58. doi:10.1016/j.cbi.2005.01.007

93. Hertz N, Lister R. Improved Survival in Patients with End-Stage Cancer Treated with Coenzyme Q10 and other Antioxidants: A Pilot Study. *Journal of International Medical Research*. 2009;37(6):1961-1971. doi:10.1177/147323000903700634

94. Lesser G, Case D, Stark N et al. A Randomized, Double-Blind, Placebo-Controlled Study of Oral Coenzyme Q10 to Relieve Self-Reported Treatment-Related Fatigue in Newly Diagnosed Patients with Breast Cancer. *J Support Oncol*. 2013;11(1):31-42. doi:10.1016/j.suponc.2012.03.003

95. National Institute of Health. Coenzyme Q10 (PDQ®). National Institute of Health. https://www.ncbi.nlm.nih.gov/books/NBK65890/. Published 2021. Accessed August 24, 2021.

96. Skubitz K, Anderson P. Oral glutamine to prevent chemotherapy induced stomatitis: A pilot study. *Journal of Laboratory and Clinical Medicine*. 1996;127(2):223-228. doi:10.1016/s0022-2143(96)90082-7

97. Pattanayak L, Panda N, Dash M, Mohanty S, Samantaray S. Management of Chemoradiation-Induced Mucositis in Head and Neck Cancers With Oral Glutamine. *J Glob Oncol*. 2016;2(4):200-206. doi:10.1200/jgo.2015.000786

98. Miraghajani M, Jolfaie N, Mirzaie S, Ghiasvand R, Askari G. The effect of glutamine intake on complications of colorectal and colon cancer treatment: A systematic review. *Journal of Research in Medical Sciences*. 2015;20(9):910-918. doi:10.4103/1735-1995.170634

99. Amara S. Oral Glutamine for the Prevention of Chemotherapy-Induced Peripheral Neuropathy. *Annals of Pharmacotherapy*. 2008;42(10):1481-1485. doi:10.1345/aph.1l179

100. Sun J, Wang H, Hu H. Glutamine for chemotherapy induced diarrhea: a meta-analysis. *Asia Pac J Clin Nutr.* 2012;21(3):380-385. https://pubmed.ncbi.nlm.nih.gov/22705427/. Accessed August 24, 2021.

101. Rubio I, Suva L, Todorova V et al. Oral Glutamine Reduces Radiation Morbidity in Breast Conservation Surgery. *Journal of Parenteral and Enteral Nutrition.* 2013;37(5):623-630. doi:10.1177/0148607112474994

102. Klek S, Scislo L, Walewska E, Choruz R, Galas A. Enriched enteral nutrition may improve short-term survival in stage IV gastric cancer patients: A randomized, controlled trial. *Nutrition.* 2017;36:46-53. doi:10.1016/j.nut.2016.03.016

103. Cluntun A, Lukey M, Cerione R, Locasale J. Glutamine Metabolism in Cancer: Understanding the Heterogeneity. *Trends Cancer.* 2017;3(3):169-180. doi:10.1016/j.trecan.2017.01.005

104. García-de-Lorenzo A, Zarazaga A, García-Luna P et al. Clinical evidence for enteral nutritional support with glutamine: A Systematic Review. *Nutrition.* 2003;19(9):805-811. doi:10.1016/s0899-9007(03)00103-5

105. Michalak K, Maćkowska-Kędziora A, Sobolewski B, Woźniak P. Key Roles of Glutamine Pathways in Reprogramming the Cancer Metabolism. *Oxid Med Cell Longev.* 2015;2015:1-14. doi:10.1155/2015/964321

106. WebMD. GLUTAMINE: Overview, Uses, Side Effects, Precautions, Interactions, Dosing and Reviews. WebMD. https://www.webmd.com/vitamins/ai/ingredientmono-878/glutamine. Published 2020. Accessed August 25, 2021.

107. Aceves C, Anguiano B, Delgado G. The Extrathyronine Actions of Iodine as Antioxidant, Apoptotic, and Differentiation Factor in Various Tissues. *Thyroid.* 2013;23(8):938-946. doi:10.1089/thy.2012.0579

108. Aceves C, Anguiano B, Delgado G. Is Iodine A Gatekeeper of the Integrity of the Mammary Gland?. *J Mammary Gland Biol Neoplasia.* 2005;10(2):189-196. doi:10.1007/s10911-005-5401-5

109. Rappaport J. Changes in Dietary Iodine Explains Increasing Incidence of Breast Cancer with Distant Involvement in Young Women. *J Cancer.* 2017;8(2):174-177. doi:10.7150/jca.17835

110. Aranda N, Sosa S, Delgado G, Aceves C, Anguiano B. Uptake and antitumoral effects of iodine and 6-iodolactone in differentiated and undifferentiated human prostate cancer cell lines. *Prostate.* 2012;73(1):31-41. doi:10.1002/pros.22536

111. Hoption Cann S, Qiu Z, van Netten C. A Prospective Study of Iodine Status, Thyroid Function, and Prostate Cancer Risk: Follow-up of the First National Health and Nutrition Examination Survey. *Nutr Cancer.* 2007;58(1):28-34. doi:10.1080/01635580701307960

112. Kargar S, Shiryazdi S, Atashi S, Neamatzadeh S, Kamali M. Urinary Iodine Concentrations in Cancer Patients. *Asian Pacific Journal of Cancer Prevention.* 2017;18(3):812-821. doi:10.22034/APJCP.2017.18.3.819

113. Rösner H, Möller W, Groebner S, Torremante P. Antiproliferative/cytotoxic effects of molecular iodine, povidone-iodine and Lugol's solution in different human carcinoma cell lines. *Oncol Lett.* 2016;12(3):2159-2162. doi:10.3892/ol.2016.4811

114. Kaczor T. Iodine and Cancer: A summary of the evidence to date. *Natural Medicine Journal*. 2014;6(6). https://www.naturalmedicinejournal.com/journal/2014-06/iodine-and-cancer. Accessed August 25, 2021.

115. WebMD. IODINE: Overview, Uses, Side Effects, Precautions, Interactions, Dosing and Reviews. WebMD. https://www.webmd.com/vitamins/ai/ingredientmono-35/iodine. Published 2020. Accessed August 25, 2021.

116. Li Y, Li S, Zhou Y et al. Melatonin for the prevention and treatment of cancer. *Oncotarget*. 2017;8(24):39896-39921. doi:10.18632/oncotarget.16379

117. Rondanelli M, Faliva M, Perna S, Antoniello N. Update on the role of melatonin in the prevention of cancer tumorigenesis and in the management of cancer correlates, such as sleep-wake and mood disturbances: review and remarks. *Aging Clin Exp Res*. 2013;25(5):499-510. doi:10.1007/s40520-013-0118-6

118. Straif K, Baan R, Grosse Y et al. Carcinogenicity of shift-work, painting, and fire-fighting. *The Lancet Oncology*. 2007;8(12):1065-1066. doi:10.1016/s1470-2045(07)70373-x

119. Ferracioli-Oda E, Qawasmi A, Bloch M. Meta-Analysis: Melatonin for the Treatment of Primary Sleep Disorders. *PLoS One*. 2013;8(5):e63773. doi:10.1371/journal.pone.0063773

120. Zhdanova I, Wurtman R, Regan M, Taylor J, Shi J, Leclair O. Melatonin Treatment for Age-Related Insomnia. *The Journal of Clinical Endocrinology & Metabolism*. 2001;86(10):4727-4730. doi:10.1210/jcem.86.10.7901

121. Liu S, Madu C, Lu Y. The Role of Melatonin in Cancer Development. *Oncomedicine*. 2018;3:37-47. doi:10.7150/oncm.25566

122. Lissoni P, Barni S, Meregalli S et al. Modulation of cancer endocrine therapy by melatonin: a phase II study of tamoxifen plus melatonin in metastatic breast cancer patients progressing under tamoxifen alone. *Br J Cancer*. 1995;71(4):854-856. doi:10.1038/bjc.1995.164

123. Mills E, Wu P, Seely D, Guyatt G. Melatonin in the treatment of cancer: a systematic review of randomized controlled trials and meta-analysis. *J Pineal Res*. 2005;39(4):360-366. doi:10.1111/j.1600-079x.2005.00258.x

124. Seely D, Wu P, Fritz H et al. Melatonin as Adjuvant Cancer Care With and Without Chemotherapy. *Integr Cancer Ther*. 2011;11(4):293-303. doi:10.1177/1534735411425484

125. Malhotra S, Sawhney G, Pandhi P. The Therapeutic Potential of Melatonin: A Review of the Science. *MedGenMed*. 2004;6(2):46. https://www.ncbi.nlm.nih.gov/pmc/articles/PMC1395802/. Accessed August 25, 2021.

126. Tailleux A, Torpier G, Bonnefont-Rousselot D et al. Daily melatonin supplementation in mice increases atherosclerosis in proximal aorta. *Biochem Biophys Res Commun*. 2002;293(3):1114-1123. doi:10.1016/s0006-291x(02)00336-4

127. Memorial Sloan Kettering Cancer Center. Melatonin. Memorial Sloan Kettering Cancer Center. https://www.mskcc.org/cancer-care/integrative-medicine/herbs/melatonin. Published 2021. Accessed August 25, 2021.

128. WebMD. MELATONIN: Overview, Uses, Side Effects, Precautions, Interactions, Dosing and Reviews. WebMD. https://www.webmd.com/vitamins/ai/ingredientmono-940/melatonin. Published 2018. Accessed August 25, 2021.

129. RxList. Melatonin. RxList. https://www.rxlist.com/melatonin/supplements.htm. Published 2021. Accessed August 25, 2021.

130. Lin P, Lee M, Wang W et al. N-acetylcysteine has neuroprotective effects against oxaliplatin-based adjuvant chemotherapy in colon cancer patients: preliminary data. *Supportive Care in Cancer*. 2006;14(5):484-487. doi:10.1007/s00520-006-0018-9

131. Moslehi A, Taghizadeh-Ghehi M, Gholami K et al. N-acetyl cysteine for prevention of oral mucositis in hematopoietic SCT: a double-blind, randomized, placebo-controlled trial. *Bone Marrow Transplant*. 2014;49(6):818-823. doi:10.1038/bmt.2014.34

132. Al-Tonbary Y, Al-Haggar M, El-Ashry R, El-Dakroory S, Azzam H, Fouda A. Vitamin E and N-Acetylcysteine as Antioxidant Adjuvant Therapy in Children with Acute Lymphoblastic Leukemia. *Adv Hematol*. 2009;2009:689639. doi:10.1155/2009/689639

133. Lomeli N, Di K, Czerniawski J, Guzowski J, Bota D. Cisplatin-induced mitochondrial dysfunction is associated with impaired cognitive function in rats. *Free Radical Biology and Medicine*. 2017;102:274-286. doi:10.1016/j.freeradbiomed.2016.11.046

134. Qanungo S, Uys J, Manevich Y et al. N-acetyl-l-cysteine sensitizes pancreatic cancers to gemcitabine by targeting the NF⊠B pathway. *Biomedicine & Pharmacotherapy*. 2014;68(7):855-864. doi:10.1016/j.biopha.2014.08.007

135. Kretzmann N, Chiela E, Matte U, Marroni N, Marroni C. N-acetylcysteine improves antitumoural response of Interferon alpha by NF-kB downregulation in liver cancer cells. *Comp Hepatol*. 2012;11(1):4. doi:10.1186/1476-5926-11-4

136. Van Schooten F, Beserati Nia A, De Flora S et al. Effects of Oral Administration of N-Acetyl-l-cysteine: A Multi-Biomarker Study in Smokers. *Cancer Epidemiology, Biomarkers & Prevention*. 2002;11:167-175. https://cebp.aacrjournals.org/content/11/2/167. Accessed August 25, 2021.

137. Omenn G. Chemoprevention of Lung Cancer Is Proving Difficult and Frustrating, Requiring New Approaches. *J Natl Cancer Inst*. 2000;92(12):959-960. doi:10.1093/jnci/92.12.959

138. Sayin V, Ibrahim M, Larsson E, Nilsson J, Lindahl P, Bergo M. Antioxidants Accelerate Lung Cancer Progression in Mice. *Sci Transl Med*. 2014;6(221):221ra15. doi:10.1126/scitranslmed.3007653

139. RxList. N-acetyl Cysteine. RxList. https://www.rxlist.com/n-acetyl_cysteine/supplements.htm. Published 2021. Accessed August 25, 2021.

140. Office of Dietary Supplements. Omega-3 Fatty Acids. Office of Dietary Supplements. https://ods.od.nih.gov/factsheets/Omega3FattyAcids-HealthProfessional/. Published 2021. Accessed August 25, 2021.

141. Gerber M. Omega-3 fatty acids and cancers: a systematic update review of epidemiological studies. *British Journal of Nutrition*. 2012;107(S2):S228-S239. doi:10.1017/s0007114512001614

142. Brasky T, Darke A, Song X et al. Plasma Phospholipid Fatty Acids and Prostate Cancer Risk in the SELECT Trial. *J Natl Cancer Inst*. 2013;105(15):1132-1141. doi:10.1093/jnci/djt174

143. Alexander D, Bassett J, Weed D, Barrett E, Watson H, Harris W. Meta-Analysis of Long-Chain Omega-3 Polyunsaturated Fatty Acids (LC⊠-3PUFA) and Prostate Cancer. *Nutr Cancer*. 2015;67(4):543-554. doi:10.1080/01635581.2015.1015745

144. Manson J, Cook N, Lee I et al. Marine n-3 Fatty Acids and Prevention of Cardiovascular Disease and Cancer. *New England Journal of Medicine*. 2019;380(1):23-32. doi:10.1056/nejmoa1811403

145. Fabian C, Kimler B, Hursting S. Omega-3 fatty acids for breast cancer prevention and survivorship. *Breast Cancer Research*. 2015;17(1):62. doi:10.1186/s13058-015-0571-6

146. Djuric Z, Turgeon D, Sen A et al. The Anti-inflammatory Effect of Personalized Omega-3 Fatty Acid Dosing for Reducing Prostaglandin E2 in the Colonic Mucosa Is Attenuated in Obesity. *Cancer Prevention Research*. 2017;10(12):729-737. doi:10.1158/1940-6207.capr-17-0091

147. Gu Z, Suburu J, Chen H, Chen Y. Mechanisms of Omega-3 Polyunsaturated Fatty Acids in Prostate Cancer Prevention. *Biomed Res Int*. 2013;2013:82463. doi:10.1155/2013/824563

148. Bougnoux P, Hajjaji N, Ferrasson M, Giraudeau B, Couet C, Le Floch O. Improving outcome of chemotherapy of metastatic breast cancer by docosahexaenoic acid: a phase II trial. *Br J Cancer*. 2009;101(12):1978-1985. doi:10.1038/sj.bjc.6605441

149. Colas S, Paon L, Denis F et al. Enhanced radiosensitivity of rat autochthonous mammary tumors by dietary docosahexaenoic acid. *Int J Cancer*. 2004;109(3):449-454. doi:10.1002/ijc.11725

150. Bonatto S, Oliveira H, Nunes E et al. Fish Oil Supplementation Improves Neutrophil Function During Cancer Chemotherapy. *Lipids*. 2011;47(4):383-389. doi:10.1007/s11745-011-3643-0

151. Gianotti L, Braga M, Nespoli L, Radaelli G, Beneduce A, Di Carlo V. A randomized controlled trial of preoperative oral supplementation with a specialized diet in patients with gastrointestinal cancer. *Gastroenterology*. 2002;122(7):1763-1770. doi:10.1053/gast.2002.33587

152. Hegde S, Kaushal N, Ravindra K et al. Δ12-prostaglandin J3, an omega-3 fatty acid-derived metabolite, selectively ablates leukemia stem cells in mice. *Blood*. 2011;118(26):6909-6919. doi:10.1182/blood-2010-11-317750

153. Chagas T, Borges D, de Oliveira P et al. Oral fish oil positively influences nutritional-inflammatory risk in patients with haematological malignancies during chemotherapy with an impact on long-term survival: a randomised clinical trial. *Journal of Human Nutrition and Dietetics*. 2017;30(6):681-692. doi:10.1111/jhn.12471

154. Abdi J, Garssen J, Faber J, Redegeld F. Omega-3 fatty acids, EPA and DHA induce apoptosis and enhance drug sensitivity in multiple myeloma cells but not in normal peripheral mononuclear cells. *J Nutr Biochem*. 2014;25(12):1254-1262. doi:10.1016/j.jnutbio.2014.06.013

155. Morland S, Martins K, Mazurak V. n-3 polyunsaturated fatty acid supplementation during cancer chemotherapy. *J Nutr Intermed Metab*. 2016;5:107-116. doi:10.1016/j.jnim.2016.05.001

156. Vaughan V, Hassing M, Lewandowski P. Marine polyunsaturated fatty acids and cancer therapy. *Br J Cancer*. 2013;108(3):486-492. doi:10.1038/bjc.2012.586

157. Begtrup K, Krag A, Hvas A. No impact of fish oil supplements on bleeding risk: a systematic review. *Dan Med J*. 2017;64(5):A5366. https://pubmed.ncbi.nlm.nih.gov/28552094/. Accessed August 25, 2021.

158. Pryce R, Bernaitis N, Davey A, Badrick T, Anoopkumar-Dukie S. The Use of Fish Oil with Warfarin Does Not Significantly Affect either the International Normalised Ratio or Incidence of Adverse Events in Patients with Atrial Fibrillation and Deep Vein Thrombosis: A Retrospective Study. *Nutrients*. 2016;8(9):578. doi:10.3390/nu8090578

159. Eritsland J, Arnesen H, Seljeflot I, Kierulf P. Long-term effects of n-3 polyunsaturated fatty acids on haemostatic variables and bleeding episodes in patients with coronary artery disease. *Blood Coagulation & Fibrinolysis*. 1995;6(1):17-22. doi:10.1097/00001721-199502000-00003

160. Hatakka K, Savilhati E, Pönkä E, Meurman J, Savelin M, Korpela R. Effect of long term consumption of probiotic milk on infections in children attending day care centres: double blind, randomised. *BMJ*. 2001;322(7298):1327. doi:10.1136/bmj.322.7298.1327

161. Jacouton E, Chain F, Sokol H, Langella P, Bermúdez-Humarán L. Probiotic Strain Lactobacillus casei BL23 Prevents Colitis-Associated Colorectal Cancer. *Front Immunol*. 2017;8:1553. doi:10.3389/fimmu.2017.01553

162. Li J, Sung C, Lee N et al. Probiotics modulated gut microbiota suppresses hepatocellular carcinoma growth in mice. *Proceedings of the National Academy of Sciences*. 2016;113(9):E1306-E1315. doi:10.1073/pnas.1518189113

163. Wang Y, Yao N, Wei K et al. The efficacy and safety of probiotics for prevention of chemoradiotherapy-induced diarrhea in people with abdominal and pelvic cancer: a systematic review and meta-analysis. *Eur J Clin Nutr*. 2016;70(11):1246-1253. doi:10.1038/ejcn.2016.102

164. Hassan H, Rompola M, Glaser A, Kinsey S, Phillips R. Systematic review and meta-analysis investigating the efficacy and safety of probiotics in people with cancer. *Supportive Care in Cancer*. 2018;26(8):2503-2509. doi:10.1007/s00520-018-4216-z

165. Wang T, Cai G, Qiu Y et al. Structural segregation of gut microbiota between colorectal cancer patients and healthy volunteers. *ISME J*. 2011;6(2):320-329. doi:10.1038/ismej.2011.109

166. Aisu N, Tanimura S, Yamashita Y et al. Impact of perioperative probiotic treatment for surgical site infections in patients with colorectal cancer. *Exp Ther Med*. 2015;10(3):966-972. doi:10.3892/etm.2015.2640

167. McFarland L. Meta-Analysis of Probiotics for the Prevention of Antibiotic Associated Diarrhea and the Treatment of Clostridium difficile Disease. *Am J Gastroenterol*. 2006;101(4):812-822. doi:10.1111/j.1572-0241.2006.00465.x

168. Surawicz C, McFarland L, Greenberg R et al. The Search for a Better Treatment for Recurrent Clostridium difficile Disease: Use of High-Dose Vancomycin Combined with Saccharomyces boulardii. *Clinical Infectious Diseases*. 2000;31(4):1012-1017. doi:10.1086/318130

169. National Health and Medical Research Council. Selenium. National Health and Medical Research Council. https://www.nrv.gov.au/nutrients/selenium. Published 2014. Accessed August 25, 2021.

170. Nuts for Life. If I eat too many Brazil nuts, will I get too much selenium?. Nuts for Life. https://www.nutsforlife.com.au/resource/if-i-eat-too-many-brazil-nuts-will-i-get-too-much-selenium/. Published 2019. Accessed August 25, 2021.

171. Clark L, Dalkin B, Krongrad A et al. Decreased incidence of prostate cancer with selenium supplementation: results of a double-blind cancer prevention trial. *BJU Int.* 1998;81(5):730-734. doi:10.1046/j.1464-410x.1998.00630.x

172. Duffield-Lillico A, Dalkin B, Reid M et al. Selenium supplementation, baseline plasma selenium status and incidence of prostate cancer: an analysis of the complete treatment period of the Nutritional Prevention of Cancer Trial. *BJU Int.* 2003;91(7):608-612. doi:10.1046/j.1464-410x.2003.04167.x

173. Lippman S, Klein E, Goodman P et al. Effect of Selenium and Vitamin E on Risk of Prostate Cancer and Other Cancers. *JAMA.* 2009;301(1):39-51. doi:10.1001/jama.2008.864

174. Algotar A, Stratton M, Ahmann F et al. Phase 3 clinical trial investigating the effect of selenium supplementation in men at high-risk for prostate cancer. *Prostate.* 2012;73(3):328-335. doi:10.1002/pros.22573

175. Muecke R, Micke O, Schomburg L, Buentzel J, Kisters K, Adamietz I. Selenium in Radiation Oncology—15 Years of Experiences in Germany. *Nutrients.* 2018;10(4):483. doi:10.3390/nu10040483

176. Puspitasari I, Abdulah R, Yamazaki C, Kameo S, Nakano T, Koyama H. Updates on clinical studies of selenium supplementation in radiotherapy. *Radiation Oncology.* 2014;9(1):125. doi:10.1186/1748-717x-9-125

177. WebMD. SELENIUM: Overview, Uses, Side Effects, Precautions, Interactions, Dosing and Reviews. WebMD. https://www.webmd.com/vitamins/ai/ingredientmono-1003/selenium. Published 2020. Accessed August 25, 2021.

178. Office of Dietary Supplements. Zinc. Office of Dietary Supplements. https://ods.od.nih.gov/factsheets/%20Zinc-HealthProfessional/. Published 2020. Accessed August 25, 2021.

179. Sandstead H, Freeland-Graves J. Dietary phytate, zinc and hidden zinc deficiency. *Journal of Trace Elements in Medicine and Biology.* 2014;28(4):414-417. doi:10.1016/j.jtemb.2014.08.011

180. Andrews R. Phytates and phytic acid. Here's what you need to know. Precision Nutrition. https://www.precisionnutrition.com/all-about-phytates-phytic-acid. Published 2021. Accessed August 25, 2021.

181. Li L, Gai X. The association between dietary zinc intake and risk of pancreatic cancer: a meta-analysis. *Biosci Rep.* 2017;37(3):BSR20170155. doi:10.1042/bsr20170155

182. Feng P, Li T, Guan Z, Franklin R, Costello L. Direct effect of zinc on mitochondrial apoptogenesis in prostate cells. *Prostate.* 2002;52(4):311-318. doi:10.1002/pros.10128

183. Costello L, Franklin R. A comprehensive review of the role of zinc in normal prostate function and metabolism; and its implications in prostate cancer. *Arch Biochem Biophys.* 2016;611:100-112. doi:10.1016/j.abb.2016.04.014

184. Iguchi K, Hamatake M, Ishida R et al. Induction of necrosis by zinc in prostate carcinoma cells and identification of proteins increased in association with this induction. *Eur J Biochem.* 1998;253(3):766-770. doi:10.1046/j.1432-1327.1998.2530766.x

185. Liang J, Liu Y, Zou J, Franklin R, Costello L, Feng P. Inhibitory effect of zinc on human prostatic carcinoma cell growth. *Prostate.* 1999;40(3):200-207. doi:10.1002/(sici)1097-0045(19990801)40:3<200::aid-pros8>3.0.co;2-3

186. Gutiérrez-González E, Castelló A, Fernández-Navarro P et al. Dietary Zinc and Risk of Prostate Cancer in Spain: MCC-Spain Study. *Nutrients.* 2018;11(1):18. doi:10.3390/nu11010018

187. Gallus S, Foschi R, Negri E et al. Dietary Zinc and Prostate Cancer Risk: A Case-Control Study from Italy. *Eur Urol.* 2007;52(4):1052-1056. doi:10.1016/j.eururo.2007.01.094

188. Mahmoud A, Al-Alem U, Dabbous F et al. Zinc Intake and Risk of Prostate Cancer: Case-Control Study and Meta-Analysis. *PLoS One.* 2016;11(11):e0165956. doi:10.1371/journal.pone.0165956

189. Age-Related Eye Disease Study Research Group. A Randomized, Placebo-Controlled, Clinical Trial of High-Dose Supplementation With Vitamins C and E, Beta Carotene, and Zinc for Age-Related Macular Degeneration and Vision Loss. *Archives of Ophthalmology.* 2001;119(10):1417-1436. doi:10.1001/archopht.119.10.1417

190. Jarrard D. Does Zinc Supplementation Increase the Risk of Prostate Cancer?. *Archives of Ophthalmology.* 2005;123(1):102-103. doi:10.1001/archopht.123.1.102

191. Abnet C, Lai B, Qiao Y et al. Zinc Concentration in Esophageal Biopsy Specimens Measured by X-Ray Fluorescence and Esophageal Cancer Risk. *J Natl Cancer Inst.* 2005;97(4):301-306. doi:10.1093/jnci/dji042

192. Yarom N, Ariyawardana A, Hovan A et al. Systematic review of natural agents for the management of oral mucositis in cancer patients. *Supportive Care in Cancer.* 2013;21(11):3209-3221. doi:10.1007/s00520-013-1869-5

193. Tian X, Liu X, Pi Y, Chen H, Chen W. Oral Zinc Sulfate for Prevention and Treatment of Chemotherapy-Induced Oral Mucositis: A Meta-Analysis of Five Randomized Controlled Trials. *Front Oncol.* 2018;8:484. doi:10.3389/fonc.2018.00484

194. Ripamonti C, Zecca E, Brunelli C et al. A randomized, controlled clinical trial to evaluate the effects of zinc sulfate on cancer patients with taste alterations caused by head and neck irradiation. *Cancer.* 1998;82(10):1938-1945. doi:10.1002/(sici)1097-0142(19980515)82:10<1938::aid-cncr18>3.0.co;2-u

195. Najafizade N, Hemati S, Gookizade A et al. Preventive effects of zinc sulfate on taste alterations in patients under irradiation for head and neck cancers: A randomized placebo-controlled trial. *Journal of Research in Medical Sciences The Official Journal of Isfahan University of Medical Sciences.* 2013;18(2):123-126. https://pubmed.ncbi.nlm.nih.gov/23914214/. Accessed August 25, 2021.

196. Halyard M, Jatoi A, Sloan J et al. Does Zinc Sulfate Prevent Therapy-Induced Taste Alterations in Head and Neck Cancer Patients? Results of Phase III Double-Blind, Placebo-Controlled Trial from the North Central Cancer Treatment Group (N01C4). *Int J Radiat Oncol Biol Phys.* 2007;67(5):1318-1322. doi:10.1016/j.ijrobp.2006.10.046

197. Lin L, Que J, Lin K, Leung H, Lu C, Chang C. Effects of Zinc Supplementation on Clinical Outcomes in Patients Receiving Radiotherapy for Head and Neck Cancers: A Double-Blinded Randomized Study. *Int J Radiat Oncol Biol Phys.* 2008;70(2):368-373. doi:10.1016/j.ijrobp.2007.06.073

198. Lin Y, Lin L, Lin S. Effects of zinc supplementation on the survival of patients who received concomitant chemotherapy and radiotherapy for advanced nasopharyngeal carcinoma: Follow-up of a double-blind randomized study with subgroup analysis. *Laryngoscope.* 2009;119(7):1348-1352. doi:10.1002/lary.20524

199. Consolo L, Melnikov P, Cônsolo F, Nascimento V, Pontes J. Zinc supplementation in children and adolescents with acute leukemia. *Eur J Clin Nutr.* 2013;67(10):1056-1059. doi:10.1038/ejcn.2013.146

200. Australian Bureau of Statistics. Australian Health Survey: Usual Nutrient Intakes, 2011-12 financial year. Australian Bureau of Statistics. https://www.abs.gov.au/ausstats/abs@.nsf/Lookup/by%20Subject/4364.0.55.008~2011–12~Main%20Features~Zinc~408. Published 2015. Accessed August 25, 2021.

201. Penttilä O, Hurme H, Neuvonen P. Effect of zinc sulphate on the absorption of tetracycline and doxycycline in man. *Eur J Clin Pharmacol.* 1975;9(2-3):131-134. doi:10.1007/bf00614009

202. Memorial Sloan Kettering Cancer Center. Zinc. Memorial Sloan Kettering Cancer Center. https://www.mskcc.org/cancer-care/integrative-medicine/herbs/zinc#msk_professional. Published 2020. Accessed August 25, 2021.

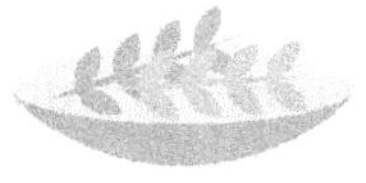

Chapter 8

Herbs and spices

'Plants love us. They help us reclaim our health and our whole selves. Plants are healers.'

— **Robin Rose Bennett**

There are many herbs and spices that can be helpful during and after cancer treatment to help with side-effects, recovery and prevention of further cancers. We'll cover a few of the most common ones. You'll notice that many of the studies are either carried out in a laboratory or on animals. Sadly, it's difficult to get finance to research herbs. Governments prioritise pharmaceutical approaches rather than natural medicine, and drug companies only research things that can be patented. However, the actions of these particular herbs are all directed at areas important to cancer patients and survivors.

A naturopath or herbalist can advise you on the most appropriate ones for your particular condition, and I strongly suggest that you consult one to get the most effective treatment. They also have easy access to many more.

The herbs in this chapter are listed in alphabetical order for ease of finding them, not order of importance.

Aloe vera (Aloe barbadensis)

Aloe vera is a plant in the lily family. It's best known for the topical use of its gel on burns to soothe and speed healing, because it's antibacterial, anti-inflammatory and antioxidant. This makes it useful for those undergoing radiotherapy.

During treatment

Patients with cancers of the head and neck, abdomen and pelvis, chest and the extremities who received a cumulative radiation dose exceeding 2,700 centigrays (cGy) found that using a mixture of mild soap followed by aloe vera **topically** had a significant effect on radiation-induced dermatitis.[1] However, there are many studies showing no benefit from aloe vera.

Radiation around the pelvic area causes symptoms such as diarrhoea, cramping, rectal bleeding and pain, known as Acute Radiation Proctitis (ARP). **Topical** aloe vera treatment is extremely effective against this, reducing symptoms, particularly diarrhoea, by about 75% in 4 weeks.[1]

Breast cancer patients receiving radiotherapy often suffer from skin dryness and sometimes burning. Sadly, aloe vera doesn't help with either skin irritation or pain in breast cancer patients receiving radiation.[1]

If you choose to use aloe vera, ensure that you use 100% pure gel without added alcohol, as alcohol could cause more irritation.

Used **topically**, though, it's generally considered to be safe.[2] It can be used as often as necessary. An important consideration is the hygiene of any gel or creams that you use. I suggest that you either buy tubes or that you use a spatula or spoon to get any product out of a container.

Astragalus (Astragalus membranaceus)

Astragalus is a herb commonly used in Chinese Traditional Medicine that's been adopted by Western herbalists.

Astragalus is an **adaptogen**, which means it supports the body when it's stressed, either physically or mentally, making it valuable for treating fatigue. This can be very helpful during and following cancer treatment.

For prevention

Rats given chemicals that induce liver cancer were treated with astragalus. It delayed the formation of liver cancer.[3]

During treatment

In laboratory tests, astragalus boosts **apoptosis**[4], so it could be valuable during cancer treatment.

It boosts the immune system by activating **B** and **T cells**, increasing antibody levels, stimulating **NK cells**, and boosting the effects of interferon, which helps the body fight viruses.[5] These actions may boost the immune systems of cancer patients, which are often depleted.

It supports the heart by opening up blood vessels and increasing cardiac output, and it helps with kidney function by its diuretic action, which reduces blood pressure. The heart and the kidneys are often badly affected by cancer treatments, so this can be helpful during recovery from chemo.

Astragalus also protects the liver from damaging chemicals.[6]

The body's helper **T cells** (Th), part of the immune system, are divided into 2 types, Th1 and Th2. The chemical messengers secreted by Th1 cells are anti-tumour and those secreted by Th2 cells are mostly immune system inhibitors, stopping the body from killing cancer cells. A study of non-small cell lung cancer patients found they have a higher level of Th2 cells and lower Th1 cells, which is related to shorter survival times.[7] A laboratory study showed that astragalus reverses the dominance of Th2 cells in lung cancer patients' blood.[8] No human studies have been conducted yet but this shows promise that astragalus could increase lung cancer survival.

Patients with advanced cancers who suffered from moderate to severe cancer-related fatigue were treated with astragalus. It significantly improved their fatigue compared with the **placebo** group.[9]

In laboratory tests and in mice with cancers implanted, astragalus together with either cisplatin or 5-fluorouracil reduced resistance to the drugs, and increased survival times of the mice.[10]

In animal studies, astragalus protected against heart damage caused by the chemo drug doxorubicin.[11]

Nausea and vomiting are side-effects commonly associated with chemotherapy treatment and seriously reduce quality of life. A **meta-analysis** of astragalus found that it reduced nausea and vomiting by 35%. A combination of *Panax ginseng* and astragalus was even more effective, reducing them by 50%.[12]

To prevent recurrence

Astragalus reduced mortality from acute myeloid leukaemia (AML) by 63% in a nationwide population based study on the use of traditional Chinese medicine in AML patients. The patients generally started using it about 7 months after diagnosis. The results improved the longer they took it, with use over more than 6 months being about 3 times more effective than 30–89 days. The study included those who had received a stem cell transplant from a donor.[13]

Dosage

You'll usually find astragalus in tablet form. Take 2.5–3.4 **g** per day.[14] If you can find the dried root, you can make a decoction instead by boiling it for 10 minutes and drinking the liquid once it's cooled. The daily dose for a decoction is 10–30 **g** of dried herb.[6]

Interactions, contraindications and side-effects

Astragalus has few side-effects but it's generally considered unwise to use it during an acute infection.

In laboratory tests, astragalus had some oestrogenic effect.[15] This suggests that it shouldn't be used if you have a hormone-sensitive cancer.

Astragalus protects against the effects of chemo on the bone marrow. However, this potentially means that it could be dangerous for anyone receiving treatment for active blood cancer. That includes anyone who's had a bone marrow transplant, until it's established that the graft has been successful. It could stimulate the growth of cancer cells and may reduce the effects of immunosuppressants.[16]

There's inconclusive evidence on whether cyclophosphamide is affected by astragalus.[16]

Since it stimulates the immune system, avoid taking astragalus if you suffer from any autoimmune disease.[16]

Astragalus is mildly diuretic and may reduce the excretion of lithium, therefore increasing its levels in your body. If you're taking lithium, you should ask your doctor to monitor you.[16]

Boswellia (Boswellia serrata)

Boswellia is a small tree or shrub that grows in the dry tropics of Asia and Africa. It produces a fragrant resin. The resin from some species of boswellia is known as frankincense, which has been used since antiquity for embalming and incense. *Boswellia serrata* is also known as Indian frankincense.

Boswellia is used by traditional healers, particularly in India, to treat a variety of inflammatory diseases. These include arthritis, chronic pain, inflammatory bowel disease and asthma. Unlike non-steroidal anti-inflammatory drugs (**NSAID**s), boswellia doesn't upset the gastrointestinal system.

During treatment

A recent review found it was anti-tumour and increased **apoptosis**.[17]

In a laboratory, extracts of boswellia were more effective at killing liver and colon cancer cells than the chemotherapy drugs doxorubicin and 5-fluorouracil.[18]

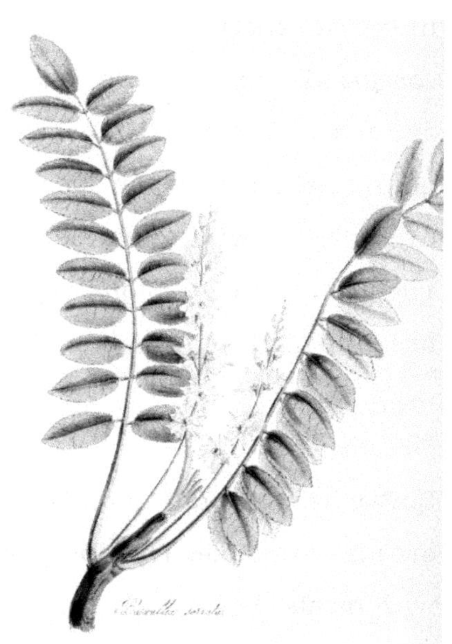

Another study implanted human colon cancer cells in mice, then treated them with a boswellia extract. They found it not only inhibited the growth of the cancers but also suppressed metastasis.[19] This paper also cited other studies showing that the extract inhibited other types of cancer cells in the laboratory, including leukaemia, prostate cancer and glioma.

Human pancreatic cancer cells were planted in mice and treated with a boswellia extract alone and in combination with gemcitabine, a drug used to treat pancreatic cancer. Boswellia inhibited growth of the tumours and sensitised them to gemcitabine, meaning that the gemcitabine was more effective. It also suppressed metastasis to the lungs, spleen and liver.[20]

Patients irradiated for brain tumours often suffer from oedema in the brain, which is usually treated with dexamethasone, which has various side-effects. Boswellia reduced oedema by more than 75% in the majority of patients receiving it, compared with 26% in patients receiving **placebo** treatment.[21]

Boswellia cream 2% used **topically** following radiation therapy in breast cancer patients reduced the intensity of skin damage compared with a **placebo**. It was used immediately after radiation and at bedtime on radiation days, and in the morning and night on non-radiation days.[22] This method is important, as the cream base can interfere with radiation treatment if it's applied too thickly. There have been occasional reports of allergic dermatitis following use of boswellia cream, though.[23] If this happens, discontinue use.

Dosage

Boswellia is generally found in tablet and capsule form but creams are also available. The dosage is 200–400 mg, 3 times per day with meals. There are no known issues with long-term use.[6]

Interactions, contraindications and side-effects

Taking warfarin with high doses of boswellia (1200 **mg** per day) has increased blood clotting time in isolated cases.[24]

In laboratory studies, boswellia stimulates the immune system. Theoretically this could reduce the effects of immunosuppressants, including azathioprine, basiliximab, cyclosporine, daclizumab, muromonab-CD3, mycophenolate, tacrolimus, sirolimus, prednisone and other corticosteroids.[6]

Because of its effects on the immune system, it is not suitable for anyone with a blood cancer.

Laboratory studies showed that boswellia increases the effects of tamoxifen, codeine, ibuprofen and treatments for reducing stomach acidity and it interacts with a wide range of other drugs. So if you are on any medication, it should only be prescribed by a healthcare practitioner trained in complementary medicine working alongside your GP or oncologist.[6]

Calendula (Calendula officinalis)

Calendula is in the marigold family. It's anti-inflammatory, antimicrobial, antiviral (**topically**), antifungal (**topically**), helps with wound healing and helps stop bleeding.

During treatment

In a human trial of breast cancer patients having radiotherapy, calendula cream containing 4% calendula was compared to trolamine, a salicylate cream believed to be effective against radiation side-effects. The calendula cream was significantly better at reducing acute dermatitis. It reduced radiation-induced pain considerably, and patients were better able to continue with radiotherapy. The patients found the particular calendula cream used in the trial more difficult to apply than the trolamine but were happier with the results.[25] Calendula creams vary: the one used in the trial was mixed with petroleum jelly, making it very thick and probably painful to apply to damaged skin. Calendula cream in a vitamin E cream base would be much easier to use.

Some studies disagree. A recent review highlighted a study that compared Weleda's calendula cream, with an unspecified percentage of calendula, with aqueous cream in breast cancer patients. It found there was no significant difference between the 2 treatment groups.[26] This may have been because the strength of the calendula was insufficient.

Calendula cream can be used as frequently as necessary. The latest advice is that it is quite safe to use a layer up to 2 mm thick just prior to radiotherapy, although thicker layers can reduce the effectiveness of the radiation.[27]

Interactions, contraindications and side-effects

A small number of people have an allergy to members of the *Compositae* family, which includes calendula, echinacea, arnica and dandelion amongst many others. When used topically, this can cause contact dermatitis. If you have a reaction to calendula cream, stop using it and consult a health professional if it persists.[149]

Ginger (Zingiber officinale)

Ginger is a pungent spice often used in food but also widely used in herbal medicine, both in the East and the West. Its uses include:

- anti-nausea, vomiting and digestive disturbances
- anti-inflammatory, especially for arthritis and rheumatism
- promoting peripheral circulation in hands and feet
- anti-microbial, particularly against *E. coli*, *Salmonella typhi* (cause of typhoid), *Candida albicans* (cause of thrush), and tuberculosis
- reducing fasting blood glucose levels
- protecting the brain
- protecting the liver
- migraine relief
- anti-tumour.[28]

There are several known active constituents in ginger: gingerol, zingerone, zerumbone, paradol, shogaol and essential oils, with gingerol being the one most researched.

For prevention

As yet there have been no human trials for its anti-cancer effects. However, animal trials and laboratory studies show that ginger's active constituents are effective against the following cancers:

- breast
- liver
- cervix
- myeloma
- colorectal area
- prostate
- pancreas
- melanoma
- glioblastoma
- leukaemia
- Burkitt Raji lymphoma.[29]

Chronic myeloid leukaemia (CML) cells treated with ginger in a laboratory were killed.[30] CML patients often progress to acute myeloid leukaemia.

People at high risk of developing colorectal cancers have higher levels of certain inflammatory chemicals in their gut tissue. Treating them with **NSAID**s causes significant side-effects in the gut. In high risk patients, 2 **g** per day of ginger significantly reduced the inflammatory markers, but in normal risk patients there was no change.[31]

During treatment

Cells from head and neck cancers were killed by ginger extracts in laboratory tests, and the effects of ginger during radiation therapy showed it was better than either therapy alone.[32]

In laboratory studies, low dosages of zerumbone extracted from ginger profoundly sensitised colorectal cancer cells to radiation.[33]

Acute lymphoblastic leukaemia (ALL) is a childhood blood cancer that's often resistant to chemo, with a poor prognosis. In laboratory studies of ALL cells resistant to methotrexate, ginger extract made the cells more sensitive to methotrexate treatment.[34]

Laboratory studies also show that ginger can protect against damage caused to heart cells by doxorubicin.[29] This means that the dosage of doxorubicin could be safely increased without the risk of heart damage.

Ginger may be helpful during chemo where the cancer is resistant. In laboratory studies, relatively low doses of ginger significantly increase sensitivity to cisplatin and/or paclitaxel in ovarian cancer cells.[35] This not only results in better survival but also means that the drugs' dosages can be reduced, with fewer side-effects.

Ginger is best known for treating nausea. Numerous studies have been done on its effects during chemo and they show that combining ginger capsules with anti-emetic drugs is very effective.[36-40]

Dosage

Standardised ginger capsules are ideal, using a dosage equivalent to 2–4 **g** of dried ginger per day, preferably divided into 3 doses per day.[41]

Interactions, contraindications and side-effects

Although ginger is known for treating digestive disturbances, it sometimes causes mild heartburn, diarrhoea, bloating or other digestive upsets. This is more likely when using ginger powder.[16]

Ginger is best avoided if you have a peptic ulcer or gallstones.[14]

In some people, ginger can have a mild sedative effect or cause dizziness. If you're affected, avoid driving or using machinery.[16]

Some women in a clinical trial experienced heavy periods when taking 1 **g** of ginger per day for 3 days.[16]

There's a theoretical concern that ginger might increase bleeding time. If you're taking anticoagulant medication this should be monitored.[16]

Some research suggests that ginger can increase insulin levels or reduce blood sugar.[16] If you're taking antidiabetic drugs, monitor your blood sugar levels.

Animal studies show that ginger can reduce blood pressure similarly to calcium channel blockers[16], so the effects of calcium channel blockers could be increased.

One animal study found that ginger juice taken 2 hours prior to cyclosporine reduced its effects, although it had no effect if taken concurrently with the cyclosporine.[16]

An animal study showed that ginger affected the metabolism of metronidazole (Flagyl).[16] It isn't known whether this happens in humans.

Nifedipine (Procardia, Adalat), used for treating angina, high blood pressure and some other conditions, significantly increased bleeding time when taken with ginger.[16]

Korean Ginseng (Panax ginseng)

There are various kinds of ginseng and they all have different properties. The one I'm covering here is Korean ginseng, as that's most relevant to cancer patients. Please don't assume that other kinds of ginseng will work in the same way. They don't necessarily.

Despite its name, Korean ginseng also grows in north-eastern China and far-eastern Siberia. The root is the part of the plant that's used. It grows in the shape of a human, leading to the Chinese name *Jen shen*, meaning 'man-root'. It's been used in Traditional Chinese Medicine for thousands of years. It comes in 2 distinct forms: red, which is prepared by steaming and then drying, and white, prepared by just drying. The 2 forms have slightly different concentrations of active compounds, with red ginseng containing more.

It's traditionally used as an **adaptogen**, to increase resistance to environmental stress and as a general tonic. It's helpful as a remedy for weakness and fatigue, both during and after cancer treatment. It's antioxidant and anti-inflammatory. It also:

- Regulates blood sugar levels.
- Improves male libido.
- Boosts mental well-being.
- Reduces **LDL cholesterol**, increases **HDL cholesterol**, and reduces blood pressure.
- Stimulates the immune system by increasing **T cells** and **NK cells.**
- Protects against some cancers. Improves cancer survival rates by inhibiting cancer growth and inducing **apoptosis**, helping

prevent **angiogenesis**, reducing metastasis, and increasing cancer sensitivity to chemo and radiation.[42]

- Reduces nausea and vomiting in chemo and radiotherapy patients.

For prevention

A large study in Korea, where Korean ginseng is often taken regularly, looked at a sample of cancer patients and compared them with healthy people from similar backgrounds, noting their ginseng intake. Regular ginseng consumption reduced the incidence of cancers by 50% overall and a startling 80% when they used red ginseng.[43] They followed this up with a large 5 year **prospective study** and found a 60% reduction in cancers in ginseng users, with particular preventive effects on gastric and lung cancers.[44]

Laboratory and animal studies show Korean ginseng's ability to prevent prostate cancers and their metastasis.[45]

In laboratory tests, extracts of Korean ginseng have anti-cancer properties against breast cancer cells, including hormone-sensitive breast cancer cells.[46-52]

In animal studies, Korean ginseng reduced benign prostatic dysplasia (enlarged prostate), which is often how prostate cancer starts. It worked by blocking testosterone receptors rather than reducing testosterone.[53]

During treatment

One of the active ingredients in Korean ginseng was used in a study of post-operative patients with Stage 2 or 3A non-small cell lung cancer. One group received chemo alone, one the chemo plus 40–50 **mg** per day of ginseng in 2 doses, and the other the same dosage of ginseng alone, with the ginseng groups continuing to take it for 6 months. The group that received combined chemo and ginseng had the best survival rates after 1, 2 and 3 years.[54]

In a 12 week trial of patients with mostly gynaecological and liver cancers, taking 3 **g** per day of sun ginseng, a type of red Korean ginseng, improved some aspects of physical and mental function.[55]

Patients with differing cancers received 800 **mg** of Korean ginseng extract capsules daily for 4 weeks. It quickly improved fatigue, pain, appetite, sleep disturbances and overall quality of life.[56]

In animal studies, Korean ginseng extract significantly reduced metastasis of colon cancer cells to the lungs.[57, 58]

Gynaecological cancer cell growth and migration were inhibited in laboratory tests by whole Korean ginseng extract.[59]

In animals, red Korean ginseng reduced nausea and vomiting during cisplatin chemo, with higher doses of ginseng proving more effective.[60]

To prevent recurrence

In laboratory tests, Korean ginseng kills breast cancer stem cells, which often cause patients to suffer recurrence of disease.[61] However, Korean ginseng has been used to help post-menopausal women with menopausal problems.[62] This suggests it has an oestrogenic effect. Even a mild oestrogenic effect could stimulate oestrogen-sensitive cancers, so don't use it if you have one. However, it could be helpful against triple negative breast cancer.

Dosage

Normal dosage for Korean ginseng is 300–500 mg per day in tablet form. This is for preventive therapy. It's best taken in the morning to avoid overstimulation and sleep disturbance.

To combat cancer-related fatigue during chemo, doses of 1–3 g per day have been used successfully in research.[63]

Interactions, contraindications and side-effects

Korean ginseng could affect how the body processes certain drugs, including some chemo drugs, corticosteroids, antifungals, calcium channel blockers, antidepressants and a number of other drug types, most likely increasing their effects. Consult a pharmacist before taking ginseng.[16]

Korean ginseng could reduce the effects of warfarin or other anticoagulant drugs, and increase bleeding time[63], so only use it under the supervision of a trained healthcare practitioner.

Alcohol could be processed more quickly when taken with Korean ginseng, reducing its effects.[16]

In some people, taking Korean ginseng with caffeine causes insomnia and agitation.[16]

Ginseng can increase the effects of anti-diabetes drugs[16], so only use it under the supervision of a trained healthcare practitioner.

Avoid Korean ginseng with any hormone-sensitive cancer, as it's known to stimulate various hormonal pathways.

Milk thistle (Silybum marianum)

Milk thistle, also known as St Mary's thistle, is native to Europe but is now grown all over the world. It's a thistle that grows up to 2 metres high, with a big, bright purple flower and lots of large spines. The milk in its name refers to the white veins on its leaves, traditionally said to carry the milk of the Virgin Mary. Its alternative name is St Mary's Thistle.

The active constituent in milk thistle is silymarin. It's antioxidant, antiviral and anti-inflammatory. It's also mildly oestrogenic. Its various uses are to:

- help prevent age-related mental decline
- protect bones
- reduce severity of hay fever when used in conjunction with an antihistamine
- boost breast milk production
- improve symptoms in men with enlarged prostates
- help maintain remission from ulcerative colitis
- reduce fasting glucose and improve insulin resistance in type 2 diabetes
- increase HDL cholesterol
- protect the liver and stimulate liver cell growth
- improve liver function in detoxification
- increase bile production
- reduce chemo and radiation side-effects.[16]

During treatment

A common side-effect of chemo is liver damage, which shows

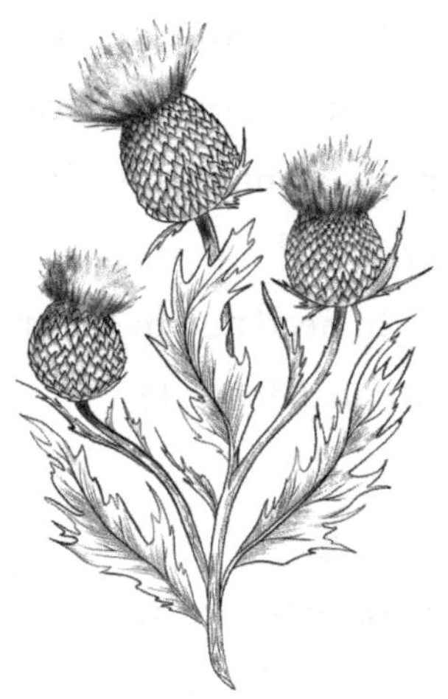

up as elevated liver enzymes. This can result in chemo being interrupted. Milk thistle is often used by cancer patients to prevent this. It's generally accepted that doses less than 5 **g** per day of silymarin are unlikely to interfere with chemo drugs[64], but please check with your healthcare practitioner first, as some drugs are affected by it. It can also be used successfully after treatment to help the liver recover from damage caused by the drugs used. Although there hasn't been any research yet on treating the effects of chemo drugs, the known effects of silymarin on the liver support the idea of using it.[65]

Milk thistle significantly reduced the incidence of liver damage in children with acute lymphoblastic leukaemia (ALL). The number of children whose chemo was suspended was fewer in those taking milk thistle. There were no adverse effects on the drugs involved, L-asparaginase and vincristine. In fact, the effects of vincristine were increased by the milk thistle.[66]

Capecitabine is a chemo drug often used for gastrointestinal cancers. One of the side-effects is 'hand-foot syndrome', where the palms of the hands and soles of the feet become very red and sore, and sometimes peel. A trial of silymarin gel 1% used twice a day on those areas delayed the onset of 'hand-foot syndrome' and reduced its severity.[67]

Use of a mainly silymarin-based cream, Leviaderm, significantly reduced radiation dermatitis in women undergoing radiation treatment for breast cancer, with 23.5% of patients not developing any dermatitis, compared with 2% of those who didn't use the cream.[68]

In head and neck cancers, taking 420 **mg** of silymarin daily in 3 divided doses delayed the onset of **mucositis** and its progression.[69]

Dosage

Dosage varies according to the purpose:

- To reduce liver toxicity of chemo drugs, take 420 **mg** of silymarin per day.[16]
- To improve liver function after treatment, take 200–400 **mg** of silymarin per day.[70]
- To prevent **mucositis** from radiotherapy, take 140 **mg** of silymarin 3 times per day.[69]
- For topical use to prevent side-effects of chemo and radiation, use a gel or cream form at 0.25–1% concentration.[67, 68]

Interactions, contraindications and side-effects

Milk thistle is well tolerated, with mild digestive issues being the main problems when taken orally.

Milk thistle can affect how some drugs are processed. If you're using any medication, consult a pharmacist before taking milk thistle. Most interactions are likely to have a minor effect. However, some could be serious, so **always** check.

Milk thistle can cause an allergic reaction in people sensitive to the daisy family (Asteraceae/Compositae).

In animal research, the active ingredient of silymarin binds to oestrogen receptors.[16] So it shouldn't be used in oestrogen-sensitive cancers.

In Type 2 diabetics, milk thistle can cause blood sugar to drop. If you're taking medication for Type 2 diabetes, your blood sugar levels should be closely monitored.[16]

In animal studies, tamoxifen levels in the blood were increased in animals given silymarin. It's not known whether this occurs in humans.[16] Advise your oncologist if you plan to take milk thistle alongside tamoxifen.

There could be interaction with warfarin, so bleeding time should be carefully monitored by your doctor.[16]

If your liver function is impaired, sirolimus levels could be increased with milk thistle[16], so advise your oncologist if you plan taking milk thistle alongside sirolimus.

Mushroom extracts

There are about 14,000 different types of mushroom and about 700 have shown medicinal properties. Many have been used in Traditional Chinese Medicine (TCM) for a long time, but some are being investigated by Western scientists for their properties, which include:

- antioxidant
- antiviral
- antimicrobial
- immuno-modulating
- anti-tumour

- anti-metastatic.[71]

One of the main active constituents is beta-glucans, which are believed to stimulate the immune system to exert anti-tumour effects. They stimulate:

- **NK cells**, which secrete chemicals that burst cancer cells' cell membranes
- **T cells**, which produce chemicals that kill cancer cells directly
- Neutrophils.[72]

Alpha-glucans are also found in some mushrooms. They're effective in fighting cancer and reducing side-effects of chemo and radiation.[73]

Other chemicals in mushrooms directly prevent growth and division of cancer cells and inhibit **angiogenesis**, which helps reduce metastasis.[74]

I'm only going to cover the types of mushrooms that have some research behind them and that are most easily available. These are: shiitake, reishi, maitake, cordyceps and turkey tail mushrooms. You might have seen some of these in the supermarket. Many more are successfully used in TCM and Western Herbal Medicine. You can access these through natural medicine practitioners.

Cordyceps (Cordyceps sinensis or Cordyceps militaris)

Cordyceps is sometimes known as the 'caterpillar fungus' because it's a parasite on the body of a moth caterpillar. Pretty gross, I know. These days, wild cordyceps is quite rare and very expensive, so it's cultivated commercially in laboratories.

It's been used for centuries in Korea and China as:

- treatment for asthma, as well as inflammation of the lungs and bronchi
- aphrodisiac
- immune modulator
- antioxidant
- painkiller
- tumour growth inhibitor.

During treatment

A review conducted on the effects of *Cordyceps sinensi* covered a number of clinical trials on humans:

- A fermented form of cordyceps, Cs-4, was used in terminal lung cancer patients, in combination with chemo and radiation. Significantly more patients were able to tolerate chemo and/or radiation therapies than those in the **control group**, and could therefore complete their treatment. The patients also suffered less bone marrow damage from the therapies.
- Cordyceps capsules in combination with chemo or other herbal treatments were used in a trial on lung cancer patients. After treatment, tumours were partially or slightly reduced in 46% of them, the patients' subjective symptoms improved and their immune systems weren't significantly affected, which is unusual after chemo.
- A fermented form was used on cancer patients undergoing chemo or radiation. In almost all of them, subjective symptoms improved, their white blood counts stayed high,

and about half of them experienced about 50% reduction in tumour size.

- Fermented cordyceps was used on patients with gentamicin toxicity. They showed an 89% recovery rate after 6 days compared with 45% recovery in the **control group**.
- Cordyceps also showed beneficial effects in 2 studies of patients with liver damage following hepatitis. Liver damage is quite common during chemo.[75]

Mice were injected with aggressive, **metastatic** human breast cancer cells and fed an extract from *Cordyceps sinensis*, either from when the cancer cells were injected or from when the tumours were removed. Although it didn't have any effect on growth of the tumours, even at high doses, it significantly reduced the incidence and numbers of **metastases** compared with controls.[76]

Human melanoma cells were implanted into mice. Once the tumours had grown substantially, half were injected subcutaneously with *Cordyceps militaris* extract near the tumour sites. The other half was a **control group**. The treated group had substantially less **angiogenesis**, and their tumours were about 20% the size and about 25% the weight of the **control group**.[77]

In vitro research found that cordyceps induced significant **apoptosis** in:

- renal cancer cells[78, 79]
- ovarian cancer cells[80]
- prostate cancer cells[81]
- oral cancer cells[82]
- colorectal cancer cells.[83]

Cordycepin is one of the active constituents of cordyceps. In laboratory tests it significantly reduced **metastasis** of liver cancer cells, and when combined with JSH-23, a treatment used in liver cancer, the 2 worked synergistically to significantly enhance the effects.[84]

A new, promising treatment for cancer is TRAIL (tumour necrosis factor **apoptosis**-inducing ligand), which can treat many types of cancers. It causes **apoptosis** with no effect on healthy cells. However, many cancer cells are resistant to it. Cordycepin works synergistically with TRAIL to significantly inhibit growth of liver cancer cells resistant to TRAIL alone.[85]

Non-small cell lung cancer (NSCLC) accounts for more than 80% of lung cancers and is resistant to radiation and most chemo drugs. Cells from NSCLC were treated with cisplatin alone or with cisplatin and a *Cordyceps sinensis* extract. After 48 hours, the combination was about twice as effective at inhibiting growth and about 25% more effective at causing **apoptosis** than cisplatin alone.[86]

Dosage

A dose of 6 **g** per day was used for 2 months in clinical studies on lung cancer patients.[87]

Interactions, contraindications and side-effects

As an immune modulator, cordyceps isn't appropriate for anyone with active blood cancer.

Cordyceps is generally well tolerated. Mild, rare side-effects include abdominal discomfort, constipation and diarrhoea, but these are minimised by taking it after food.[16]

Theoretically, there's a risk that cordyceps could increase bleeding if taken with anti-platelet drugs, such as warfarin. Monitor bleeding time carefully if you're taking these medications.[16]

There's a theoretical concern that cordyceps could interact with immunosuppressant drugs[16] but this hasn't been demonstrated.

There's a risk that cordyceps might increase the effects of monoamine oxidase inhibitors (MAOI), which are sometimes used to treat depression.[87] Therefore use only under the supervision of a qualified healthcare practitioner.

In theory, cordyceps could increase the effects of antiviral drugs and drugs used to lower blood sugar levels.[87]

Maitake (Grifola frondosa)

The name maitake is Japanese, where '*mai*' means dance and '*take*' means mushroom, making 'dancing mushroom'. It isn't known whether it got its name because the fruiting bodies look like nymphs or butterflies wildly dancing or if it came from the happy dance that mushroomers did if they found it. Maitake was very valuable in Japan.

Maitake has been used medicinally in Japan, India, Korea and China for centuries to enhance the immune system and as a tonic or **adaptogen**. More recent research shows that it:

- lowers blood sugar and possibly increases insulin sensitivity
- reduces blood pressure and prevents it rising
- assists with liver function

- can help with weight control
- has anti-tumour actions.[88]

For prevention

Research into maitake is in the early stages. Most studies have been performed on human cancer cells in a laboratory or in animals. One human study was conducted on breast cancer patients following surgery and other treatment, and currently in remission. They found that the most effective dose of liquid maitake extract for improving immune function was around 5 **mg** per **kg** of body weight per day, split into 2 doses.[89]

Extracts from maitake improve immune function by increasing the numbers of **NK cells**, macrophages (a type of white blood cell) and cytotoxic **T cells**. It can also activate **genes** that cause breast cancer cells to undergo **apoptosis.**[90, 91]

During treatment

Triple-negative breast cancer is particularly malignant and prone to **metastasis**. Researchers tested maitake extract on triple-negative breast cancer cells and found it caused **apoptosis** and reduced their **metastatic** potential. They then implanted human triple-negative breast cancer cells in mice and treated them with maitake extract. The result was slower tumour growth and reduced lung **metastasis.**[92]

A study using maitake extract on 4 different gastric cancer cell types found they underwent **apoptosis**, in one case causing 90% of the cells to die in 3 days.[93]

In a laboratory study, a combination of interferon-α and maitake extract reduced growth of bladder cancer cells by about 75%. This was better than interferon-α could achieve alone, and at a lower dose.[94]

In mice treated with paclitaxel, damage to bone marrow recovered quickly with oral maitake extract. It was as effective as G-CSF, the usual treatment.[95] Paclitaxel affects the ability of white blood cells to kill infectious agents. G-CSF treatment doesn't restore that, but maitake increased white blood cells' ability, reducing the likelihood of infection.[95]

Dosage

In the human trial, 5–7 **mg** per **kg** body weight, per day of liquid extract split into 2 doses improved immune function.[89]

Commercially, maitake is available as capsules, powder or liquid extract.

For disease prevention, the recommended doses are either:

- 12–25 **mg** of the extract plus 200–250 **mg** of whole powder per day, or
- 500– 2,500 **mg** of whole powder per day.[96]

Interactions, contraindications and side-effects

Maitake isn't appropriate for anyone with active blood cancer because it increases immune system activity.

Maitake can cause mild nausea, diarrhoea, stomach ache, joint swelling or a mild skin rash.[16]

Maitake can lower blood glucose. If you're on diabetic medication you should monitor your blood glucose carefully.[16]

In animals, maitake can lower blood pressure. If you're on blood pressure lowering medication, monitor your blood pressure carefully and contact your doctor if it drops.[16]

In one case report, a patient on warfarin and taking maitake had increased clotting time. This suggested that it increased warfarin's effects, but there have been no other cases reported.[97] If you're taking warfarin, advise your health practitioner before you take maitake.

Reishi (Ganoderma lucidum)

Reishi mushrooms have been used in Traditional Chinese Medicine for over 2,000 years to treat a variety of illnesses, including:

- autoimmune diseases
- diabetes
- respiratory diseases
- gastrointestinal diseases
- high blood pressure
- migraine
- kidney and liver diseases
- some cardiovascular problems
- high cholesterol
- fatigue
- insomnia
- prevention and treatment of cancer
- immune system support.

For prevention

Laboratory studies show reishi can help prevent development of breast, liver, prostate and bladder cancers.[98]

By the age of 60, about 40% of men have enlarged prostates, known as benign prostatic hyperplasia (BPH). This rises to about 90% of men between the age of 80 and 90. The condition is caused by dihydrotestosterone, a male hormone that can't easily be broken down. Although there's no conclusive evidence that BPH is linked to prostate cancer, medications that lower dihydrotestosterone reduce the risk of prostate cancer but come with significant side-effects. In an 8 week study of men over 50 suffering from BPH with lower urinary tract symptoms, 6 **mg** of reishi in tablets once daily resulted in higher urine output and an improvement in their International Prostate Symptom Score with only minor adverse reactions.[99]

During treatment

A Cochrane **systematic review** and **meta-analysis** found reishi made chemo work 25% better. It also helped counteract immunosuppression and improved quality of life in the patients, with only a few minor side-effects.[100]

It slows growth of breast and prostate cancer cells in laboratory studies. In animal studies, transplanted colon cancer cells grew more slowly when treated with reishi. It also reduces the likelihood of **metastasis** by affecting the **genes** that control part of the process.[98]

The high rate of mortality in breast cancer patients is usually because of **metastasis**. One study on mice implanted them with a particularly invasive type of human breast cancer. They were treated with reishi after the tumours had grown. At the end of the study, they found about 30% fewer **metastases** to the lungs in the reishi group compared with controls.[101]

Inflammatory breast cancer is a particularly aggressive form of breast cancer. In both laboratory and animal testing, reishi reduced the weight of tumours by 45% and the volume by more than 50% compared with the **placebo** group. The dose used was equivalent to twice the normal dose given to human patients but caused no ill effects.[102]

Osteosarcoma is the most common bone cancer found in children and adults. It's a highly malignant cancer and often **metastasises**, so it has a poor prognosis. Laboratory studies show that reishi slows the growth of osteosarcoma cells.[103]

Breast cancer patients who had completed or were undergoing endocrine therapy were given reishi for 4 weeks. They had significant improvements in their physical well-being and fatigue levels. They suffered less anxiety and depression, and had a better quality of life compared with the **placebo** group.[104]

Dosage

Recommended dosage is one of the following:

- dried mushroom: 1.5–9 **g** per day, or
- powder: 1–1.5 **g** per day, or
- tincture: 1 **ml** per day.[105]

Interactions, contraindications and side-effects

Reishi isn't appropriate for anyone with active blood cancer because it increases immune system activity.

Some studies found that reishi increases the effect of blood thinning medications, suggesting it could cause bleeding, particularly following surgery. This seems to be a question of dosage:

- A study using 3 **g** per day of reishi capsules found evidence that it increases bleeding time.[106]
- Another study using 1.5 **g** per day (the standard dosage) found it didn't increase bleeding time.[107]

Provided that you don't exceed 1.5 **g** per day, there shouldn't be a problem.

The evidence around interactions between reishi and antidiabetic drugs is inconsistent: Type II diabetics don't find reishi reduces fasting glucose levels, and studies on reishi's effects on HbA1C, which measures long-term blood glucose, disagree on whether it has an effect or not.[16] If you take antidiabetic drugs, monitor your blood sugar levels.

There's evidence that some, but not all, people with hypertension have a reduction in blood pressure if they take reishi.[16] If you take medication to reduce blood pressure, reishi might lower it even more, so monitor it carefully.

Shiitake (Lentinus edodes)

For prevention

Shiitake mushrooms contain high levels of alpha-glucans. An extract is made from them, called 'active hexose-correlated compound'

(AHCC). In Japan particularly, it's been used for many years to enhance the immune system. It's been tested in clinical trials and found to have anti-cancer effects. In humans, twice the normal dose only caused minor side-effects in most people, including nausea, bloating, diarrhoea, fatigue, headache and foot cramps.[108]

During treatment

In a **meta-analysis** of patients suffering from advanced cancer of different types, lentinan, a beta-glucan extract of shiitake, was given alongside chemo. The lentinan group had an increased survival rate at one year and a reduction in disease progression compared with the **placebo** group.[109]

Gastric or colon cancer patients ranging from Stage I to Stage IV were recruited to a trial after surgery and alongside chemo. They were given AHCC orally 3 times per day, and their survival was tracked for 5 years. For patients with Stage I to Stage IB gastric cancer, 5 year survival was 100%, with Stage II, IIIA, IIIB and IV being 92.3%, 82.7%, 35.7% and 14.3% respectively. Most Stage I colon cancer patients survive for 5 years anyway, but in the study 5 year survival rates for Stage II, Stage IIIA, IIIB and Stage IV were 100%, 95.2%, 73.3% and 7.1% respectively. In both gastric and colon cancer, these results are significantly better than average.[110]

In a small study on head and neck cancer patients, AHCC was given along with chemo. Most of the patients had significantly fewer side-effects like vomiting, nausea, reduction in white blood cells, constipation or diarrhoea. Some had experienced a loss of red blood cells prior to chemo, before taking the AHCC, requiring blood transfusions. The rate of loss with AHCC was reduced, although chemo often results in higher rates of loss. Almost all of them experienced an increase in appetite and said they felt stronger.[111]

Breast cancer patients undergoing chemo who took AHCC had fewer problems with low white blood cells (**neutrophils**), which are often reduced by chemo. This allowed the intensity of the chemo to be increased. It also helped keep cholesterol and triglyceride levels stable. Rises in these are a common problem in chemo patients. The overall data suggested liver toxicity was reduced too.[112]

To prevent recurrence

Liver cancer patients are often diagnosed at a late stage, with a poor prognosis. One group who'd undergone surgery were treated with AHCC. They had significantly lower recurrence and an improved survival rate over those who hadn't received it.[113]

Another study looked at patients with inoperable liver cancer. The group that received AHCC had a median survival about twice as long as the **placebo** group. After 3.5 months none of the **placebo** group had survived, whereas in the AHCC group 18% survived for 7 months and one survived for over 2 years. The AHCC group also reported a higher quality of life.[114]

Dosage

All of the studies here used 1 **g**, taken 3 times per day, after meals.

Interactions, contraindications and side-effects

Shiitake protects bone marrow cells, so don't use it during active blood cancers.

Because shiitake stimulates the immune system, avoid it if you're taking immune suppressant medication.

Doses of 4 **g** per day of shiitake powder increased eosinophils, a type of white blood cell usually associated with allergies or parasitic infections.[115] This is probably because of stimulation of the bone marrow, where these cells grow. At very high levels, increased eosinophils can cause organ damage. However, there's no evidence that the doses used in the studies can cause this.

Turkey tail (Coriolus versicolor or Trametes versicolor)

During treatment

The turkey tail mushroom has been used for centuries in China and Japan to promote strength, health and longevity. More recently, laboratory testing suggests it also has antiviral, antimicrobial and anti-tumour properties. In both China and Japan, it's been approved for use in cancer patients alongside chemo and radiation therapies.[116] Japan has been using one extract, PSK, since 1977 and China has been using another, PSP, since 1987.

Turkey tail extract helps colon cancer patients receiving treatment following surgery by increasing cytotoxic **T cells** (which destroy 'foreign' cells like cancer cells and bacteria), helper **T cells** (which help the cytotoxic **T cells** identify the foreign cells), and

NK cells. It reduced the recurrence rate from 36.5% in the **control group** to 23.3% in the turkey tail group and this was particularly pronounced in patients with Stage II or Stage III cancers. It also reduced **metastasis** to the lungs, a common site in colon cancer. Disease-free survival for 5 years was 73% compared with 58.8% in the **control group.**[117]

Following curative surgery, turkey tail extract was tested alongside chemo on gastric cancer patients, compared with a **control group** who received only chemo. The group receiving turkey tail extract had a better 5 year disease-free survival rate (70.7% instead of 59.4% in the **control group**) and the 5 year survival rate with recurrence was also significantly better (73% instead of 60% in the control).[118]

Non-small cell lung cancer (NSCLC) accounts for about 80% of all lung cancers and about 60% of them are Stage IIIb or Stage IV because it's usually diagnosed once cancer has really taken hold. PSP, an extract of turkey tail, was used on NSCLC patients who'd completed treatment, either chemo or radiation or nothing, at least 4 weeks prior to the trial. They were given 1020 **mg,** 3 times per day for 4 weeks and then their tumours and their blood tests were compared against those done before the trial. There was no change in the size of the tumours between the test and **placebo** groups, but there was a significant increase in the IgG and IgM levels in the test group, whereas they'd dropped in the **placebo** group. These immunoglobulins (Ig) are antibodies, and higher levels of them in NSCLC patients lead to longer survival and fewer chest infections, so this is a positive difference.[119]

The same paper highlights another study on patients receiving turkey tail alongside chemo that showed a significant reduction in vomiting, anorexia, pain and fatigue compared with **placebo.**[119]

Dosage

Studies show that 3 **g** of extract per day spread over 3 doses is effective.[117, 118, 119]

Interactions, contraindications and side-effects

Turkey tail isn't appropriate for anyone with active blood cancer because of its effects on the immune system.

Patients using turkey tail often report dark coloured stools, although stool tests don't show any evidence of blood[120], so it isn't from damage to the digestive system.

Occasionally, there may be darkening of the fingernails.[121]

Turmeric (Curcuma longa)

Turmeric is the spice that gives curry its yellow colour. It's in the ginger family and looks very much like ginger apart from its colour. It's been widely used for centuries in the Indian sub-continent, both in cooking and in Ayurvedic medicine, which is Indian traditional medicine.

In Western Herbal Medicine, it's used as an:

- anti-inflammatory
- antioxidant
- antibacterial and antifungal
- antiplatelet

- cholesterol reducer
- digestive stimulant
- liver stimulant
- anti-cancer herb.

Its main active constituent is curcumin and this is often sold on its own.

For prevention

Taking 4 **g** of curcumin for 30 days prevents the development and spread of the early signs of colon cancer.[122] It also helps prevent the relapse of ulcerative colitis, which is a precursor to colon cancer.[122]

During treatment

In a study on mice with grafted human colon cancer cells, curcumin inhibited **metastasis** as well as tumour growth.[123]

Colon cancer patients taking curcumin lost less weight, had lower inflammatory markers, and there was more cancer cell **apoptosis** than in the **control group.**[124]

Patients with castration-resistant prostate cancer and a rising PSA tested the chemo combination of docetaxel and prednisone with 6 **g** of curcumin a day. The PSA dropped in 59% of patients with no adverse effects.[125]

In animal studies of lung cancer, curcumin prevented **carcinogenesis**, increased **apoptosis**, reduced tumour growth, and inhibited **angiogenesis** and **metastasis**. It may reduce resistance to chemo and improve its efficiency. It improved the effects of radiotherapy and reduced scar tissue formation caused by it.[126]

In laboratory tests, curcumin has an anti-**carcinogenic** effect on cells from leukaemia, lymphoma, multiple myeloma, melanoma, and cancers in the digestive tract, pancreas, cervix and colon. It also suppresses growth of ovarian, prostate, breast, liver, bladder, stomach, lung and colon cancers. It reduced **carcinogenesis** of breast cancers, tumour growth and **angiogenesis**, and was effective on both hormone-sensitive and other types of breast cancer.[127]

Curcumin taken orally, 2 **g**, 3 times per day, reduced the severity of radiation dermatitis in breast cancer patients having radiation therapy without chemo. However, it wasn't effective for those who had a total mastectomy before radiation, possibly because their radiation dosage was higher.[128]

A **systematic review** showed that topical application of turmeric or curcumin, either in a gel or a mouthwash, delayed the onset of oral **mucositis** in patients receiving chemo, radiotherapy or a combination of the 2. The severity, pain and ulceration were also reduced.[129]

Curcumin isn't well absorbed on its own. It's better absorbed with fat, together with piperine, which is extracted from black pepper. It has a good safety profile, with a review of toxicity studies showing that 6 **g** per day over 4–7 weeks was safe for humans. Adverse effects at this dosage were mainly limited to digestive problems, such as constipation and reflux.[130]

Dosage

Turmeric is usually found as a capsule that is standardised to a certain level of curcumin. The dosage of curcumin depends on why you're taking it:

- For cancer prevention, the equivalent of 400—600 **mg** curcumin, 3 times per day.
- For active cancer, the equivalent of 4— 6 **g** curcumin per day, but stop using it for a week before and a week after chemo.
- For prevention and/or treatment of oral **mucositis**, various different formulae in different doses are effective:
  - In gels, 10 **mg** of curcumin within the gel or a concentration of 0.5% were both found to reduce **mucositis**.
  - As a mouthwash, either 400 **mg** of turmeric in 80 **ml** water or 1.5 **g** of turmeric powder in 50 **ml** were effective.

This suggests that the dosage for preventing **mucositis** doesn't need to be particularly high. The mouthwash is more convenient. The gel is messier and needs to maintain contact with the affected areas.

Interactions, contraindications and side-effects

Turmeric can affect the way some chemo drugs work. Laboratory testing shows it can reduce their effectiveness, and animal studies found it reduced the effects of cyclophosphamide. However, some research suggests it can increase the effects of these drugs. It's suggested that this may be dose-related. In low doses, turmeric has an antioxidant effect, whereas higher doses may be pro-oxidant.[16] This isn't unusual: vitamin C does it, as do a number of other antioxidant nutrients and herbs. This is why the suggested doses for treating active cancer are significantly higher than those for preventing it. But don't take it within a week before or a week after chemo, to allow the drugs to work unimpeded.

Turmeric thins the blood. If you're using blood thinners it's possible that higher doses of turmeric could cause bleeding[16], so ensure that you advise your health practitioner before you take it.

In diabetics, turmeric reduces blood glucose levels and HbA1C. If you're on diabetic medication, it could increase the possibility of hypoglycaemia.[16] Monitor your blood glucose levels carefully.

Quite a few medications, including some chemo drugs have their effects either increased or reduced by turmeric. If you take anything at all, check with your pharmacist to see if it is affected.[16] I recommend that you only use turmeric under the care of a healthcare practitioner who is trained in complementary therapies.

In high doses, turmeric might affect hormone replacement therapy, but the effects are likely to be minor and mild.[16]

Some laboratory and animal testing shows turmeric can bind with iron. This hasn't been shown to happen in humans with dietary turmeric, but it's theoretically possible at high doses.[16] If your iron levels drop after taking high doses of turmeric, you may need a supplement.

Turmeric could worsen gallstones or gastro-oesophageal reflux (heartburn).[16] If you find symptoms increase, stop taking it.

Stop taking turmeric 2 weeks before surgery.[16]

Withania, aka Ashwagandha (Withania somnifera)

Withania is a small evergreen shrub native to the dry parts of the Middle East, India and some parts of Africa. It's been used in Ayurvedic medicine for over 3,000 years. It's also used in Western

Herbal Medicine as a:

- tonic
- adaptogen
- mild sedative
- anti-inflammatory
- immune modulator
- aphrodisiac for both men and women and to boost fertility in men
- liver support
- cancer support.

For prevention

Withania protected against colon cancers in an animal study. It significantly reduced the number and size of polyps compared with the controls that didn't receive withania.[131] This is especially important to anyone who has a family history of colon cancer which can be connected to a **genetic mutation**, or anybody with inflammatory bowel disease, which often leads to polyps.

Animal studies show withania is effective at preventing cancers of the head and neck, breast and skin when the animals were exposed to **carcinogens.**[132]

During treatment

In laboratory studies, withania causes **apoptosis** of cancer cells, inhibits **angiogenesis**, reduces inflammation and regulates the immune system.[132] They also show that one of its constituents helps protect liver cells.[133]

In animal and laboratory tests, withania caused **apoptosis** of cancer cells from:

- kidney[134]
- glioma, a type of brain cancer[135, 136]
- breast[137]
- lung[137]
- colon[137]
- liver[138]
- cervix[139]
- head and neck cancers.[140]

Paclitaxel is often used in triple negative breast cancer but cancer cells are often resistant to it, and it's highly toxic, so high doses are normally avoided. Withania was found to sensitise breast cancer cells to paclitaxel, increasing its effectiveness, so that lower doses could be used.[141]

An animal study showed withania's protective effects against the suppression of bone marrow cells, the origin of much of our immune system. In the group treated with paclitaxel alone, levels of white blood cells significantly decreased, whereas in the group treated with withania too, the reverse happened: red and white blood cells and haemoglobin were significantly increased.[142]

In animal studies withania also reduced tumour weight or volume in prostate, breast, medullary thyroid, cervical, lung and colon cancers.[132]

Withania's effects on cancer-related fatigue were studied in breast cancer patients, mainly Stage II or III. Fatigue was significantly reduced, physical and role functioning improved, insomnia was reduced, pain was significantly less, and emotional and social functioning was much higher in the group that received withania. The 24 month survival rate was 72% in the withania group compared with 56% in the **control group.**[143] This wasn't an ideal trial:

- The groups weren't randomly selected, just allocated alternately, although the 2 groups were relatively similar in terms of their cancer staging and types, and whether they had received radiotherapy or surgery prior to the study.
- The **control group** didn't receive **placebo** treatment, so the group receiving withania was aware that they were the study group, which might have affected their scoring.
- They received 2 different chemo regimes.
- It was relatively small.

However, the results were significant, and confirmed the expected **adaptogenic** effects of withania.

A big problem with cancer patients is the sudden loss of fat and muscle known as **cachexia**. It leads to poor outcomes and significant loss of quality of life. A laboratory study examined the effects of withania on the inflammatory markers associated with **cachexia** and found it reduces them.[144] So it may help you maintain your weight if you're currently suffering from active cancer.

One of the effects of radiotherapy is an increase in liver enzymes, indicating the liver's struggle to remove toxins generated by radiation. An animal study showed using withania before radiotherapy reduced liver enzyme numbers significantly.[145]

Dosage

Dosage depends on the reason for taking it:

- For chemo-related fatigue, take 2 **g,** 3 times per day, throughout treatment, with food or milk.
- To protect the liver from radiotherapy, take 5 **g** before treatment with food or milk.
- For protecting against cancer, take 1 **g,** 3 times per day with food or milk.

Interactions, contraindications and side-effects

Withania should not be used by anyone with active blood cancer because it stimulates the immune system.

Its immunostimulating effect could theoretically reduce the effects of immunosuppressant drugs. Avoid taking withania with them.

At doses of 6 **g** per day, about 1% of people experienced digestive problems: gastritis, nausea, flatulence.

Some early evidence suggests withania may lower blood sugar.[146] If you're taking anti-diabetic medication, monitor your blood sugar carefully.

Some animal evidence indicates withania could lower blood pressure.[147] If you're taking blood pressure lowering medication monitor your blood pressure.

Withania has a sedative effect, so it may have an additive effect with barbiturates, sedatives and anxiety-reducing medication.

There's some evidence that withania stimulates the thyroid.[148] If your thyroid is overactive (Graves' disease) withania could potentially make it worse. If you're taking thyroid hormones for an underactive thyroid, their dosage may need adjusting.

References

1. Farrugia C, Burke E, Haley M, Bedi K, Gandhi M. The use of aloe vera in cancer radiation: An updated comprehensive review. *Complement Ther Clin Pract*. 2019;35:126-130. doi:10.1016/j.ctcp.2019.01.013
2. Mayo Clinic. Aloe. Mayo Clinic. https://www.mayoclinic.org/drugs-supplements-aloe/art-20362267. Published 2020. Accessed August 25, 2021.
3. Cui R, He J, Wang B et al. Suppressive effect of Astragalus membranaceus Bunge on chemical hepatocarcinogenesis in rats. *Cancer Chemother Pharmacol*. 2003;51(1):75-80. doi:10.1007/s00280-002-0532-5
4. Auyeung K, Law P, Ko J. Astragalus saponins induce apoptosis via an ERK-independent NF-⊠B signaling pathway in the human hepatocellular HepG2 cell line. *Int J Mol Med*. 2009;23(2):189-196. doi:10.3892/ijmm_00000116
5. Block K, Mead M. Immune System Effects of Echinacea, Ginseng, and Astragalus: A Review. *Integr Cancer Ther*. 2003;2(3):247-267. doi:10.1177/1534735403256419
6. Bone K, Mills S. *Principles And Practice Of Phytotherapy*. 2nd ed. Edinburgh: Churchill Livingstone/Elsevier; 2013.
7. Li J, Wang Z, Mao K, Guo X. Clinical significance of serum T helper 1/T helper 2 cytokine shift in patients with non-small cell lung cancer. *Oncol Lett*. 2014;8(4):1682-1686. doi:10.3892/ol.2014.2391
8. Wei H, Sun R, Xiao W et al. Traditional Chinese medicine Astragalus reverses predominance of Th2 cytokines and their up-stream transcript factors in lung cancer patients. *Oncol Rep*. 2003:1507-1512. doi:10.3892/or.10.5.1507
9. Chen H, Lin I, Chen Y et al. A novel infusible botanically-derived drug, PG2, for cancer-related fatigue: A phase II double-blind, randomized placebo-controlled study. *Clinical & Investigative Medicine*. 2012;35(1):E1-E11. doi:10.25011/cim.v35i1.16100
10. Phacharapiyangkul N, Wu L, Lee W et al. The extracts of Astragalus membranaceus enhance chemosensitivity and reduce tumor indoleamine 2, 3-dioxygenase expression. *Int J Med Sci*. 2019;16(8):1107-1115. doi:10.7150/ijms.33106
11. Lin J, Fang L, Li H et al. Astragaloside IV alleviates doxorubicin induced cardiomyopathy by inhibiting NADPH oxidase derived oxidative stress. *Eur J Pharmacol*. 2019;859:172490. doi:10.1016/j.ejphar.2019.172490
12. Chen M, May B, Zhou I, Zhang A, Xue C. Integrative Medicine for Relief of Nausea and Vomiting in the Treatment of Colorectal Cancer Using Oxaliplatin-Based Chemotherapy: A Systematic Review and Meta-Analysis. *Phytotherapy Research*. 2016;30(5):741-753. doi:10.1002/ptr.5586
13. Fleischer T, Chang T, Chiang J, Sun M, Yen H. Improved Survival With Integration of Chinese Herbal Medicine Therapy in Patients With Acute Myeloid Leukemia: A

Nationwide Population-Based Cohort Study. *Integr Cancer Ther.* 2016;16(2):156-164. doi:10.1177/1534735416664171

14. Bone K. *The Ultimate Herbal Compendium*. 1st ed. Warwick, QLD: Phytotherapy Press; 2007.

15. Zhang C, Wang S, Zhang Y, Chen J, Liang X. In vitro estrogenic activities of Chinese medicinal plants traditionally used for the management of menopausal symptoms. *J Ethnopharmacol.* 2005;98(3):295-300. doi:10.1016/j.jep.2005.01.033

16. Therapeutic Research Center. Natural Medicines Database. Therapeutic Research Center. https://naturalmedicines.therapeuticresearch.com/#. Published 2021. Accessed August 25, 2021.

17. Khan M, Ali R, Parveen R, Najmi A, Ahmad S. Pharmacological evidences for cytotoxic and antitumor properties of Boswellic acids from Boswellia serrata. *J Ethnopharmacol.* 2016;191:315-323. doi:10.1016/j.jep.2016.06.053

18. Ahmed H, Abd-Rabou A, Hassan A, Kotob S. Phytochemical Analysis and Anti-cancer Investigation of Boswellia Serrata Bioactive Constituents In Vitro. *Asian Pacific Journal of Cancer Prevention.* 2015;16(16):7179-7188. doi:10.7314/apjcp.2015.16.16.7179

19. Yadav V, Prasad S, Sung B et al. Boswellic acid inhibits growth and metastasis of human colorectal cancer in orthotopic mouse model by downregulating inflammatory, proliferative, invasive and angiogenic biomarkers. *Int J Cancer.* 2011;130(9):2176-2184. doi:10.1002/ijc.26251

20. Park B, Prasad S, Yadav V, Sung B, Aggarwal B. Boswellic Acid Suppresses Growth and Metastasis of Human Pancreatic Tumors in an Orthotopic Nude Mouse Model through Modulation of Multiple Targets. *PLoS One.* 2011;6(10):e26943. doi:10.1371/journal.pone.0026943

21. Kirste S, Treier M, Wehrle S et al. Boswellia serrata acts on cerebral edema in patients irradiated for brain tumors. *Cancer.* 2011;117(16):3788-3795. doi:10.1002/cncr.25945

22. Togni S, Maramaldi G, Bonetta A, Giacomelli L, Di Pierro F. Clinical evaluation of safety and efficacy of Boswellia-based cream for prevention of adjuvant radiotherapy skin damage in mammary carcinoma: a randomized placebo controlled trial. *Eur Rev Med Pharmacol Sci.* 2015;19(8):1338-1344. https://pubmed.ncbi.nlm.nih.gov/25967706/. Accessed August 25, 2021.

23. Memorial Sloan Kettering Cancer Center. Boswellia. Memorial Sloan Kettering Cancer Center. https://www.mskcc.org/cancer-care/integrative-medicine/herbs/boswellia. Published 2021. Accessed August 25, 2021.

24. Anticoagulants/herbal medicines interaction. *Reactions Weekly.* 2011;(1347):9. doi:10.2165/00128415-201113470-00024

25. Pommier P, Gomez F, Sunyach M, D'Hombres A, Carrie C, Montbarbon X. Phase III Randomized Trial of Calendula Officinalis Compared With Trolamine for the Prevention of Acute Dermatitis During Irradiation for Breast Cancer. *Journal of Clinical Oncology.* 2004;22(8):1447-1453. doi:10.1200/jco.2004.07.063

26. Kodiyan J, Amber K. A Review of the Use of Topical Calendula in the Prevention and Treatment of Radiotherapy-Induced Skin Reactions. *Antioxidants.* 2015;4(2):293-303. doi:10.3390/antiox4020293

27. Perelman School of Medicine. Cancer patients can now use skin creams during radiation therapy. Medical Xpress. https://medicalxpress.com/news/2018-10-cancer-patients-skin-creams-therapy.html. Published 2018. Accessed August 25, 2021.

28. Rahmani A, Al shabrmi A, Aly S. Active ingredients of ginger as potential candidates in the prevention and treatment of diseases via modulation of biological activities. *Int J Physiol Pathophysiol Pharmacol*. 2014;6(2):125-136. https://www.ncbi.nlm.nih.gov/pmc/articles/PMC4106649/. Accessed August 25, 2021.

29. de Lima R, dos Reis A, de Menezes A et al. Protective and therapeutic potential of ginger (Zingiber officinale) extract and [6]-gingerol in cancer: A comprehensive review. *Phytotherapy Research*. 2018;32(10):1885-1907. doi:10.1002/ptr.6134

30. Tiber P, Sevinc S, Kilinc O, Orun O. Biological effects of whole Z.Officinale extract on chronic myeloid leukemia cell line K562. *Gene*. 2019;692:217-222. https://pubmed.ncbi.nlm.nih.gov/30684525/. Accessed August 25, 2021.

31. Jiang Y, Turgeon D, Wright B et al. Effect of ginger root on cyclooxygenase-1 and 15-hydroxyprostaglandin dehydrogenase expression in colonic mucosa of humans at normal and increased risk for colorectal cancer. *European Journal of Cancer Prevention*. 2013;22(5):455-460. doi:10.1097/cej.0b013e32835c829b

32. Kotowski U, Kadletz L, Schneider S et al. 6-shogaol induces apoptosis and enhances radiosensitivity in head and neck squamous cell carcinoma cell lines. *Phytotherapy Research*. 2018;32(2):340-347. doi:10.1002/ptr.5982

33. Deorukhkar A, Ahuja N, Mercado A et al. Zerumbone, a Sesquiterpene from Southeast Asian Edible Ginger Sensitizes Colorectal Cancer Cells to Radiation Therapy. *Int J Radiat Oncol Biol Phys*. 2010;78(3):S654. doi:10.1016/j.ijrobp.2010.07.1522

34. Babasheikhali S, Rahgozar S, Mohammadi M. Ginger extract has anti-leukemia and anti-drug resistant effects on malignant cells. *J Cancer Res Clin Oncol*. 2019;145(8):1987-1998. doi:10.1007/s00432-019-02949-5

35. Ben-Arye E, Lavie O, Samuels N et al. Safety of herbal medicine use during chemotherapy in patients with ovarian cancer: a "bedside-to-bench" approach. *Medical Oncology*. 2017;34(4):1-6. doi:10.1007/s12032-017-0910-9

36. Ryan J, Heckler C, Roscoe J et al. Ginger (Zingiber officinale) reduces acute chemotherapy-induced nausea: a URCC CCOP study of 576 patients. *Supportive Care in Cancer*. 2011;20(7):1479-1489. doi:10.1007/s00520-011-1236-3

37. Pillai A, Sharma K, Gupta Y, Bakhshi S. Anti-emetic effect of ginger powder versus placebo as an add-on therapy in children and young adults receiving high emetogenic chemotherapy. *Pediatr Blood Cancer*. 2011;56(2):234-238. doi:10.1002/pbc.22778

38. Ansari M, Mohammadianpanah M, Omidvari S et al. 381P Efficacy of ginger (G) in control of chemotherapy induced nausea and vomiting (CINV) in breast cancer patients (BCPs) receiving doxorubicin-based chemotherapy (DBCT). *Annals of Oncology*. 2015;26(S9):IX111. doi:10.1093/annonc/mdv531.14

39. Arslan M, Ozdemir L. Oral Intake of Ginger for Chemotherapy-Induced Nausea and Vomiting Among Women With Breast Cancer. *Clin J Oncol Nurs*. 2015;19(5):E92-E97. doi:10.1188/15.cjon.e92-e97

40. Sanaati F, Najafi S, Kashaninia Z, Sadeghi M. Effect of Ginger and Chamomile on Nausea and Vomiting Caused by Chemotherapy in Iranian Women with Breast Cancer.

Asian Pacific Journal of Cancer Prevention. 2016;17(8):4125-4129. https://pubmed.ncbi.nlm.nih.gov/27644672/. Accessed August 25, 2021.

41. Stargrove M, Treasure J, McKee D. *Herb, Nutrient And Drug Interactions*. St Louis, Missouri: Mosby; 2008.

42. Choi J, Chun K, Kundu J, Kundu J. Biochemical basis of cancer chemoprevention and/or chemotherapy with ginsenosides (Review). *Int J Mol Med*. 2013;32(6):1227-1238. doi:10.3892/ijmm.2013.1519

43. Yun T, Choi S. Preventive effect of ginseng intake against various human cancers: a case-control study on 1987 pairs. *Cancer Epidemiology, Biomarkers and Prevention*. 1995;4(4):401. https://pubmed.ncbi.nlm.nih.gov/7655337/. Accessed August 25, 2021.

44. Yun T, Choi S. Non-organ specific cancer prevention of ginseng: a prospective study in Korea. *Int J Epidemiol*. 1998;27(3):359-364. doi:10.1093/ije/27.3.359

45. Wang W, Qin J, Li X et al. Prevention of prostate cancer by natural product MDM2 inhibitor GS25: in vitro and in vivo activities and molecular mechanisms. *Carcinogenesis*. 2018;39(8):1026-1036. doi:10.1093/carcin/bgy063

46. Kang J, Song K, Woo J et al. Ginsenoside Rp1 from Panax ginseng Exhibits Anti-cancer Activity by Down-regulation of the IGF-1R/Akt Pathway in Breast Cancer Cells. *Plant Foods for Human Nutrition*. 2011;66(3):298-305. doi:10.1007/s11130-011-0242-4

47. Kwak J, Park J, Lee D et al. Inhibitory effects of ginseng sapogenins on the proliferation of triple negative breast cancer MDA-MB-231 cells. *Bioorg Med Chem Lett*. 2014;24(23):5409-5412. https://pubmed.ncbi.nlm.nih.gov/25453798/. Accessed August 25, 2021.

48. Liu Y, Fan D. Ginsenoside Rg5 induces apoptosis and autophagy via the inhibition of the PI3K/Akt pathway against breast cancer in a mouse model. *Food Funct*. 2018;9(11):5513-5527. doi:10.1039/c8fo01122b

49. Duan Z, Wei B, Deng J et al. The anti-tumor effect of ginsenoside Rh4 in MCF-7 breast cancer cells in vitro and in vivo. *Biochem Biophys Res Commun*. 2018;499(3):482-487. https://pubmed.ncbi.nlm.nih.gov/29596831/. Accessed August 25, 2021.

50. Chen X, Qian L, Jiang H, Chen J. Ginsenoside Rg3 inhibits CXCR4 expression and related migrations in a breast cancer cell line. *Int J Clin Oncol*. 2011;16(5):519-523. doi:10.1007/s10147-011-0222-6

51. Li L, Wang Y, Qi B et al. Suppression of PMA-induced tumor cell invasion and migration by ginsenoside Rg1 via the inhibition of NF-⊠B-dependent MMP-9 expression. *Oncol Rep*. 2014;32(5):1779-1786. doi:10.3892/or.2014.3422

52. Choi S, Oh J, Kim S. Ginsenoside Rh2 induces Bcl-2 family proteins-mediated apoptosis in vitro and in xenografts in vivo models. *J Cell Biochem*. 2011;112(1):330-340. doi:10.1002/jcb.22932

53. Bae J, Park H, Park J, Li S, Chun Y. Red ginseng and 20(S)-Rg3 control testosterone-induced prostate hyperplasia by deregulating androgen receptor signaling. *J Nat Med*. 2011;66(3):476-485. doi:10.1007/s11418-011-0609-8

54. Lu P, Su W, Miao Z, Niu H, Liu J, Hua Q. Effect and mechanism of ginsenoside Rg3 on postoperative life span of patients with non-small cell lung cancer. *Chin J Integr Med*. 2008;14(1):33-36. doi:10.1007/s11655-007-9002

55. Kim J, Park C, Lee S. Effects of Sun Ginseng on subjective quality of life in cancer patients: a double-blind, placebo-controlled pilot trial. *J Clin Pharm Ther.* 2006;31(4):331-334. doi:10.1111/j.1365-2710.2006.00740.x

56. Yennurajalingam S, Reddy A, Tannir N et al. High-Dose Asian Ginseng (Panax Ginseng) for Cancer-Related Fatigue. *Integr Cancer Ther.* 2015;14(5):419-427. doi:10.1177/1534735415580676

57. Seo E, Kim W. Red Ginseng Extract Reduced Metastasis of Colon Cancer Cells In Vitro and In Vivo. *J Ginseng Res.* 2011;35(3):315-324. doi:10.5142/jgr.2011.35.3.315

58. Kee J, Han Y, Mun J, Park S, Jeon H, Hong S. Effect of Korean Red Ginseng extract on colorectal lung metastasis through inhibiting the epithelial–mesenchymal transition via transforming growth factor-β1/Smad-signaling-mediated Snail/E-cadherin expression. *J Ginseng Res.* 2019;43(1):68-76. doi:10.1016/j.jgr.2017.08.007

59. Park K, Hwang D, Lee J, Jang J, Lee K, Lee C. Inhibitory effect of Panax ginseng C. A. Meyer on gynecological cancer. *Orient Pharm Exp Med.* 2013;13(3):217-223. doi:10.1007/s13596-013-0128-0

60. Haniadka R, Popouri S, Palatty P, Arora R, Baliga M. Medicinal Plants as Antiemetics in the Treatment of Cancer. *Integr Cancer Ther.* 2012;11(1):18-28. doi:10.1177/1534735411413266

61. Mai T, Moon J, Song Y et al. Ginsenoside F2 induces apoptosis accompanied by protective autophagy in breast cancer stem cells. *Cancer Lett.* 2012;321(2):144-153. doi:10.1016/j.canlet.2012.01.045

62. Ghorbani Z, Mirghafourvand M, Charandabi S, Javadzadeh Y. The effect of ginseng on sexual dysfunction in menopausal women: A double-blind, randomized, controlled trial. *Complement Ther Med.* 2019;45:57-64. doi:10.1016/j.ctim.2019.05.015

63. Choi M, Song I. Interactions of ginseng with therapeutic drugs. *Arch Pharm Res.* 2019;42(10):862-878. doi:10.1007/s12272-019-01184-3

64. Comelli M, Mengs U, Schneider C, Prosdocimi M. Toward the Definition of the Mechanism of Action of Silymarin: Activities Related to Cellular Protection From Toxic Damage Induced by Chemotherapy. *Integr Cancer Ther.* 2007;6(2):120-129. doi:10.1177/1534735407302349

65. Federico A, Dallio M, Loguercio C. Silymarin/Silybin and Chronic Liver Disease: A Marriage of Many Years. *Molecules.* 2017;22(2):191. doi:10.3390/molecules22020191

66. Ladas E, Kroll D, Oberlies N et al. A randomized, controlled, double-blind, pilot study of milk thistle for the treatment of hepatotoxicity in childhood acute lymphoblastic leukemia (ALL). *Cancer.* 2010;116(2):506-513. doi:10.1002/cncr.24723

67. Elyasi S, Shojaee F, Allahyari A, Karimi G. Topical Silymarin Administration for Prevention of Capecitabine-Induced Hand-Foot Syndrome: A Randomized, Double-Blinded, Placebo-Controlled Clinical Trial. *Phytotherapy Research.* 2017;31(9):1323-1329. doi:10.1002/ptr.5857

68. Becker-Schiebe M, Mengs U, Schaefer M, Bulitta M, Hoffmann W. Topical Use of a Silymarin-Based Preparation to Prevent Radiodermatitis: results of a prospective study in breast cancer patients. *Strahlentherapie und Onkologie.* 2011;187(8):485-491. doi:10.1007/s00066-011-2204-z

69. Elyasi S, Hosseini S, Moghadam M, Aledavood S, Karimi G. Effect of Oral Silymarin Administration on Prevention of Radiotherapy Induced Mucositis: A Randomized, Double-Blinded, Placebo-Controlled Clinical Trial. *Phytotherapy Research*. 2016;30(11):1879-1885. doi:10.1002/ptr.5704

70. Drugs.com. Milk Thistle Uses, Benefits & Dosage. Drugs.com. https://www.drugs.com/npp/milk-thistle.html. Published 2021. Accessed August 25, 2021.

71. Joseph T, Chanda W, Padhiar A et al. A Preclinical Evaluation of the Antitumor Activities of Edible and Medicinal Mushrooms: A Molecular Insight. *Integr Cancer Ther*. 2017;17(2):200-209. doi:10.1177/1534735417736861

72. De Silva D, Rapior S, Fons F, Bahkali A, Hyde K. Medicinal mushrooms in supportive cancer therapies: an approach to anti-cancer effects and putative mechanisms of action. *Fungal Divers*. 2012;55(1):1-35. doi:10.1007/s13225-012-0151-3

73. AHCC® Research Association. What is AHCC®. AHCC® Research Association. https://www.ahcc.net/pages/what-is-ahcc/. Accessed August 25, 2021.

74. Patel S, Goyal A. Recent developments in mushrooms as anti-cancer therapeutics: a review. *3 Biotech*. 2011;2(1):1-15. doi:10.1007/s13205-011-0036-2

75. Holliday J, Cleaver M. Medicinal Value of the Caterpillar Fungi Species of the Genus Cordyceps (Fr.) Link (Ascomycetes). A Review. *Int J Med Mushrooms*. 2008;10(3):219-234. https://www.researchgate.net/publication/247854986_Medicinal_Value_of_the_Caterpillar_Fungi_Species_of_the_Genus_Cordyceps_Fr_Link_Ascomycetes_A_Review. Accessed August 25, 2021.

76. Jordan J, Nowak A, Lee T. Activation of innate immunity to reduce lung metastases in breast cancer. *Cancer Immunology, Immunotherapy*. 2009;59(5):789-797. doi:10.1007/s00262-009-0800-x

77. Ruma I, Putranto E, Kondo E et al. Extract of Cordyceps militaris inhibits angiogenesis and suppresses tumor growth of human malignant melanoma cells. *Int J Oncol*. 2014;45(1):209-218. doi:10.3892/ijo.2014.2397

78. Park S, Jang H, Hwang I et al. Cordyceps militaris Extract Inhibits the NF-⊠B pathway and Induces Apoptosis through MKK7-JNK Signaling Activation in TK-10 Human Renal Cell Carcinoma. *Nat Prod Commun*. 2018;13(4):1934578X1801300. doi:10.1177/1934578X1801300422

79. Yamamoto K, Shichiri H, Uda A et al. Apoptotic Effects of the Extracts of Cordyceps militaris via Erk Phosphorylation in a Renal Cell Carcinoma Cell Line. *Phytotherapy Research*. 2015;29(5):707-713. doi:10.1002/ptr.5305

80. Jo E, Jang H, Yang K et al. Cordyceps militaris induces apoptosis in ovarian cancer cells through TNF-α/TNFR1-mediated inhibition of NF-⊠B phosphorylation. *BMC Complement Med Ther*. 2020;20(1). doi:10.1186/s12906-019-2780-5

81. Lee H, Park C, Jeong J et al. Apoptosis induction of human prostate carcinoma cells by cordycepin through reactive oxygen species-mediated mitochondrial death pathway. *Int J Oncol*. 2013;42(3):1036-1044. doi:10.3892/ijo.2013.1762

82. Wu W, Hsiao J, Lian Y, Lin C, Huang B. The apoptotic effect of cordycepin on human OEC-M1 oral cancer cell line. *Cancer Chemother Pharmacol*. 2007;60(1):103-111. doi:10.1007/s00280-006-0354-y

83. Seo H, Song J, Kim M, Han D, Park H, Song M. Cordyceps militaris Grown on Germinated Soybean Suppresses KRAS-Driven Colorectal Cancer by Inhibiting the RAS/ERK Pathway. *Nutrients*. 2018;11(1):20. doi:10.3390/nu11010020

84. Guo Z, Chen W, Dai G, Huang Y. Cordycepin suppresses the migration and invasion of human liver cancer cells by downregulating the expression of CXCR4. *Int J Mol Med*. 2020;45(1):141-150. doi:10.3892/ijmm.2019.4391

85. Lee H, Jeong J, Lee J et al. Cordycepin increases sensitivity of Hep3B human hepatocellular carcinoma cells to TRAIL-mediated apoptosis by inactivating the JNK signaling pathway. *Oncol Rep*. 2013;30(3):1257-1264. doi:10.3892/or.2013.2589

86. Ji N, Yao L, Li Y, He W, Yi K, Huang M. Polysaccharide of Cordyceps sinensis Enhances Cisplatin Cytotoxicity in Non–Small Cell Lung Cancer H157 Cell Line. *Integr Cancer Ther*. 2011;10(4):359-367. doi:10.1177/1534735410392573

87. Drugs.com. Cordyceps Uses, Benefits & Dosage. Drugs.com. https://www.drugs.com/npp/cordyceps.html. Published 2020. Accessed August 26, 2021.

88. Mayell M. Maitake Extracts and Their Therapeutic Potential – A Review. Alternative Medicine Review. https://altmedrev.com/wp-content/uploads/2019/02/v6-1-48.pdf. Published 2011. Accessed August 26, 2021.

89. Deng G, Lin H, Seidman A et al. A phase I/II trial of a polysaccharide extract from Grifola frondosa (Maitake mushroom) in breast cancer patients: immunological effects. *J Cancer Res Clin Oncol*. 2009;135(9):1215-1221. doi:10.1007/s00432-009-0562-z

90. Soares R, Meireles M, Rocha A et al. Maitake (D Fraction) Mushroom Extract Induces Apoptosis in Breast Cancer Cells by BAK-1 Gene Activation. *J Med Food*. 2011;14(6):563-572. doi:10.1089/jmf.2010.0095

91. Alonso E, Orozco M, Nieto A, Balogh G. Genes Related to Suppression of Malignant Phenotype Induced by Maitake D-Fraction in Breast Cancer Cells. *J Med Food*. 2013;16(7):602-617. doi:10.1089/jmf.2012.0222

92. Alonso E, Ferronato M, Fermento M et al. Antitumoral and antimetastatic activity of Maitake D-Fraction in triple-negative breast cancer cells. *Oncotarget*. 2018;9(34):23396-23412. doi:10.18632/oncotarget.25174

93. Shomori K, Yamamoto M, Arifuku I, Teramachi K, Ito H. Antitumor effects of a water-soluble extract from Maitake (Grifola frondosa) on human gastric cancer cell lines. *Oncol Rep*. 2009;22(3):615-620. doi:10.3892/or_00000480

94. Louie B, Rajamahanty S, Won J, Choudhury M, Konno S. Synergistic potentiation of interferon activity with maitake mushroom d-fraction on bladder cancer cells. *BJU Int*. 2010;105(7):1011-1015. doi:10.1111/j.1464-410x.2009.08870.x

95. Lin H, de Stanchina E, Zhou X et al. Maitake beta-glucan promotes recovery of leukocytes and myeloid cell function in peripheral blood from paclitaxel hematotoxicity. *Cancer Immunology, Immunotherapy*. 2010;59(6):885-897. doi:10.1007/s00262-009-0815-3

96. Drugs.com. Maitake Uses, Benefits & Dosage. Drugs.com. https://www.drugs.com/npp/maitake.html. Published 2020. Accessed August 26, 2021.

97. Hanselin M, Vande Griend J, Linnebur S. INR Elevation with Maitake Extract in Combination with Warfarin. *Annals of Pharmacotherapy*. 2010;44(1):223-224. doi:10.1345/aph.1M510

98. Kladar N, Gavarić N, Božin B. Ganoderma: insights into anticancer effects. *European Journal of Cancer Prevention*. 2016;25(5):462-471. doi:10.1097/cej.0000000000000204

99. Noguchi M, Kakuma T, Tomiyasu K et al. Effect of an extract of Ganoderma lucidum in men with lower urinary tract symptoms: a double-blind, placebo-controlled randomized and dose-ranging study. *Asian J Androl*. 2008;10(4):651-658. doi:10.1111/j.1745-7262.2008.00336.x

100. Jin X, Beguerie J, Sze D, Chan G. Ganoderma lucidum (Reishi mushroom) for cancer treatment. *Cochrane Database of Systematic Reviews*. 2016;5(4):4. doi:10.1002/14651858.cd007731.pub3

101. Loganathan J, Jiang J, Smith A et al. The mushroom Ganoderma lucidum suppresses breast-to-lung cancer metastasis through the inhibition of pro-invasive genes. *Int J Oncol*. 2014;44(6):2009-2015. doi:10.3892/ijo.2014.2375

102. Suarez-Arroyo I, Rosario-Acevedo R, Aguilar-Perez A et al. Anti-Tumor Effects of Ganoderma lucidum (Reishi) in Inflammatory Breast Cancer in In Vivo and In Vitro Models. *PLoS One*. 2013;8(2):e57431. doi:10.1371/journal.pone.0057431

103. Zhang Q, Hu Q, Xie D et al. Ganoderma lucidum Exerts an Anticancer Effect on Human Osteosarcoma Cells via Suppressing the Wnt/β-Catenin Signaling Pathway. *Integr Cancer Ther*. 2019;18(1):1534735419890917. doi:10.1177/1534735419890917

104. Zhao H, Zhang Q, Zhao L, Huang X, Wang J, Kang X. Spore Powder of Ganoderma lucidum Improves Cancer-Related Fatigue in Breast Cancer Patients Undergoing Endocrine Therapy: A Pilot Clinical Trial. *Evidence-Based Complementary and Alternative Medicine*. 2012;2012:1-8. doi:10.1155/2012/809614

105. Medscape. Reishi (Herb/Suppl). Medscape. https://reference.medscape.com/drug/ganoderma-lucidum-ling-chih-reishi-344488#0. Published 2021. Accessed August 26, 2021.

106. Tao J, Feng K. Experimental and clinical studies on inhibitory effect of Ganoderma lucidum on platelet aggregation. *Journal of Tongji Medical University*. 1990;10(4):240-243. doi:10.1007/bf02887938

107. Kwok Y, Ng K, Li C, Lam C, Man R. A Prospective, Randomized, Double-Blind, Placebo-Controlled Study of the Platelet and Global Hemostatic Effects of Ganoderma Lucidum (Ling-Zhi) in Healthy Volunteers. *Anesthesia & Analgesia*. 2005;101(2):423-426. doi:10.1213/01.ane.0000155286.20467.28

108. Spierings E, Fujii H, Sun B, Walshe T. A Phase I Study of the Safety of the Nutritional Supplement, Active Hexose Correlated Compound, AHCC, in Healthy Volunteers. *J Nutr Sci Vitaminol (Tokyo)*. 2007;53(6):536-539. doi:10.3177/jnsv.53.536

109. Wang H, Cai Y, Zheng Y, Bai Q, Xie D, Yu J. Efficacy of biological response modifier lentinan with chemotherapy for advanced cancer: a meta-analysis. *Cancer Med*. 2017;6(10):2222-2233. doi:10.1002/cam4.1156

110. Kawaguchi Y. Improved Survival of Patients with Gastric Cancer or Colon Cancer when treated with Active Hexose Correlated Compound (AHCC): Effect of AHCC on digestive system cancer. *Natural Medicine Journal*. 2009;1(1):1-6. http://ahccpublishedresearch.com/articles/wp-content/uploads/2016/07/I.J.-AHCC-2009-Kawaguchi-Human.pdf. Accessed August 26, 2021.

111. Parida D, Wakame K, Nomura T. Integrating Complimentary (sic) and Alternative Medicine in Form of Active Hexose Co-Related Compound (AHCC) in the Management of Head & Neck Cancer Patients. *Int J Clin Med*. 2011;2(5):588-592. https://www.scirp.org/journal/PaperInformation.aspx?paperID=8530. Accessed August 26, 2021.

112. Hangai S, Iwase S, Kawaguchi T et al. Effect of Active Hexose-Correlated Compound in Women Receiving Adjuvant Chemotherapy for Breast Cancer: A Retrospective Study. *The Journal of Alternative and Complementary Medicine*. 2013;19(11):905-910. doi:10.1089/acm.2012.0914

113. Matsui Y, Uhara J, Satoi S et al. Improved prognosis of postoperative hepatocellular carcinoma patients when treated with functional foods: a prospective cohort study. *J Hepatol*. 2002;37(1):78-86. doi:10.1016/s0168-8278(02)00091-0

114. Cowawintaweewat S, Manoromana S, Sriplung H et al. Prognostic improvement of patients with advanced liver cancer after active hexose correlated compound (AHCC) treatment. *Asian-Pacific Journal of Allergy and Immunology*. 2006;24(1):33-35. https://pubmed.ncbi.nlm.nih.gov/16913187/. Accessed August 26, 2021.

115. Levy A, Kita H, Phillips S et al. Eosinophilia and gastrointestinal symptoms after ingestion of shiitake mushrooms. *Journal of Allergy and Clinical Immunology*. 1998;101(5):613-620. doi:10.1016/s0091-6749(98)70168-x

116. Saleh M, Rashedi I, Keating A. Immunomodulatory Properties of Coriolus versicolor: The Role of Polysaccharopeptide. *Front Immunol*. 2017;8:1087. doi:10.3389/fimmu.2017.01087

117. Ohwada S, Ikeya T, Yokomori T et al. Adjuvant immunochemotherapy with oral Tegafur/Uracil plus PSK in patients with stage II or III colorectal cancer: a randomised controlled study. *Br J Cancer*. 2004;90(5):1003-1010. doi:10.1038/sj.bjc.6601619

118. Nakazato H. Efficacy of immunochemotherapy as adjuvant treatment after curative resection of gastric cancer. *The Lancet*. 1994;343(8906):1122-1126. doi:10.1016/s0140-6736(94)90233-x

119. Tsang K, Lam C, Yan C et al. Coriolus versicolor polysaccharide peptide slows progression of advanced non-small cell lung cancer. *Respir Med*. 2003;97(6):618-624. doi:10.1053/rmed.2003.1490

120. Shiu W, Leung T, Tao M. A clinical study of PSP on peripheral blood counts during chemotherapy. *Phytotherapy Research*. 1992;6(4):217-218. doi:10.1002/ptr.2650060410

121. Kidd P. The Use of Mushroom Glucans and Proteoglycans in Cancer Treatment. *Alternative Medicine Review*. 2000;5(1):4-27. https://pubmed.ncbi.nlm.nih.gov/10696116/. Accessed August 26, 2021.

122. Carroll R, Benya R, Turgeon D et al. Phase IIa Clinical Trial of Curcumin for the Prevention of Colorectal Neoplasia. *Cancer Prevention Research*. 2011;4(3):354-364. doi:10.1158/1940-6207.capr-10-0098

123. Li M, Yue G, Tsui S, Fung K, Lau C. Turmeric extract, with absorbable curcumin, has potent anti-metastatic effect in vitro and in vivo. *Phytomedicine*. 2018;46:131-141. doi:10.1016/j.phymed.2018.03.065

124. He Z, Shi C, Wen H, Li F, Wang B, Wang J. Upregulation of p53 Expression in Patients with Colorectal Cancer by Administration of Curcumin. *Cancer Invest*. 2011;29(3):208-213. doi:10.3109/07357907.2010.550592

125. Mahammedi H, Planchat E, Pouget M et al. The New Combination Docetaxel, Prednisone and Curcumin in Patients with Castration-Resistant Prostate Cancer: A Pilot Phase II Study. *Oncology*. 2016;90(2):69-78. doi:10.1159/000441148

126. Mehta H, Patel V, Sadikot R. Curcumin and lung cancer—a review. *Target Oncol*. 2014;9(4):295-310. doi:10.1007/s11523-014-0321-1

127. Nagaraju G, Aliya S, Zafar S, Basha R, Diaz R, El-Rayes B. The impact of curcumin on breast cancer. *Integrative Biology*. 2012;4(9):996-1007. doi:10.1039/c2ib20088k

128. Ryan J, Heckler C, Ling M et al. Curcumin for Radiation Dermatitis: A Randomized, Double-Blind, Placebo-Controlled Clinical Trial of Thirty Breast Cancer Patients. *Radiat Res*. 2013;180(1):34-43. doi:10.1667/rr3255.1

129. Normando A, de Menêses A, de Toledo I et al. Effects of turmeric and curcumin on oral mucositis: A systematic review. *Phytotherapy Research*. 2019;33(5):1318-1329. doi:10.1002/ptr.6326

130. Soleimani V, Sahebkar A, Hosseinzadeh H. Turmeric (Curcuma longa) and its major constituent (curcumin) as nontoxic and safe substances: Review. *Phytotherapy Research*. 2018;32(6):985-995. doi:10.1002/ptr.6054

131. Chandrasekaran B, Pal D, Kolluru V et al. The chemopreventive effect of withaferin A on spontaneous and inflammation-associated colon carcinogenesis models. *Carcinogenesis*. 2018;39(12):1537-1547. doi:10.1093/carcin/bgy109

132. Palliyaguru D, Singh S, Kensler T. Withania somnifera: From prevention to treatment of cancer. *Mol Nutr Food Res*. 2016;60(6):1342-1353. doi:10.1002/mnfr.201500756

133. Saxena M, Faridi U, Srivastava S et al. A Cytotoxic and Hepatoprotective Agent from Withania somnifera and Biological evaluation of its Ester Derivatives. *Nat Prod Commun*. 2007;2(7). https://www.researchgate.net/publication/220000116_A_Cytotoxic_and_Hepatoprotective_Agent_from_Withania_somnifera_and_Biological_evaluation_of_its_Ester_Derivatives. Accessed August 26, 2021.

134. Um H, Min K, Kim D, Kwon T. Withaferin A inhibits JAK/STAT3 signaling and induces apoptosis of human renal carcinoma Caki cells. *Biochem Biophys Res Commun*. 2012;427(1):24-29. doi:10.1016/j.bbrc.2012.08.133

135. Kataria H, Kumar S, Chaudhary H, Kaur G. Withania somnifera Suppresses Tumor Growth of Intracranial Allograft of Glioma Cells. *Mol Neurobiol*. 2015;53(6):4143-4158. doi:10.1007/s12035-015-9320-1

136. Marlow M, Shah S, Véliz E, Ivan M, Graham R. Treatment of adult and pediatric high-grade gliomas with Withaferin A: antitumor mechanisms and future perspectives. *J Nat Med*. 2016;71(1):16-26. doi:10.1007/s11418-016-1020-2

137. Dar P, Mir S, Bhat J et al. An anti-cancerous protein fraction from Withania somnifera induces ROS-dependent mitochondria-mediated apoptosis in human MDA-MB-231 breast cancer cells. *Int J Biol Macromol*. 2019;135:77-87. doi:10.1016/j.ijbiomac.2019.05.120

138. Nagalingam A, Bok J, Khurana S, Sharma D, Saxena N. Su1579 Withaferin a: an Active Ingredient From Withania Sominifera Inhibits HCC Growth via up-Regulating ERK-ELK1 Axis. *Gastroenterology*. 2012;142(5):S-970. doi:10.1016/s0016-5085(12)63759-7

139. Munagala R, Kausar H, Munjal C, Gupta R. Withaferin A induces p53-dependent apoptosis by repression of HPV oncogenes and upregulation of tumor suppressor

proteins in human cervical cancer cells. *Carcinogenesis*. 2011;32(11):1697-1705. doi:10.1093/carcin/bgr192

140. Park J, Min K, Kim D, Kwon T. Withaferin A induces apoptosis through the generation of thiol oxidation in human head and neck cancer cells. *Int J Mol Med*. 2014;35(1):247-252. doi:10.3892/ijmm.2014.1983

141. Hahm E, Lee J, Abella T, Singh S. Withaferin A inhibits expression of ataxia telangiectasia and Rad3-related kinase and enhances sensitivity of human breast cancer cells to cisplatin. *Mol Carcinog*. 2019;58(11):2139-2148. doi:10.1002/mc.23104

142. Senthilnathan P, Padmavathi R, Banu S, Sakthisekaran D. Enhancement of antitumor effect of paclitaxel in combination with immunomodulatory Withania somnifera on benzo(a)pyrene induced experimental lung cancer. *Chem Biol Interact*. 2006;159(3):180-185. doi:10.1016/j.cbi.2005.11.003

143. Biswal B, Sulaiman S, Ismail H, Zakaria H, Musa K. Effect of Withania somnifera (Ashwagandha) on the Development of Chemotherapy-Induced Fatigue and Quality of Life in Breast Cancer Patients. *Integr Cancer Ther*. 2012;12(4):312-322. doi:10.1177/1534735412464551

144. Naidoo D, Chuturgoon A, Phulukdaree A, Guruprasad K, Satyamoorthy K, Sewram V. Withania somnifera modulates cancer cachexia associated inflammatory cytokines and cell death in leukaemic THP-1 cells and peripheral blood mononuclear cells (PBMC's). *BMC Complement Altern Med*. 2018;18(1):126. doi:10.1186/s12906-018-2192-y

145. Mansour H, Hafez H. Protective effect of Withania somnifera against radiation-induced hepatotoxicity in rats. *Ecotoxicol Environ Saf*. 2012;80:14-19. doi:10.1016/j.ecoenv.2012.02.003

146. Andallu B, Radhika B. Hypoglycemic, Diuretic and Hypocholesterolemic Effect of Winter Cherry (Withania Somnifera, Dunal) Root. *Indian J Exp Biol*. 2000;38(6):607-609. https://pubmed.ncbi.nlm.nih.gov/11116534/. Accessed August 26, 2021.

147. Ahumada F, Aspee F, Wikman G, Hancke J. Withania somnifera extract. Its effect on arterial blood pressure in anaesthetized dogs. *Phytotherapy Research*. 1991;5(3):111-114. doi:10.1002/ptr.2650050305

148. Sharma A, Basu I, Singh S. Efficacy and Safety of Ashwagandha Root Extract in Subclinical Hypothyroid Patients: A Double-Blind, Randomized Placebo-Controlled Trial. *The Journal of Alternative and Complementary Medicine*. 2018;24(3):243-248. doi:10.1089/acm.2017.0183

149. Oakley A. Compositae allergy. DermNet NZ. https://dermnetnz.org/topics/compositae-allergy/. Published 2009. Accessed August 26, 2021.

Author Note

I hope that you've found this book informative and helpful and that it will help you to live a longer, healthier life, as it has me.

Don't forget to sign up for my newsletter at https://www.naturallysupportingcancertreatment.com.au/, to ensure that you receive regular updates on new research findings. You'll get a free ebook called Guide to the Best Anticancer Foods as a thank you gift. I also encourage you to follow me on Facebook at https://www.facebook.com/NaturallySupportingCancerTreatment. You can message me from there if you have any questions.

If the book has helped you, it would be much appreciated if you would leave a review at the following sites so that other people can also benefit:

https://www.goodreads.com/book/show/59510959-naturally-supporting-cancer-treatment

https://www.facebook.com/NaturallySupportingCancerTreatment

Index of cancers and related research

Type of cancer	Research	Page number
Chemotherapy side effects (cont)	Hair loss	236
	Hand-foot syndrome	295
	Heart damage	221, 235, 279, 280, 288
	Immunosuppression	226, 245, 279, 299, 303, 304, 306, 309, 310, 312, 319
	Infections	259-261
	Insomnia	Chapter 5, 320
	Kidney damage	280
	Liver damage	239, 240, 280, 286, 294, 295, 300, 302, 310, 318, 320
	Mucositis	224-226, 240, 260, 296, 315
	Nausea	78, 205,280, 286, 288, 291, 292, 309
	Neuropathy	226, 227, 240
	Pain	205, 227, 234, 240, 278, 285, 292, 313, 315, 320
	Platelet loss	212, 236, 240
	Skin dryness	202
	Vomiting	224, 280, 286, 291, 292, 309, 313
Colon and bowel	Alcohol	29
	Alkalising diet	53
	Alpha-tocopheryl succinate	212
	Boswellia	283
	Calcium	216
	Cocoa	33
Colon and bowel (cont)	Cordyceps	300

Type of cancer	Research	Page number
	Melatonin	234
	Pesticides	150
	Red meat and processed meat	16
	Vegetables and fruit	13
Fibrosarcoma	Fermented foods	34
Gallbladder	Gerson diet	47
	Ketogenic diet	45
Gastro-intestinal tract	Milk thistle	295
	Omega 3 fatty acids	245
	Turmeric	314, 315
Glioblastoma (a brain cancer)	Calorie restriction diet	51
	Ginger	287
	Ketogenic diet	44
Glioma (a brain cancer)	Alkalising diet	54
	Boswellia	283
	Withania	319
Gynaecological	Korean ginseng	292
	Selenium	253
Head and neck	Aloe vera	278
	Ginger	288
	Glutamine	225
	Milk thistle	296
	N-acetyl cysteine (NAC)	241
	Selenium	253
	Shiitake	309
	Vitamin A	198
	Vitamin E	196
	Withania	318, 319
	Zinc	260
Hodgkin disease	Pesticides	149

Type of cancer	Research	Page number
Liver	Alcohol	29
	Arsenic	139
	Astragalus	279
	Boswellia	283
	Coffee	27
	CoQ10	221, 222
	Cordyceps	300
	Fermented foods	34
	Ginger	287
	Green tea	28
	Ketogenic diet	45
	Korean ginseng	293
	N-acetyl cysteine (NAC)	241
	Non-stick pans	39
	Pesticides	150
	Probiotics	249
	Reishi	306
	Riboflavin (vitamin B2)	202
	Shiitake	310
	Sleep	108
	TCE/PCE	154
	Turmeric	315
	Vitamin C	13, 205
	Vitamin K2	215
	Withania	319
Lung	Acrylamides	19
	Alpha-tocopheryl succinate (Vitamin E)	212
	Arsenic	139
	Asbestos	139
	Astragalus	280
	Beta-carotene	198
	Cadmium	141
	CoQ10	220, 222

Type of cancer	Research	Page number
Melanoma (cont)	Iodine	232
	Ketogenic diet	44
	Mineral oils	147
	Turmeric	315
Mesothelioma	Alpha-tocopheryl succinate	212
	Asbestos	139
Myeloma	Ginger	287
	Omega 3 fatty acids	246
	Pesticides	150
	TCE/PCE	154
	Turmeric	315
Neuroblastoma	Folate (vitamin B9)	203
Non-Hodgkin lymphoma	Gerson diet	47
	Hair colourants	159
	Omega 3 fatty acids	246
	Pesticides	12, 149, 150
	Red meat and processed meat	16
	TCE/PCE	154
Oesophagus	Acrylamides	19
	Alcohol	29
	Folate (vitamin B9)	203
	Green tea	28
	Hot drinks	28
	Polystyrene	42
	Red meat and processed meat	16
	Riboflavin (vitamin B2)	202
	Vegetables and fruit	13
	Vitamin C	13
	Vitamin E	211
	Zinc	259
Oral	Acrylamides	19
	Cordyceps	300

Type of cancer	Research	Page number
Stomach	Acrylamides	19
	Folate (vitamin B9)	203
	Glutamine, arginine and omega-3s	227
	Green tea	28
	Iodine	232
	Korean ginseng	291
	Maitake	303
	Pesticides	149, 150
	Red meat and processed meats	16
	Shiitake	309
	Turkey tail	312
	Turmeric	315
	Vegetables and fruit	13
	Vitamin C	13
Surgery side effects	Calorie restriction	52
	Co Q10	221
	Delta-tocotrienol (Vitamin E)	213
	Exercise	96
	Glutamine	224, 226, 227
	Grounding	83
	Omega 3 fatty acids	246, 247
	Probiotics	249
	Reishi	308
	Vitamin A	197, 199
	Vitamin C	205, 206
	Vitamin E	213
Testicles	Cadmium	141
	Mobile phones	183
	Non-stick pans	39
	Pesticides	150
Throat	Alcohol	29
	Folate (vitamin B9)	203
	Vegetables and fruit	13

Acknowledgements

Firstly, I'd like to thank Carla Wrenn, who wrote the wonderful Foreword and contributed some valuable input into the book content. Carla, your support was so important to me and really boosted my self-confidence with the book. Thank you so much.

Next, my thanks go to Lynne Scacco and Edward Enever, both naturopathic colleagues, who took the time to read through the manuscript and give me their feedback. Each of you helped enormously in different ways by helping to shape the book into something more useful.

A big shout out to Anne Cullinan, my editor, for making some very helpful suggestions around wording and content. I'm immensely grateful.

Thank you to Muriel Crawford, without whom I would never have even thought about writing a book. I don't know whether you were serious at the time, as I was in hospital and fighting some huge battles. But you planted a seed that took root. A bit like the mighty oak, it's taken a while to grow but I got there in the end.

I wouldn't have been able to write this book if it hadn't been for my sister, Liz Jackson, who saved my life by donating her stem cells to me, despite the best efforts of the Icelandic volcano! Liz, I will be eternally grateful to you. I know how difficult it was for you to cope with all those needles. Thank you so much.

I really appreciate the support that my family and friends have given me along the way. Your encouragement really helped, especially when I was finding some of the research difficult.

I would like to thank Granny Stone, my great-grandmother. I only met her once when I was a baby and she died when I was 4 months old. But she was the 'wise woman' of the village, skilled in herbs. In an earlier time, she would probably have been burned as a witch. I'm glad that she wasn't, as I like to think that I inherited some of her genes. Granny, I hope that you're looking down and are proud of what I've done with that inheritance.

Lastly, but by no means least, I'd like to say a huge thank you to my husband, Peter. You shared with me your experience in health matters, helped me with picking up typos, made me endless cups of tea, and gave me a massive amount of support. Your wisdom was invaluable to me. I love you very much and will always be grateful.

www.ingramcontent.com/pod-product-compliance
Lightning Source LLC
Chambersburg PA
CBHW072045020426
42334CB00017B/1390
9780645293203